International Practice Development in Nursing and Healthcare

D0886478

International Practice Development in Nursing and Healthcare

Edited by

Kim Manley

Brendan McCormack

Val Wilson

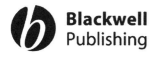

Blackwell Publishing

4\09

Library of Congress Cataloging-in-Publication Data

International practice development in nursing and healthcare / edited by Kim Manley, Brendan McCormack, Val Wilson.
   p. ; cm.
Includes bibliographical references and index.
    ISBN-13: 978-1-4051-5676-9 (pbk. : alk. paper)
    ISBN-10: 1-4051-5676-7 (pbk. : alk. paper) 1. Nursing.   2. Nurse practitioners.
    3. Nursing–International cooperation. I. Manley, Kim, MN.   II. McCormack, Brendan.
    III. Wilson, Val.
    [DNLM: 1. Nursing Research.   2. Clinical Competence.   3. Evidence-Based Medicine.
    4. International Cooperation.   5. Nurse's Role.   6. Patient-Centered Care. WY 20.5 I6185 2008]

RT82.8.I56 2008
610.73–dc22

                                                                                    2007039587

A catalogue record for this book is available from the British Library.

Set in 9.5/11.5pt Palatino by Aptara Inc., New Delhi, India
Printed in Singapore by C.O.S. Printers Pte Ltd

1   2008

Contents

Contents

Contributors

Christine Boomer, Research Officer, Belfast Health and Social Care Trust, The Royal Hospitals Nursing Development Centre, Belfast, Northern Ireland, UK

Christine's clinical experience has been in Neurosciences Nursing, holding a variety of positions within the field. Within the last 7 years Christine has been actively involved in a variety of practice development (PD) roles and programmes of work. In her current role Christine is involved in both the research evaluation of PD activity within the organisation and the facilitation of PD programmes, including the development of facilitation skills within the trust's nursing community. She is also a member of the International Practice Development Colloquium and is involved in national and international research and PD activity.

Bob Brown, Assistant Director of Nursing, Southern Eastern Health and Social Care Trust, Trust HQ Thompson House Hospital, Lisburn, Northern Ireland, UK

Bob has extensive experience as a practice development facilitator throughout NI and internationally. He is an accredited RCN Facilitator and is a member of the International Practice Development Colloquium. Bob has held a number of positions during the last 10 years; firstly in a joint appointment between University of Ulster and Newry and Mourne Trust, then as an Intermediate Care Facilitator and Nurse Commissioner. Recently, he has been a Senior Professional Officer at the Northern Ireland Practice and Education Council for Nursing and Midwifery. Bob's main research interest is in the field of palliative, supportive and end-of-life care.

Tracey Bucknall, Professor of Nursing, Deakin University, Head, Cabrini-Deakin Centre for Nursing Research, Cabrini Health, Malvern, Australia

Prior to her appointment at Cabrini Health and Deakin University, Tracey was an Associate Professor at the University of Melbourne and Director of Nursing Research and Development at Western Health. Tracey has held a variety of clinical, educational and research appointments in both private and public hospitals, and in the tertiary sector. Her primary research interests have been clinical decision making and research implementation. Tracey has obtained research funding from NHMRC, State and Federal Health Departments, and private and professional organisations. She has published and presented her research nationally and internationally and is an Associate Editor for *Worldviews on Evidence Based Nursing*.

Shirley Burke, Practice Development Lead, Royal Children's Hospital, Melbourne, Australia. Honorary Lecturer, School of Nursing and Midwifery, Monash University, Victoria, Australia

Shirley is a paediatric nurse with significant experience in paediatric nursing education. She has been involved in utilising practice development facilitation principles in her work since 2003. Her present role is a new position at the Royal Children's Hospital, Melbourne and she has been in this position for 1 year. This year has been spent developing the new role and working with healthcare teams to raise awareness about practice development, and to contribute to developing a strategic plan for practice development within the organization.

Jane Canny, Head of Patient Quality, Barts and The London NHS Trust, The Royal London Hospital, Whitechapel, London, UK

Jane has been working at Barts and London Trust since 1993 and held a number of senior nursing positions. She specialised in HIV / AIDS nursing and held posts managing nursing services in in-patient, out-patient and day care environments and developing services to meet the changing healthcare needs of an increasingly diverse patient population. As the trust Senior Nurse, Practice Development, she has worked collaboratively with the Royal College of Nursing in developing and implementing a practice development strategy for the trust. Her current role focuses on patient and public involvement and feedback – including the corporate complaints service, together with coordinating clinical effectiveness and audit activity.

Jane Chittenden, Registered New Zealand Nurse, Bachelor Health Science. Manager, Tokoroa Hospital and Family Health Team, Tokoroa Hospital, Waikato District Health Board, Tokoroa, New Zealand

Jane has been involved with nursing and health delivery professionally for 20 years. Her clinical history of generalist practice in rural hospitals and urban settings has enabled a broad understanding of health issues and systems. She currently manages a rural hospital that provides both community and hospital services. Her passion is quality patient care and supporting, enabling and challenging staff to provide that quality care.

Charlotte L. Clarke, Professor of Nursing, Practice Development Research, Associate Dean (Research), School of Health, Community and Education Studies, Northumbria University, Newcastle upon Tyne, UK

Charlotte Clarke works at Northumbria University as Professor of Nursing Practice Development Research and Associate Dean for Research. She worked with older people and people with dementia since qualifying as a nurse in the late 1980s. After several years working clinically, she has concentrated on teaching and multi-disciplinary applied research. Among many research projects, her PhD study focused on carers of people with dementia and a more recent study focused on the ways in which risk is constructed and managed in dementia care. Charlotte has published widely in this field, the most recent edited book on community-based care for people with dementia having been published by the Open University in July 2007.

Jacqueline Clarke, Practice Development Facilitator, Southern Health and Social Care Trust, Newry, Northern Ireland, UK

Following qualification as a Registered General Nurse, Jacqueline has mainly worked in cardiology. She then completed her Midwifery and Health Visiting Training. She completed her academic studies through the University of Ulster achieving a BSc (Hons) Professional Development in Nursing with the Community option in Health Visiting. Presently, Jacqueline is working as a Practice Development Facilitator within the Southern Health and Social Care Trust.

Karen Cox, Clinical Chair, the Knowledge Centre for Evidence Based Practice, Faculty of Nursing, Fontys University of Applied Science, Eindhoven, The Netherlands

Karen holds a Clinical Chair at the Knowledge Centre for Evidence Based Practice at Fontys University School of Nursing. The vision of this Knowledge Centre is to work with patients and key stakeholders to achieve effective, person-centred and evidence-based care. Karen facilitates staff members of the Knowledge Centre in a range of projects. Among these projects are practice development projects (e.g. developing lecturer–practitioner roles), education projects (e.g. Masters of Advanced Nursing Practice) and several international collaborations (e.g. International Practice Development Collaborative).

Margaret Devlin, RN, PG Cert BSc [Hons] Dip Nursing. Nurse Education Coordinator, Belfast Health and Social Care Trust, The Royal Hospital Nursing Development Centre, Belfast, Northern Ireland, UK

Margaret's background was in cardiac nursing before moving into the area of clinical education and practice development, where she led a major project to develop a new Clinical Career Framework (REACH) for nursing in the trust. In her current post, she is responsible for pre- and post-registration nurse education on site, but still continues her involvement in practice development.

Jan Dewing, Independent Consultant Nurse, Honorary Research Fellow, University of Ulster and Visiting Fellow, Northumbria University, Newcastle upon Tyne, UK

Jan works on a range of emancipatory and transformational practice development initiatives mainly in the United Kingdom and Ireland, particularly in services for older people. She is especially interested in how practice developers enable active learning, learning in the work place and ultimately learning cultures to be developed.

Jill Down, Senior Nurse, Nursing Project Office, Addenbrooke's Hospital, Cambridge University Hospitals, NHS Foundation Trust, Cambridge, UK

Jill has held clinical and leadership posts in critical care, workforce development and acute medicine that have informed and developed a passion for helping staff to improve patient care. She has worked in partnership with the Royal College of Nursing to deliver and evaluate practice development activities in an acute trust. She is particularly interested in working with staff to develop a culture of effectiveness and achieve sustainable change within the realities of everyday practice.

Mary FitzGerald, Professor of Nursing, James Cook University, Cairns, Australia

Mary worked in Oxford in the 1980s where she was able to work with a talented team of nurses to develop practice on a general medical ward. Since leaving the United Kingdom to study and work in Australia she has maintained her interest in practice development. As Professor of Nursing at Central Coast Health in New South Wales, she facilitated the development of an area wide practice development strategy. Currently, she is Director of Research at James Cook University in Far North Queensland.

Donna Frost, Quality and Innovation Manager, WZH Nieuw Berkendael Nursing Home, Den Haag, The Netherlands

Donna gained her nursing registration in New Zealand. She believes in the transforming power of practice development and participative research methods. Since beginning work in The Netherlands in 2003 She has been involved with nurses and managers who are working to develop nursing practice in long-term care settings.

Jane-Marie Hamill, Clinical Nurse Leader, Chelsea and Westminster Intensive Care Nursing Development Unit, Chelsea and Westminster Foundation Hospital, London, UK

Jane-Marie has worked in intensive care for the last 17 years and her current role involves the operational and clinical management of the unit. The unit is a charter mark holder. She has a particular interest in quality initiatives, especially finding out about users, experiences through focus groups and developing ways to improve the service delivered to patients and their significant others.

Sally Hardy, Director of Research and Practice Development, The Royal Children's Hospital, Melbourne, Australia

Sally trained as a general nurse, then moved into mental health nursing. Her desire to inform practice led her towards education and research and is currently working with the Royal Children's Hospital in Melbourne utilizing PD to support, prepare and enable practitioners for contemporary practice. She is an Honorary Associate Professor with Monash University in promoting a new Masters in PD, engagement in a PD round table and in sharing her experience of PD with practitioners of all levels to bring about transformation through human-flourishing.

Liz Henderson, Network Nurse Director, Northern Ireland Cancer Network (NICaN), UK

Liz has worked in cancer nursing for the past 25 years. In her current role she provides nursing leadership in the strategic development of cancer services across Northern Ireland. In partnership with colleagues in the network team she contributed to the establishment and development of the Cancer Network. Her particular focus is around improving the patient experience. She serves on a number of regional committees and has been involved in a series of practice development programmes.

Lucienne Hoogwerf, Head of Department, Fontys University of Applied Science Faculty of Nursing, Eindhoven, The Netherlands

Lucienne became an RN in 1980. She specialised in gerontology nursing. In this interesting nursing speciality she held several positions such as clinical nurse manager, educator and consultant. She obtained her PhD in 2002 at the University of Utrecht. She now holds the position of Head of Department, Faculty of Nursing, at Fontys University of Applied science. Her research interests are patient participation, relocation and dementia.

Bridie Kent, Associate Professor, Director of Clinical Nurse Research, School of Nursing, Faculty of Medical and Health Sciences, University of Auckland, Auckland, New Zealand

Bridie is a clinically focused nurse academic who specialised in adult critical care nursing. I gained a PhD in 1998. She has extensive experience in health services practice, education and research in the United Kingdom and New Zealand, where She is also the Director of the Centre of Evidence Based Nursing Aotearoa (CEBNA).

Marja Legius, Senior Lecturer, Fontys University of Professional Education, Eindhoven, The Netherlands

Marja has been a senior lecturer at Fontys University of Professional Education (Eindhoven, The Netherlands), Nursing Faculty, since 1996. She has also been a member of the Knowledge Center 'Evaluation and Implementation of Evidence Based Practice' for the last 2 years. In the early 1980s she graduated as a paediatric nurse, and is still passionate about children and paediatric nursing. She is an active advisory board member of the National Paediatric Nursing Association, and National Nursing Association in The Netherlands. After several studies in education, paediatrics and nursing science, she now enjoys working with students (just grown up children really). She has recently completed a project entitled 'Care in dialogue', about patient-centred care. As a member of the Knowledge Centre she co-facilitates the PD and EBP courses run within the faculty. The courses have been held in English and Dutch. In January 2006 she started the first phase of her PhD study. The subject matter being 'facilitation' and in particular the 'Critical Companionship model'.

Elaine Manderson, Clinical Nurse Specialist, Intensive Care, Chelsea and Westminster Hospital NHS Foundation Trust, London, UK

Elaine has worked in the field of intensive care for the past 13 years in a variety of settings including general, liver and cardiothoracic. Her interests lie with the development of nursing language in critical care, the experience of weaning from ventilation for nurses and patients and the development of an evidence-based, patient-centred culture.

Kim Manley, Learning and Development Manager, Resources for Learning and Improving, Royal College of Nursing, UK

Kim, previously Head of Practice Development at the Royal College of Nursing, has a long history of working in practice, with practitioners and practice teams nationally and internationally to help them become more person centred and effective in their work. Her particular interests are approaches to research, inquiry, learning and development that are transformational and make a difference to the care experienced by users and patients. Developing workplace cultures where the patient is at the centre, staff are clinically effective, shared governance principles are realised and services continually improved is her passion. Kim is Visiting Professor, Bournemouth University, and Visiting Fellow, Brighton University. She was the founding co-editor of *Nursing in Critical Care.*

Charlotte McArdle, Director of Primary Care and Older People, Executive Director of Nursing, South Eastern Health and Social Services Trust, Northern Ireland, UK

Charlotte joined South Eastern Trust from the Royal Hospitals Trust, Belfast, where she was the Acting Director of Nursing having been the Deputy Director of Nursing for 2 years. Her current responsibilities include the professional leadership of nursing and midwifery, training and development for nurses and the provision of services for Primary Care and Older People. Charlotte has extensive experience in nursing clinical leadership, practice development and senior nursing management.

Tanya McCance, Co-Director for Nursing R&D, Belfast Trust/Mona Grey Professor for Nursing R&D, University of Ulster, Northern Ireland, UK

Tanya currently holds a joint appointment between the University of Ulster and the Belfast Health and Social Care Trust. She has been a registered nurse since 1990 and throughout her career has gained experience in a range of posts within higher education and the health service that have focused on practice, education and research. Tanya has been involved in a variety of research and practice development projects, but her main areas of interest are the development of person-centred practice and the use of practice development to promote this concept within clinical settings, and also the strategic development of nursing and midwifery R&D.

Brendan McCormack, Professor of Nursing Research, Institute of Nursing Research/School of Nursing, University of Ulster, Newtownabbey, Belfast, Northern Ireland, UK

Brendan leads a variety of practice development and research projects in Ireland, the United Kingdom, Europe and Australia that focus on the development of person-centred practice. In addition, he is the leader of the Institute of Nursing Research 'Working with Older People' Recognised Research Group, coordinating research and development activity in this area. He has a particular focus on the use of arts and creativity in healthcare research and development. He is the co-editor of the *International Journal of Older People Nursing*.

Joanna McCormick, Nurse Consultant, Critical Care, Belfast Health and Social Services Trust, Royal Hospitals, Belfast, Northern Ireland, UK

Joanna has worked within critical care settings for the past 20 years and has been in her current post for 5 years. Joanna's work focuses on improving outcomes for critically ill patients and staff caring for them through initiatives such as early warning scoring systems, critical care outreach services and organisation of patient care. This work is carried out within a PD framework.

Sandra McKillop, Network Director, Northern Ireland Cancer Network (NICaN), UK

Sandra is the Network Director of the cancer network in Northern Ireland (NICaN). In partnership with clinical leads, she was responsible for establishing and developing the Cancer Network, the first regional managed network within health and social care in Northern Ireland. Before joining the health service in 2004, Sandra worked for over 12 years in Queens University, Belfast, in both teaching and management positions; her latter post setting up a network to support innovation in learning for students across the further and higher education institutions in Northern Ireland.

Rob McSherry, Principal Lecturer, Practice Development, School of Health and Social Care, University of Teesside, Middlesbrough, UK

Rob holds an honorary contract for the post of Practice Development Advisor within the Division of Medicine, James Cook, University Hospital, Middlesbrough. Following nurse registration in 1988 Rob pursued a career in Care of the Older Person and Acute Medical Nursing until in 1994 when he became a Practice Development Advisor/Lecturer in Medical Specialties for Chesterfield and North Derbyshire Royal Hospitals NHS Trust and the University of Sheffield. Rob joined the University of Teesside in 1999 as a Senior Lecturer in practice development, which has remained his focus of expertise since. Rob was the founder member of the North East and Yorkshire Developing Practice Network and in June 2005 was elected as the Chair of the Developing Practice Network United Kingdom. In March 2007 Rob was appointed Clinical Associate Professor with the Australian Catholic University, Brisbane, Australia. Rob's main interest is seeing research being utilized at a clinical level where nurses, midwives, nurse specialists and other allied health professionals are equipped with the essential skills and knowledge to aid this process.

Natalie Moroney, Previously Senior Sister, Colorectal Surgical Ward. Barts and The London NHS Trust, The Royal London Hospital, Whitechapel, London, UK

Cheryle Moss, Associate Professor, Graduate School Nursing, Midwifery and Health, Victoria University of Wellington, Wellington, New Zealand

Cheryle is interested in practice development and in how health professionals learn and progress their practice in the context of workplace environments. Cheryle also has a role as a practice development facilitator at Thames Hospital in New Zealand.

Jenny Newton, Post Doctoral Industry Fellow, Australian Research Council, School of Nursing and Midwifery, Monash University, Melbourne, Australia

Jenny is the coordinator for the international Master's of Practice Development offered in partnership with the University of Ulster. She is a proactive researcher in the field of clinical nurse education and practice development and maintains her clinical practice skills on a cardiothoracic/cardiology unit.

Helen O'Neal (Crisp), Practice Development Sister, Intensive Care, Addenbrookes NHS Trust, Cambridge, UK

Helen's practice development and facilitation skills have developed since qualifying as a nurse in 1994. Whilst working in various clinical areas, but now specialising in critical care, She has participated in advancing clinical practice through developing staff skills and knowledge or promoting evidence-based practice. She became an accredited facilitator as a result of learning and involvement as a researcher practitioner in a trust-wide action research project supported by the Royal College of Nursing.

Alyce A. Schultz, Clinical Professor, Phoenix Children's Hospital, College of Nursing and Healthcare Innovation, Arizona State University, Phoenix, AZ, USA

Alyce is a Clinical Professor at Arizona State University with a joint appointment at Phoenix Children's Hospital. For 12 years, she was the Director of the Center for Nursing Research and Quality Outcomes at Maine Medical Center, in Portland, Maine. In collaboration with staff nurses, faculty, physicians, social workers and dietitians, she was funded by six external grants, three internal grants, and has written over 25 peer-reviewed publications. She and her colleagues at Maine Medical Center have been honored national and internationally for their work in clinical research and evidence-based practice. She is currently a co-investigator on a Robert Wood Johnson study with an international team of researchers studying the characteristics in a work environment that promote and sustain evidence-based practice. She is a participant in the international interdisciplinary Knowledge Utilization colloquium that meets annually face-to-face with continual work during the year via the internet. Dr Schultz had been an appraiser for the American Nurses Association Magnet Recognition Program since its inception in 1994. She is currently Vice President on the Board of Directors for Sigma Theta Tau International.

She was inducted as a Fellow into the American Academy of Nursing for her work in developing the Clinical Scholar Mentorship Model.

Theresa Shaw, Chief Executive, Foundation of Nursing Studies, London, UK

As CEO and PD facilitator at the FoNS, Theresa is committed to enabling practice-based development and research with the ultimate purpose of transforming patient care and nursing practice. She has worked with a wide range of nursing and health-care teams and views facilitation as key to enabling transformation towards more person-centred thinking and practice.

Paul Slater, Research Fellow, Institute of Nursing Research, University of Ulster, Newtownabbey, Belfast, Northern Ireland, UK

Paul's background is in psychology, having completed an undergraduate and Master's degree in Applied Psychology at the University of Ulster. In 2006 he completed my PhD with a focus on the development and psychometric testing of an instrument to measure nurse practice environment. He has worked as a researcher since 1998 in the university, and conducted research on smoking behaviour, the assessment of older peoples' capacities, person-centred nursing and measurement of the healthcare work environment.

Annette Solman, Adjunct Professor, Director of Nursing, The Children's Hospital, Westmead, Sydney, Australia

Annette has extensive experience and credentials in education and training within nursing and the broader healthcare context. She has worked in senior roles within health focusing on leadership development, organisational culture change and practice development.

Debra Thoms, Adjunct Professor, Chief Nursing Officer, Department of Health, Sydney, Australia

Debra has worked in several states in Australia and held senior roles in nursing management for a number of years. Her interests are in organisational change and the creation of a culture that supports nursing and midwifery practice. Her current role is to provide statewide leadership and advice on nursing and midwifery professional issues in NSW. She is also an Adjunct Professor of Nursing with the University of Technology, Sydney.

Angie Titchen, Clinical Chair, Knowledge Centre for Evidence-Based Practice, Fontys University of Applied Science, Eindhoven, The Netherlands; Visiting Professor, University of Ulster, Belfast, Northern Ireland, UK

Nationally and internationally Angie collaborates with nursing, health professional and higher education colleagues to investigate person-centred healthcare, evidence-based practice, professional artistry and practitioner research. She undertakes philosophical, theoretical and methodological development in qualitative research and practice development, including processes, outcomes and evaluation through research that is creative, person centred and action orientated. Angie designs, delivers and evaluates work-based programmes for practice development, specifically facilitation programmes. She can be contacted at a.titchen@fontys.nl

Ken Walsh, Clinical Professor of Nursing, Graduate School of Nursing, Midwifery and Health, Victoria University of Wellington, Wellington, New Zealand; Director, Nursing Research and Development Unit, Waikato District Health Board, Hamilton, New Zealand

Ken has extensive nursing experience as both a clinician and academic. His research activities and interests revolve around clinical practice research, with a particular focus on nurse–patient interactions and the implementation and evaluation of practice development initiatives. Ken has developed a large portfolio of work related to clinical practice change and quality improvement in the healthcare environment. His fresh, innovative and dynamic approach to nursing research and development is well respected and recognised at an international level.

Raelene Walsh, Nurse Unit Manager, Special Care Nursery, Dandenong Hospital, Melbourne, Australia

Raelene completed her Bachelor of Nursing at Latrobe University. She gained experience on an adult medical ward, a cardiothoracic surgical ward, then worked as a Clinical Nurse Educator. Completed her Neonatal Intensive Care course at Monash University and then travelled overseas for 12 months, which included working as a Neonatal Nurse in London. She left nursing for 3 years and worked for a large insurance firm as a claims assessor and Training Manager. She returned to nursing as a Nurse Unit Manager of the Special Care Nursery and has been in this position for 5 years. It was during this time that she was involved with practice development and also completed studies in Business Management. She has currently on maternity leave and have an 11-month-old son, Oliver.

Val Wilson, Director of Nursing, Research and Practice Development, The Children's Hospital, Westmead, Australia; Professor of Nursing, Research and Practice Development, The University of Technology, Sydney, Australia

Val works with clinicians and practice developers to develop person-centred approaches to care, which are both evidenced based and take into account the needs of patients and families. The evaluation of this work, together with a number of local, state and international projects form the basis of her research work.

Helen Young, Clinical Manager Neurological Rehabilitation, Bedfordshire Primary Care Trust, UK

Helen qualified in Swindon in 1994 and has since held a variety of nursing positions in general medicine, orthopaedics, research, care of older people and rehabilitation (both neurological and general), working up to holding management positions. Within management positions held, Helen has led on service redesign and implementation of new projects to benefit patients. Helen is passionate about her job and a firm believer in lifelong learning, especially the role of practice development within nursing. Helen became involved in an RCN expert practice pilot project whilst working as a nurse manager on the Stroke and Neurological Rehabilitation Unit at Addenbrookes Hospital, Cambridge.

Roz Young, Senior Nurse, Emergency Assessment Unit, Northampton General Hospital Trust, Northampton, MA, USA

Roz trained in Manchester, and since qualifying She has predominantly worked in Emergency Care and Medicine. After her children were born she became a Practice Development (PD) Nurse. Though she is now back in practice she strongly believes that you can take the girl out of PD, but you can't take PD out of the girl.

Preface

At a time when healthcare is undergoing major transformation, it is a privilege to be involved with this book with its focus on changing the workplace cultures of healthcare systems. *Practice Development in Nursing* (2004, edited by McCormack, Manley & Garbett) presented a first attempt at bringing together a variety of perspectives on practice development (PD). Contributors to the book came from a variety of UK nursing specialities and with a diverse range of views and perspectives about PD. This book (like all books) represented the perspectives of the day and an articulation of the collective knowledge about PD at that time. The editors were conscious of their responsibility to faithfully represent the empirical, experiential, creative and tacit knowledge of PD and to do so in a way that represented the culture of healthcare of the period. *Practice Development in Nursing* has been a highly successful book and is used internationally to inform a variety of initiatives under the umbrella term of PD. A significant focus of the book was the articulation of two distinct methodologies for PD – technical and emancipatory – and to articulate these methodologies in action as well as their evaluation.

Four years later, it is fair to say that our thinking about PD has developed substantially and PD has established itself on an international platform. The body of published literature has grown enormously and we have greater clarity about the overall direction of travel – we could even suggest that PD has come of age! This coming of age is happening at a time when the discourse of person centredness dominates in healthcare and when clinical redesign is the order of the day. PD is at the heart of this agenda. With its focus on developing person-centred and evidence-based workplaces and enabling human-flourishing, it offers a coherent approach to unravelling the complexity of workplaces and enabling person centredness to be realised. A distinct shift in thinking in this volume is less emphasis on arguing the differences between technical and emancipatory approaches to the development of practice. Instead, the book offers a coherency in thinking about methodological perspectives that are considered to be effective in transforming the cultures of workplaces in healthcare services. Centred on a new and contemporary definition of PD, each chapter provides a rigorous articulation and critique of theoretical, methodological, strategic and practical frameworks and approaches to PD. Because of this approach, the book provides a valuable source of information for academics, managers, researchers and clinicians alike. It challenges our thinking about PD, unravels assumptions, exposes blind spots, and offers practical solutions to changing workplace cultures.

Preface

Part 1 of *International Practice Development in Nursing* explores the knowledge base for PD encompassing the following: using and generating evidence in PD work; collaborative working to enable effective PD work; the role of PD in the modernisation of healthcare services; the theory and practice of facilitation; critical creativity and active learning; and approaches to evaluating PD.

Part 2 focuses on the critical application of PD in practice exploring the following: the development of facilitation expertise and knowledge; using and generating evidence; changing the culture and context of practice; leadership development; active learning; person-centred outcomes; cultural change; and frameworks for accrediting PD.

International Practice Development in Nursing challenges perceptual boundaries of what counts as valid evidence from a variety of perspectives and worldviews. It advances new understandings of PD concepts and theories in order to inform the international development of rigorous frameworks that will further develop knowledge and understanding. This is not without its challenges however. It remains the case that PD is poorly understood outside of the nursing profession and that critics of PD regard it as a 'nurse-centric' approach that has little relevance outside of nursing practice per se. We cannot afford for this view to dominate at a time when our evidence of effectiveness in undertaking PD is greater than ever. We have for the first time a body of evidence underpinning our work and a variety of international scholarly outputs that demonstrate the imagination, creativity and rigour of the work undertaken. This book makes an important contribution to this agenda and it demonstrates the impact of PD on healthcare practice generally.

Brendan McCormack
Kim Manley
Val Wilson

Acknowledgements

This book would not have happened without considerable support and help from a variety of people. We would like to sincerely thank the following:

- All those who have contributed to each of the chapters. Each of the authors accepted the challenge of writing complex chapters that in many cases are breaking new ground in the theory and practice of PD. We are grateful for their commitment to working with challenging deadlines and for accepting critique with grace and thoughtfulness.
- Sinead Kelly, Administrative Assistant, Royal Hospitals, Belfast, and Tricia Berhardt, Administrative Assistant, Royal College of Nursing, London, who provided us with administrative support, maintained systems, organised meetings and maintained contact with authors. We could not have worked so effectively without them.
- Anne-Marie Davis, Nursing and Practice Development Unit, The Children's Hospital, at Westmead, Sydney, who undertook a final critique of the completed chapters. Her attention to detail in critiquing the final manuscript and giving so generously her time to do so is greatly appreciated.
- Beth Knight and Adam Burbage at Wiley-Blackwell whose commitment to spreading the word about PD has enabled this project to be brought to fruition.
- Our respective partners, families, friends and colleagues who tolerated our burning of the midnight oil and supplied endless support in the final stages of the project.

1. *Introduction*

Kim Manley, Brendan McCormack and Val Wilson

Introduction

For more than 20 years, practice development (PD) has been used as a term to describe a variety of methods for developing healthcare practice. In particular, the term has been used in the context of nursing development. Over the past 10 years significant conceptual, theoretical and methodological advances have been made in the development of frameworks to guide PD activities. Of most significance has been our increased understanding of key concepts underpinning PD work irrespective of the methodological perspective being adopted – for example, workplace culture (Manley, 2004), person centredness (McCormack, 2004; Dewing, 2004; Titchen, 2000; Nolan et al., 2004), practice context (McCormack et al., 2002), evidence (Rycroft-Malone et al., 2003), evidence implementation (Rycroft-Malone, 2004), values (Manley, 2001; Wilson et al., 2005; Wilson, 2005) and approaches to learning for sustainable practice (Dewar et al., 2003; Wilson et al., 2005; Wilson et al., 2006; Hardy et al., 2006). A number of researchers have explored the meaning of PD through conceptual analysis (Garbett & McCormack, 2002, 2004; Unsworth, 2000), action inquiry (Binnie & Titchen, 1999; Manley, 1997; Clarke et al., 2004; Clarke & Wilcockson, 2001; Gerrish, 2001) and evaluation (McCormack et al., 2004; Wilson & McCormack, 2006; Tolson, 1999).

In a concept analysis of PD, Garbett and McCormack (2004) articulated the interconnected and synergistic relationships between the development of knowledge and skills, enablement strategies, facilitation and systematic, rigorous and continuous processes of emancipatory change in order to achieve the ultimate purpose of evidence-based person-centred care. Manley and McCormack (2004) articulated these elements of PD in a model called 'emancipatory PD', drawing on previous theoretical developments in action research (Grundy, 1982). Emancipatory PD explicitly uses critical social scientific concepts on the basis that the emphasis on the development of individual practitioners, cultures and contexts within which they work, will result in sustainable change. Whilst one of the key distinctions between action research and emancipatory PD has been the explicit intent of developing transferable knowledge in action research, this increased PD literature also articulates transferable principles for action and thus demonstrates the 'coming of age' of PD and its potential as a systematic process of transformative action. In a recent systematic review of the evidence underpinning PD, McCormack et al. (2007a) identified a range of outcomes that have been achieved from systematic PD work, including the following:

- Implementation of patient care knowledge utilisation projects.
- Development of research knowledge and skills of participating staff.
- Development of facilitation skills among staff.
- Development of new services.
- Increased effectiveness of existing services or expansion of more effective services.
- Changing workplace cultures to ones that are more person centred.
- Developing learning cultures.
- Increased empowerment of staff.
- Role clarity and shared understanding of role contributions.
- Development of greater team capacity.
- Development of frameworks to guide ongoing development (e.g. competency frameworks, integrated care pathways).

Whilst these outcomes are evident in the published literature, it is also evident that much work is needed to develop strategic level evaluation frameworks that reflect the complex and multi-faceted nature of PD interventions.

International collaborations are emerging that will enable these advances to happen. Take for example this book; each chapter has a number of authors who are drawn from across the world with differing workplace contexts and cultures, with a multiplicity of professional roles from a diverse range of clinical and academic backgrounds. This of itself has been a major achievement in crossing international boundaries with PD. The issue of language is of course at times confusing across international boundaries; to ensure consistency throughout this text we have used the universal term practitioner, which in the Australia and New Zealand context denotes a clinician.

To date a number of collaboration endeavours have developed across different contexts, providing wider and more sophisticated understandings of PD to be developed. An example of this work can be drawn from the International Practice Development Colloquium (IPDC), a group of practice developers from the United Kingdom, The Netherlands New Zealand, and Australia that meet and work together to develop PD, theory and practice. The IPDC have established a number of focus areas in which they wish to advance PD. Three of these groups have contributed to work within this book (Chapters 4, 7 and 8). Each of these chapters is a collaborative endeavour to unpick, understand and advance our thinking about PD.

Collaborative research links have also been established to provide a platform for systematic studies that not only evaluate complex interventions, but also do so across borders and contexts. An example of this work is a project titled 'The development of person-centred cultures through an integrated practice development and work-based learning program'. This project takes place in number of clinical units in four area health services across two countries (UK and Australia) and involves a partnership with two universities. Interventions are multi-faceted and are developed within particular contexts. Data are collected and analysed within each area health service and cross-comparisons will take place between these sites. The project is layered in such a way as to establish a range of outcomes for patients, staff, units and organisations in each context (area health service) as well as to develop outcomes for the overall project. Through a strategic evaluation framework the investigators hope to make explicit the transformations that are occurring for individuals (patients, families and staff), teams, and organisations as a result of PD interventions.

The conceptual, theoretical and methodological advances that are being operationalised through national and international collaborations are reflected throughout this book, demonstrating advancements in PD since the first volume of work presented in *Practice Development in Nursing* (2004, edited by McCormack, Manley & Garbett). Since 2004 these advances have contributed to the development of a PD knowledge base and helped in articulating the key principles underpinning PD.

Practice development principles

With this increasing advancement in our understanding of PD come both increasing complexity with regard to the theoretical ideas surrounding it, and at the same time increasing clarity about how these theoretical ideas inform PD activity as a specific approach in the workplace. This paradox leads to the need for a set of principles that articulate the practical activity involved in PD in a way that also integrates the theoretical and philosophical ideas that are emerging.

Nine key principles are proposed as identifying the primary elements of PD activity. They are particularly intended to help other stakeholders (in particular commissioners, research funders, policy makers) to be clear about what PD is and what it is not. These principles provide the criteria or standards by which any activity presented as PD could be judged as such and differentiated from any other activity that may be similar or different. Similarities and differences with, for example, service development are cogently illustrated in Chapter 16, where PD is articulated as an approach that focuses on changing people and practice rather than just systems and processes, although both are integrated as illustrated in Chapter 3.

Whilst there are demonstrable outcomes from PD as illustrated above, there is an urgent need for articulating the outcomes of PD in a way that

- matches current and future healthcare needs in the context of global healthcare trends that will become the future driver for policy makers and healthcare commissioners, and
- is recognised by policymakers and commissioners as an approach that is worth investing in because it can assist with addressing the above in a sustainable way.

The outcomes of PD therefore need to be constructed in messages that important stakeholders can not only recognise but also need to be linked to a specific set of principles that encompass and guide the methods and activity used.

Nine PD principles are identified that inform all PD activity, themed in relation to the following:

- Purpose
- Level
- Learning
- Evidence use and evidence development
- Creativity
- Methodology and methods

The principles (Box 1.1) are described overleaf, and whilst every principle may be reflected implicitly in each chapter, those chapters that illustrate the principles most clearly are identified.

Purpose

> **Principle 1.** *PD aims to achieve person-centred and evidence-based care that is manifested through human-flourishing and a workplace culture of effectiveness in all healthcare settings and situations.*

The aim of PD is to develop effective workplace cultures that have embedded within them person-centred processes, systems and ways of working. Chapter 2 of this book explores person-centred systems and processes and the impact these hold for care delivery as well as for patients, families and staff. Person-centred processes take into account the individual's cultural perspective as well as the prevailing workplace culture that exists and the impact this may hold for people experiencing this culture. The relevance of this for PD is explored in detail in Chapter 9, which takes us on a cultural journey through the authors' engagement with the broader cultural context of living and working within New Zealand. This chapter helps the reader explore the importance of being culturally sensitive in PD work.

A manifestation of effective workplace cultures is the use of evidence to inform decision-making and the development of practice in context. Within PD evidence this includes a broader scope than is often found within the evidence-based care movement and is sourced from four key areas: research; clinical experience; patients, clients and carers; and local context and environment (Rycroft-Malone et al., 2004). A broader discussion of evidence and its relevance to decision-making is captured in Chapter 5 of this book.

Understanding the relationship between the delivery of person-centred care and the resultant outcomes is an integral component of PD work. We are interested not only in the outcomes for patients, families and staff, but also the impact that person-centred care has on the evolving workplace culture. Chapters 10 and 11 explore through evaluations of PD initiatives the relationship between PD, person-centred

Box 1.1 Principles of practice development

Principles Practice development	Focus	Chapter(s)
1. It aims to achieve person-centred and evidence-based care that is manifested through human-flourishing and a workplace culture of effectiveness in all healthcare settings and situations.	Purpose	2, 5, 9, 10, 11
2. It directs its attention at the micro-systems level – the level at which most healthcare is experienced and provided, but requires coherent support from interrelated mezzo- and macro-systems levels.	Level	2, 3, 16
3. It integrates work-based learning with its focus on active learning and formal systems for enabling learning in the workplace to transform care.	Learning	6, 14
4. It integrates and enables both the development of evidence from practice and the use of evidence in practice.	Evidence use and development	5, 15
5 It integrates creativity with cognition in order to blend mind, heart and soul energies, enabling practitioners to free their thinking and allow opportunities for human-flourishing to emerge.	Creativity	4
6. It is a complex methodology that can be used across healthcare teams and interfaces to involve all internal and external stakeholders.	Methodology and methods	2, 17
7. It uses key methods that are utilised according to the methodological principles being operationalised and the contextual characteristics of the PD programme of work.		All
8. It is associated with a set of processes including skilled facilitation that can be translated into a specific skill-set required as near to the interface of care as possible.		8, 12, 13
9. It integrates evaluation approaches that are always inclusive, participative and collaborative.		7

practice, changes in workplace culture and the potential for human-flourishing to occur. It is through this type of exploration that we can hope to understand more fully the potential we have in achieving the stated purpose of PD.

Level

> **Principle 2.** *PD directs its attention at the micro-systems level – the level at which most healthcare is experienced and provided, but requires coherent support from interrelated mezzo- and macro-systems levels.*

From its inception PD has long been recognised as needing to dovetail with supportive and enabling organisational frameworks for its potential to be fulfilled (McCormack et al., 1999). Subsequently, the importance of executive sign up and support has been recognised as essential for PD to achieve success (Manley & Webster, 2006). Whilst other approaches to developing quality services may emphasise organisational approaches to achieving change and innovation, the primary focus of PD is at the level of healthcare practice. This level (the 'micro-systems level') is where healthcare services most closely interact with patients and users through practitioners, practice teams and patient pathways. There are a number of assumptions that drive this specific focus in PD:

- Staff providing care and services to patients and users are most likely to be able to recognise the barriers to change, where improvements can be made and the innovations that can be introduced when supported to do so.
- It is at this level that care is experienced by users and therefore positive change has most potential for impacting on the user's experience and outcome.
- Involving, supporting and enabling practitioners and practice teams with users to lead change will more likely achieve internalised and embedded change that is self-sustaining.
- Developing practitioners to think and work in a person-centred and evidence-based way will help them to work more smartly as well as be self-sustaining and self-sufficient in their own problem-solving and learning for the future.

PD is an approach that can help practitioners to work with patients, users and colleagues in a person-centred way regardless of the issue or topic that may be in vogue at any one time. These ideas are further developed in Chapter 2, where the contribution of PD to developing person-centred systems that achieve integration and continuity of care for patients and users through structures, processes and patterns, manifested in behaviour, are explored in depth. Whilst the development of person-centred systems at the micro-systems level is the focus of PD, the need for cultures of effectiveness at every level of the organisation is recognised through the integration necessary between micro-, mezzo- and macro-systems levels. The success of micro-systems rely on organisational systems that actively support practitioners and practice teams to deliver on organisational values; something that is seen very effectively in the Magnet Hospital Programme and subsequently demonstrated through its outcomes (Aiken et al., 2002) (see Chapter 17).

Learning

> **Principle 3**. *PD integrates work-based learning with its focus on active learning and formal systems for enabling learning in the workplace to transform care.*

Learning in and from practice is a major component of PD identified in the original concept analysis work (Garbett & McCormack, 2004). Since then our understanding has continued to grow about how work-based learning approaches enable the transformation of individuals, teams and practice within workplaces (Dewar & Sharp, 2006; Wilson et al., 2006; Hardy et al., 2006). The role of skilled facilitation and formal systems for enabling learning as well as its assessment, implementation and evaluation in the workplace are gaining increasing recognition as being instrumental, together with a genuine learning culture and other factors, in developing and maintaining individual, team and organisational effectiveness (Manley et al., 2007).

Work-based learning is integral to PD. Learning in PD arises from developing self knowledge and awareness through structured and intentional reflection about the impact of our actions or inactions on others within the context of our workplace. Learning in PD is not only fostered through specific processes but also through the implementation of systems such as mechanisms for clinical supervision that sustain and transform it in the workplace (Hardy et al., 2006). Processes include critical analysis and reflection, which act as motivators for action, enabling practitioners to continue to be self-sufficient in their learning approaches for life. The range of approaches used to support learning in PD, termed *active learning*, are presented in Chapter 6. Active learning is a new but broader concept for approaches to learning that build on the formal approaches usually associated with PD such as action learning and clinical supervision. Active learning encompasses all the varied formal and informal approaches that enable and sustain learning in the workplace, learning that forms the basis of ongoing effectiveness in practice. Chapter 14 shares the experiences of practitioners involved in active learning in the workplace as an integrated part of their PD. Chapter 17 identifies the role of a masters programme using PD principles in developing PD expertise.

Evidence use and evidence development

> **Principle 4.** *PD integrates and enables both the development of evidence from practice and the use of evidence in practice.*

The original drivers for PD included the research implementation agenda, the systematic implementation of practice change and innovation as well as the need to provide a person-centred approach (McCormack et al., 1999). From the research implementation agenda grew the evidence-based practice movement (Chapter 5) and subsequently now the growth in translation science defined as the 'investigation of methods, interventions, and variables that influence adoption of evidence-based practices by individuals and organisations to improve clinical and operational decision-making in healthcare' (Titler et al., in press).

The Promoting Action on Research Implementation in Health Services (PARIHS) framework (Rycroft-Malone, 2004), a key framework for guiding evidence-based practice, identified how pivotal

- skilled facilitation and a context that includes effective cultures, enabling leadership and evaluation are for successful research implementation in the workplace;
- integration of research evidence with evidence from other sources such as professional expertise and the patients, own experience and expertise are for providing effective care.

All the components of the PARIHS framework are integrated within the methodology of PD, but PD is more than the PARIHS framework. This is because its aim is to achieve not just evidence use and the blending of different types of evidence so that care is experienced by users as meeting healthcare needs, but also, the systematic development of evidence from practice and the achievement of a specific culture that sustains these endeavours as well as enabling all to flourish. Chapter 5 updates readers on the evidence-based practice movement as well as strategies for systematically developing evidence from practice. Chapter 15 provides practical examples about how practitioners and practice teams have developed their practice using evidence-based practice frameworks and Chapter 7 presents insights into how PD work can continue to be systematic in its inquiry processes so that evidence for its impact can be further developed. Chapter 17 presents a scholars, programme for developing evidence based practice expertise in Magnet Hospitals at the practice level.

As the translation science movement grows, it is vital that PD is recognised as a methodology for achieving evidence-based practice but one that not only achieves evidence implementation and development but also sustains a culture of ongoing evidence use and development at individual and team levels.

Creativity

> **Principle 5.** *PD integrates creativity with cognition in order to blend different energies, enabling practitioners to free their thinking and allow opportunities for human-flourishing to emerge.*

Introduction

Developments in PD have resulted in further critique of the often-cited definition of PD (Garbett & McCormack, 2002, p. 88, 2004, p. 29), which suggested that

> *Practice development is a continuous process of improvement towards increased effectiveness in patient centred care. This is brought about by helping healthcare teams to develop their knowledge and skills and to transform the culture and context of care. It is enabled and supported by facilitators committed to systematic, rigorous continuous processes of emancipatory change that reflect the perspectives of service users.*

Whilst this definition makes explicit the interconnected and synergistic relationships between the development of knowledge and skills, enablement strategies, facilitation and systematic, rigorous and continuous processes of emancipatory change, the definition fails to capture the more contemporary developments in PD that have creativity at their core, and indeed it is commonplace to see artistic processes embedded in PD programmes. Contemporary PD has embraced creativity with much enthusiasm and indeed some of the exciting advances in PD relate to the way creative and cognitive processes are integrated in development strategies. McCormack and Titchen (2006) recognised the need to provide theoretical and methodological frameworks to guide this integration and developed a paradigmatic synthesis of the assumptions and theories underpinning critical social theory with creative imagination. This synthesis, called 'critical creativity', brings together the cognitive and the creative in PD through the articulation of philosophical, theoretical and methodological dimensions (see McCormack and Titchen [2006] for further detail). To develop this work, the assumptions underpinning the critical paradigm (Fay, 1987) were critiqued in order to articulate the unique philosophical, theoretical and methodological assumptions of critical creativity. In the methodology of critical creativity, McCormack and Titchen (2006) propose an elaboration and alteration of Fay's sub-theory 10, that is, the theory of creativity. Creativity blends the art forms used in PD with reflexivity located in the critical paradigm. This is facilitated through the blending and weaving that is evident in skilled facilitation in order to achieve the outcome of human-flourishing. With these new developments in the integration of the creative and the cognitive, a new definition of PD is proposed here:

> *Practice development is a continuous process of developing person-centred cultures. It is enabled by facilitators who authentically engage with individuals and teams to blend personal qualities and creative imagination with practice skills and practice wisdom. The learning that occurs brings about transformations of individual and team practices. This is sustained by embedding both processes and outcomes in corporate strategy.[1]*

---

[1] This definition has been refined and developed through critical dialogue with members of the International Practice Development Colloquium – a cooperative inquiry of practice developers, practitioner researchers and educators from healthcare who share and critique work dedicated

9

This definition continues to hold central the outcomes from PD (person-centred cultures, human-flourishing and effective workplaces), and these are further articulated in Chapters 3, 9, 10 and 11. However, it emphasises the need to blend different qualities of persons, including the creative dimension, in order to achieve effective outcomes, i.e. the transformation of self and work practices. The methodology of critical creativity is evident in many chapters in this book and many authors articulate a variety of artistic and creative processes in their work that are consistent with this methodology. However in Chapter 4, Angie Titchen and Brendan McCormack bring alive their previous theoretical writings on critical creativity (McCormack & Titchen, 2006) and present a detailed reflexive analysis of the experience of critical creativity in action. Through this reflexive analysis, the methods of critical creativity are made explicit and the challenges associated with this way of working articulated. We suggest that contemporary methodological developments need to consider these methods and their location within the theory of critical creativity.

Methodology and methods

> **Principle 6.** *PD is a complex methodology that can be used across healthcare teams and interfaces to involve all internal and external stakeholders.*

Whilst the purpose and impetus of PD are simple, namely improving care for the users of healthcare in a way that enables all to flourish by working with practitioners and healthcare teams, its methodology is complex. The complexity stems from working with a number of complementary methodologies and a set of associated methods in a systematic and intentional way. The complexity arises because PD is not a single intervention but a collection of interventions based on specific philosophical principles drawn from a number of methodologies that inform it, with a particular stance about how people change, develop, learn and transform their practice in a way that is sustainable and continues to be effective.

Many published PDs explicitly focus on *emancipatory approaches* to the development of practice, i.e. the facilitation of a culture that sees all things as 'possible' by confronting oppression at whatever level it occurs. However, many practice developers struggle to identify particular methodologies in their work and this lack of methodological focus has been evident in the PD literature for many years. Indeed Garbett and McCormack (2002) identified this as a key challenge to the

---

to deepening our understandings of practice development through critically creative practice, learning and research. As our understanding of critically creative practice grows and develops, we anticipate that this definition will change also, thus reflecting the dynamic nature of practice development.

sustainability of PD, i.e. the focus on 'ad hoc' PD as opposed to the utilisation of a systematic methodologically located approach. PD is focused on developments at the patient interface (micro-systems level), i.e. changes in practice at the point of care delivery and therefore is contextually bound. In Chapter 2 it is argued that PD needs to consider the way whole systems operate and to pay attention to this kind of systems thinking. In addition, the influences of policy and strategy on PD methodologies are particularly highlighted in Chapter 18. However, the difficulties associated with designing an effective methodology for PD projects need to be kept in mind, including the challenges associated with 'keeping plates spinning', the need to develop complex social networks within an organisation, speaking the language of differing stakeholders and establishing credibility with different groups. Finding the balance between designing a coherent methodology and ensuring that practice developers are 'free' to address issues as they arise is a key challenge. The evidence in the literature is not particularly strong in terms of informing methodological perspectives for PD (McCormack et al., 2007a, 2007b). The evidence suggests that there are three dominant methodologies in use: 'participatory models', action research oriented models, and pedagogical models. Whilst these methodologies are not mutually exclusive and indeed they overlap, it is their intent that is of most significance. For example, participatory models capture a broad range of systems and processes that focus on maximising opportunities for participation and inclusivity in development work without following a specific methodology. Action research in contrast, whilst also being participatory and inclusive, makes more explicit the cycles of action and reflection. Pedagogical models view teaching and learning as the dominant activities for bringing about change. However, McCormack et al. have argued that 'pinning' PD to a particular methodological perspective may not best serve our collective purpose but instead three broad methodological principles should be used to guide PD decisions. These principles are participation, collaboration and inclusivity. These principles are in evidence throughout this book and thus further reinforce their relevance to the advancement of PD knowledge.

Principle 7. *PD uses key methods that are utilised according to the methodological principles being operationalised and the contextual characteristics of the PD programme of work.*

There is growing consensus concerning the PD methods that are effective in ensuring participatory engagement and in bringing about changes in the culture and context of practice. McCormack et al. (2007a) suggest that the complexity of PD as is evident throughout this book militates against the correlation of any one method with PD outcomes. However, the systematic review undertaken by McCormack et al. identified a range of methods that are consistent across the PD literature and as reported by practice developers themselves (McCormack et al., 2007a, 2007b; RCN, 2007), including the following:

- Agreeing ethical processes
- Analysing stakeholder roles and ways of engaging stakeholders
- Being person centred
- Clarifying the development focus
- Clarifying values
- Clarifying workplace culture
- Collaborative working relationships
- Continuous reflective learning
- Developing a shared vision
- Developing critical intent
- Developing participatory engagement
- Developing a reward system
- Evaluation
- Facilitating transitions
- Giving space for ideas to flourish
- Good communication strategies
- Implementing processes for sharing and disseminating
- High challenge and high support
- Knowing 'self' and participants

These methods are in evidence throughout this book and again highlight the dynamic and creative nature of PD work. In addition, the articulation of these methods provides further evidence of the consistency in methods employed in PD that has emerged over the past 10 years.

Principle 8. *PD is associated with a set of processes including skilled facilitation that can be translated into a specific skill-set required as near to the interface of care as possible.*

Whilst PD is now associated with the specific set of methods identified above, practitioners and practice teams require help in developing their expertise in the use of these methods in practice (Manley & Webster, 2006). Once this expertise is developed, practitioners and practice teams become self-sufficient in their ongoing use of PD methods. This is because methods integrate the self-sustaining skills of learning in and from practice, evidence use, evidence development and systematic evaluation of practice change and innovation necessary for a changing healthcare context. The specific skill-set required as near to the practice interface as possible is outlined in Box 1.2.

The primary process for enabling practitioners to develop the skills needed to use PD methods in practice is facilitation. Skilled facilitation has been identified as an important factor for enabling evidence use, learning in and from practice, person-centred nursing (Titchen, 2000) and the achievement of an effective workplace culture where individual and team effectiveness prevails (Manley et al., 2007).

Box 1.2 Skills needed for practice development (Manley & Webster, 2006)

> - Working collectively with users and others, and representing different stakeholder groups.
> - Developing an effective culture, including transformational leadership. Transformational leaders can change the culture in the workplace.
> - Work-based learning encompassing approaches that include reflective practice. Work-based learning means learning in and from practice so that practitioners change how they and their team work.
> - Using and developing knowledge and policy.
> - Evaluating practice at individual and team levels.
> - Helping individuals and teams achieve the above skill-set.

In the first practice development book (McCormack, Manley & Garbett, 2004), critical companionship was presented as a helping relationship for PD (Titchen, 2000). Since then, further work has been completed on developing evidence-based standards for explicating the role of the facilitator (RCN, 2007), against which evidence can be collected to support professional accreditation. In this book, Chapter 8 provides further insights into our understanding of the concepts of facilitation and enablement. In Chapter 12 practitioners share their experiences of a journey that illustrates how they developed their facilitation skills and evidence of achieving professional accreditation against the RCN facilitation standards.

Facilitation skills in the workplace are closely linked to leadership, particularly transformational leadership. Leadership is not only necessary for developing an effective workplace culture but also for developing capacity in PD work. Chapter 13 therefore explores the development of future leaders to this end.

> **Principle 9.** *PD integrates evaluation approaches that are always inclusive, participative and collaborative.*

Being systematic in PD work differentiates it from ad hoc ways of changing practice and emphasises the need for evaluation in all PD work (Garbett & McCormack, 2004). Evaluation, often an afterthought in other approaches, is a cornerstone in PD; it guides our thinking proactively in advance of practice change. Evaluation enables us to answer such questions as whether something works, why it works, for whom it works, under what circumstance it works, as well as enabling us to implement learning from a systematic review of what we do at the individual and team level (McCormack et al., 2004). Building on the broad range of evaluation approaches and considerations identified in *Practice Development in Nursing* (2004, edited by McCormack, Manley & Garbett), our understanding has become further refined. We can now articulate that the principles of participation, collaboration and inclusivity always underpin evaluation activity in PD (McCormack et al., 2007b). Further too, our thinking has progressed; in Chapter 7, Val Wilson, Sally Hardy and Bob Brown have unpicked the concept of evaluation in relation to PD, and propose new insights encompassed by the term 'praxis evaluation'.

Evaluation of practice underpins any activity involving the gathering of evidence against standards with the intention of improving practice. In this context, standards are used as benchmarks against which a service can be evaluated or aspired to and also as a mechanism for both demonstrating achievement and progress. Chapter 17 illustrates how using *standards for an effective workplace culture* to evaluate practice can also transform it.

Evaluation for the next era will be the single most important priority for demonstrating the impact and outcomes of PD.

Conclusion

This introductory chapter has provided a set of principles for articulating what it is that characterises PD. These principles have been based on research that articulates clearly the methods and outcomes of PD. The principles are presented in a framework that will help different stakeholders recognise its relevance, specifically how the purpose of PD would equate with the policy and commissioning agenda; and how its focus directed at the micro-systems level aims to have maximum impact on the patient's experience; its role in work-based learning and developing and using evidence in practice; its focus on creativity – a prerequisite for finding new ways in challenging times; and its underlying methods and methodology for those interested in further researching its contribution and concepts. The chapters of this book further illustrate these principles in action.

Since the publication of *Practice Development in Nursing* (2004, edited by McCormack, Manley & Garbett) there has been a growing international understanding about the relevance of PD in enabling healthcare systems to be experienced as person centred and effective by patients and users as well as simultaneously developing the potential of healthcare staff. This book builds on this body of literature and further advances the theories, frameworks and methods that have developed since 2004. All of these advances have involved and resulted from collaboration that has crossed not just different countries and continents, but also different disciplines as well. This book reflects this collaboration in its title *International Practice Development in HealthCare* and the subsequent contributions made by chapter authors.

References

Aiken, L.H., Clarke, S.P. & Sloane, D.M. (2002) Hospital, staffing, organization and quality of care: cross-national findings. *Nursing Outlook.* **50**(5), 187–194. (Reprinted from (2002) *International Journal for Quality in Health Care.* **14**.)

Binnie, A. & Titchen, A. (1999) *Freedom to Practise: The Development of Patient-Centred Nursing.* Butterworth-Heinemann, Oxford.

Clarke, C., Reed, J., Wainwright, D., McClelland, S., Swallow, V., Harden, J., Walton, G. & Walsh, A. (2004) The discipline of improvement: something old, something new? *Journal of Nursing Management.* **12**(2), 85–96.

Clarke, C. & Wilcockson, J. (2001) Professional and organizational learning: analysing the relationship with the development of practice. *Journal of Advanced Nursing.* **34**(2), 264–272.

Dewar, B. & Sharp, C. (2006) Using evidence: how action learning can support the individual and organisational learning through action research. *Educational Action Research.* **14**(2), 219–237.

Dewar, B., Tocher, R. & Watson, W. (2003) *Using Work-Based Learning to Enable Practice Development,* Foundation of Nursing Studies Dissemination Series 2003, 2, 3, 1–4. Foundation of Nursing Studies, London. (www.fons.org/projects/projects)

Dewing, J. (2004) Concerns relating to the application of frameworks to promote person-centredness in nursing with older people. *International Journal of Older People Nursing.* **13**(3a), 39–44.

Fay, B. (1987) *Critical Social Science.* Polity Press, Cambridge.

Garbett, R. & McCormack, B. (2002) A concept analysis of practice development. *NT Research.* **7**(2), 87–100.

Garbett, R. & McCormack, B. (2004) A concept analysis of practice development. In: *Practice Development in Nursing* (eds B. McCormack, K. Manley & R. Garbett), pp. 10–32. Blackwell, Oxford.

Gerrish, K. (2001) A pluralistic evaluation of nursing/practice development units. *Journal of Clinical Nursing.* **10**(1), 109–118.

Grundy, S. (1982) Three modes of action research. *Curriculum Perspectives.* **2**(3), 23–34.

Hardy, S, Garbarino, L., Titichen, A. & Manley, K. (2006) A framework for work-based learning. In: *Royal College of Nursing, Workplace Resources for Practice Development,* pp. 8–56. RCN, London.

Manley, K. (1997) A conceptual framework for advanced practice: an action research project operationalizing an advanced practitioner/consultant nurse role. *Journal of Clinical Nursing.* **6**(3), 179–190.

Manley, K. (2001) *Consultant Nurse: Concept, Processes, Outcomes.* University of Manchester/RCN Institute, London.

Manley, K. (2004) Transformational culture: a culture of effectiveness. In: *Practice Development in Nursing* (eds B. McCormack, K. Manley & R. Garbett), pp. 51–82. Blackwell, Oxford.

Manley, K. & McCormack, B. (2004) Practice development: purpose, methodology, facilitation and evaluation. In: *Practice Development in Nursing* (eds B. McCormack, K. Manley & R. Garbett), pp. 33–50. Blackwell, Oxford.

Manley, K., Sanders, K., Cardiff, S., Garbarino, L. & Davren, M. (2007) Effective workplace culture: draft concept analysis. In: *Royal College of Nursing, Workplace Resources for Practice Development,* pp. 6–10. RCN, London.

Manley, K. & Webster, J. (2006) Can we keep quality alive? *Nursing Standard.* **21**(3), 12–15.

McCormack, B. (2004) Person-centredness in gerontological nursing: an overview of the literature. *International Journal of Older People Nursing.* **13**(3a), 31–38.

McCormack, B., Kitson, A., Harvey, G., Rycroft-Malone, J., Titchen, A. & Seers, K. (2002) Getting evidence into practice: the meaning of 'context'. *Journal of Advanced Nursing.* **38**(1), 94–104.

McCormack, B., Manley, K., Kitson, A., Titchen, A. & Harvey, G. (1999) Towards practice development – a vision in reality or a reality without vision? *Journal of Nursing Management*. **7**, 255–264.

McCormack, B., Manley, K. & Wilson, V. (2004) Evaluating practice developments. In: *Practice Development in Nursing* (eds. B. McCormack, K. Manley & R. Garbett), pp. 83–117. Blackwell, Oxford.

McCormack, B. & Titchen, A. (2006) Critical creativity: melding, exploding, blending. *Educational Action Research: An International Journal*. **14**(2), 239–266. (http://www.tandf.co.uk/journals)

McCormack, B., Wright, J., Dewar, B., Harvey, G. & Ballantine, K. (2007a) A realist synthesis of the evidence relating to practice development: findings from telephone interviews and synthesis of the data. *Practice Development in Health Care*. **6**(1), 56–75.

McCormack, B., Wright, J., Dewar, B., Harvey, G. & Ballantine, K. (2007b) A realist synthesis of the evidence relating to practice development: findings from the literature analysis. *Practice Development in Health Care*. **6**(1), 25–55.

Nolan, M., Davies, S., Brown, J., Keady, J. & Nolan, J. (2004) Beyond 'person-centred' care: a new vision for gerontological nursing. *International Journal of Older People Nursing*. **13**(3a), 45–53.

RCN (2007) *Workplace Resources for Practice Development*. Royal College of Nursing, London.

Rycroft-Malone, J. (2004) Research implementation: evidence, context and facilitation–the PARIHS framework. In: *Practice Development in Nursing* (eds B. McCormack, K. Manley & R. Garbett), pp. 118–147. Blackwell, Oxford.

Rycroft-Malone, J., Harvey, G., Seers, K., Kitson, A., McCormack, B. & Titchen, A. (2004) An exploration of the factors that influence the implementation of evidence into practice. *Journal of Clinical Nursing*. **13**(8), 913–924.

Rycroft-Malone, J., Seers, K., Titchen, A., Harvey, G., Kitson, A. & McCormack, B. (2003) What counts as evidence in evidence-based practice. *Journal of Advanced Nursing*. **47**(1), 81–90.

Titchen, A. (2000) *Professional Craft Knowledge in Patient-Centred Nursing and the Facilitation of its Development*. Ashdale Press Tackley, Oxfordshire.

Titler Marita, G., Daly, J., DiCenso, A., Manley, K., Reigle, B., Shih, F.J., Sousa, K. & Stringer, L. *Translation Research* Sigma Theta Tau International. (In press)

Tolson, D. (1999) Practice innovation: a methodological maze. *Journal of Advanced Nursing*. **30**(2), 381–390.

Unsworth, J. (2000) Practice development: a concept analysis. *Journal of Nursing Management*. **6**, 317–322.

Wilson, V. (2005) Developing a vision for teamwork. *Practice Development in Health Care*. **4**(1), 40–48.

Wilson, V. & McCormack, B. (2006) Critical realism as emancipatory action: the case for realistic evaluation in practice development. *Nursing Philosophy*. **7**, 45–57.

Wilson, V., McCormack, B. & Ives, G. (2005) Understanding the workplace culture of a special care nursery. *Journal of Advanced Nursing*. **50**(1), 27–38.

Wilson, V., McCormack, B. & Ives, G. (2006) Replacing the 'self' in learning. *Learning in Health and Social Care*. **5**(2), 90–105.

2. Person-Centred Systems and Processes

Brendan McCormack, Kim Manley and Ken Walsh

Introduction

There is little doubt that in contemporary health and social care, placing the person at the centre of decision-making has now become an accepted norm. Whilst much of the effort to reform health services has been focused at the level of organisational change, systems redesign, strategy development and person-centred policy-making, practice development (PD) has a key role to play in the modernisation of health services. This may seem like an obvious statement. However, despite over 25 years of consistent advancement of PD theory and methodology, there is little evidence of PD strategies and processes featuring explicitly in much of the healthcare modernisation literature. PD is of course different to organisational development. However, as has also been argued, cultures of effectiveness are needed at all levels of an organisation in order to enable person-centred outcomes. The central focus of PD is that of creating effective person-centred care and the cultures needed to enable person centredness to happen. Person-centred systems and processes are embedded in the same principles as person-centred care, i.e. maximising opportunities to enable continuity by keeping the person at the centre of decision-making and bringing about systems redesign to minimise opportunities for discontinuity.

This chapter will work with these agendas of person-centred systems and processes and the place of PD within them. The chapter will provide an overview of systems theory and how person centredness within a systems context contributes to the agendas of continuity and integration. Drawing upon this background, principles of effective working will be explored. In particular, the interrelationship between system structures, processes and patterns will be examined. The need for the integration of different systems at different levels of an organisation in order for effective person-centred care to be realised will be emphasised. Tools and approaches to integration will be offered and the place of PD in developing modern integrated care services explored. It will be argued that PD strategies have a key role to play in modernising health services and that these strategies have the

17

potential to translate complex organisational and strategic agendas into practical reality for clinicians and patients.

Global drivers, systems and complexity

Throughout the world, modernisation of healthcare services is focusing on developing greater continuity of experience for services users, reducing costs associated with duplication of services/service components and removing barriers to integration of services. Table 2.1 presents an example of health reform agencies and their mission statements. Central to the mission of all these reform agencies is the focus on the development of healthcare delivery models.

There has been an increased awareness of the need to avoid thinking about the world of healthcare as a collection of separate entities, parts or components

Table 2.1 Healthcare reform agencies

Country	Organisation	Mission
Australia	The Australian Council on Healthcare Standards http://www.achs.org.au/	'[T]o improve the quality and safety of healthcare'
Canada	The Public Health Agency of Canada http://www.phac-aspc.gc.ca/	'To promote and protect the health of Canadians through leadership, partnership, innovation and action in public health'
United Kingdom	The NHS Institute for Innovation and Improvement (http://www.institute.nhs.uk/) (supersedes the previous 'NHS Modernisation Agency')	'[I]mprove health outcomes and raise the quality of delivery in the NHS by accelerating the uptake of proven innovation and improvements in healthcare delivery models and processes, medical products and devices and healthcare leadership'
United States	Institute for Healthcare Improvement (http://www.ihi.org)	'[I]mprove the lives of patients, the health of communities, and the joy of the healthcare workforce. We will accelerate the measurable and continual progress of healthcare systems throughout the world toward: safety, effectiveness, patient-centredness, timeliness, efficiency and equity'

that have little connection with each other. This is overtly manifested in health-care reform programmes, where large organisations have been created to coordi-nate healthcare delivery with the intention of fewer organisational boundaries to be navigated by service users and providers. Over time, the reductionist view of the world that viewed healthcare as comprising separate systems has proven to be limited as it has not helped us to understand how different parts of a system work together. Simplifying the world of healthcare into separate en-tities in a way that can be done, for example, behavioural sciences, fails to recognise the dynamic interconnections that exist between different systems. We need to pay attention to these dynamics if we are to understand how health-care delivery systems are interconnected and interrelated. Think about the SARS (severe acute respiratory syndrome) outbreak as an illustrative case. At a re-ductionist level of analysis, this could be understood as a biological process of infection, but a wider view alerts us to a number of other factors, including public health policies, animal husbandry practices, community relations, national screening strategies, and social and psychological responses that led to the scale and outcome of the outbreak. Understanding SARS and its global transmission and impact is not simply a matter of understanding precise biological mecha-nisms, but of understanding the whole system in which infections such as SARS exist.

The concept of a system embodies the idea that a set of elements are connected together to form a whole, and that the system will demonstrate properties that are more than and distinct from the properties of its separate component parts. A systems approach generally assumes that the world contains structured wholes that despite their interactions or organisation continue to exhibit certain general principles that retain their identity as a whole (Baecker, 2001). However, for most of us we cannot conceive of the world as a whole – it is too big! As Checkland (2001) has argued, we cannot cope with the world as a complex system, and think about it in that form, and so we reduce it to manageable parts that can be examined separately. Checkland argues that these parts are constructed by people, are arbi-trary divisions that enable us to cope with the enormity of the world in which we live and as such our thinking is naturally reductionist. However, when we think about contemporary healthcare reform, there has been a continuous drive to get inside the complexity of healthcare delivery systems and encourage professionals to de-emphasise their own particular 'simple' view of the organisation, but instead to embrace the complexity. Little wonder then that many professionals yearn for the 'simple days' of healthcare bygone years!

System elements

All systems comprise a number of common elements and are characterised by properties such as integration and interaction, which allow flow and continuity across their (socially constructed) boundaries. The elements of systems are a col-lection of structures and processes organised around a purpose with each system embedded in other systems. In addition, a third element, pattern, is also recognised

Table 2.2 Systems elements: structures, processes, patterns

Structures	Processes	Patterns (after Plsek, 2001)
• Organisation boundaries • Layout of equipment, facilities, departments • Roles, responsibilities • Teams, committees and working groups • Targets, goals	• Patient journeys, care pathways • Supporting processes such as requesting, ordering, delivering, dispensing • Funding flows, recruitment of staff, procurement of equipment	• *Decision-making:* rapid by experts vs hierarchy and position bound • *Relationships:* generate energy for new ideas vs draining of energy • *Conflict:* opportunities to embrace ideas vs negative and destructive feedback • *Power use:* power to enable vs power over • *Learning:* Eager to learn and improve vs learning that is threatening and risky to the status quo

as influential (Capra, 2002). Table 2.2 outlines examples of these different elements of systems.

Patterns are often ignored or go unchallenged despite changes to structures and processes (Plsek, 2001). This is because patterns are associated with distinctive behavioural norms that manifest specific values, beliefs and assumptions within a workplace. These aspects together by definition are termed 'culture' (Schein, 2004) where implicit emphasis is placed on how things are done and what counts as important. To bring about fundamental change in complex systems requires the recognition of patterns that drive thinking and behaviour (Plsek, 2001). Working with behavioural norms and developing common values, beliefs and a shared purpose provides a powerful way of achieving sustainable changes in systems that are associated with the methodology of PD (McCormack et al., 2006). PD develops shared values, beliefs and purpose through collaboration, participation and inclusion of all stakeholders, and these then inform the behavioural norms required and the structures and processes necessary to deliver on agreed purposes. It is the integration of changes across structures, processes and patterns that enables transformational change to occur (Plsek, 2001).

Characteristics of systems: interaction, relationship, flow, integration

Systems historically have been defined as 'open or closed'. Von Bertanlanffy (1968) suggested that open systems are open because they allow a flow between the system and the context in which it exists, whereas closed systems do not, i.e. they have unchanging components. No social systems are closed, as social systems largely comprise people who engage in ways that are not always dictated by established boundaries. How a system is controlled enables us to look at how closed or open it is. Healthcare is characterised by its 'openness' as a system. Flows may be physical, e.g. materials, people, machines, money, or abstract, e.g. information, energy or influences (McGuire, 1999). Much of the development in contemporary healthcare focuses on streamlining the 'flows' between and among systems (e.g. streamlining the transfer of patients from acute hospital to community care) and subsystems (e.g. streamlining patients' journeys from the accident and emergency department and onwards through other departments of the hospital).

This focus on 'flow' in healthcare is consistent with The World Health Organization's Framework for Integration (Grone & Garcia-Barbero, 2002), which suggests that integration is a means to improve services in relation to access, quality, user satisfaction and efficiency. Four main foci for integration are highlighted:

- **Horizontal integration** – strategies linking similar levels of care (e.g. overcoming professional and departmental boundaries).
- **Vertical integration** – strategies linking different levels of care (e.g. primary, secondary, tertiary).
- **Continuity of care** – strategies highlighting the patient's experience (e.g. models of care).
- **Integrated care** – a broad term encompassing the bringing together of different aspects of services (e.g. technological, managerial and economic integration).

Working to improve service delivery requires an understanding of healthcare systems and the different levels at which they operate.

Macro, mezzo, micro health systems

Health systems comprise many systems organised at different levels. At the highest level are macro-systems that interrelate other macro-systems, such as, social, political, education and economic systems (Murray & Frenk, 2000). The World Health Organization (WHO) describes macro health systems as a set of elements and their relations in a complex whole, designed to serve the healthcare needs of the population and reflected by three goals (purposes):

- Health – the primary goal.
- Responsiveness – to meet people's 'legitimate non-health expectations about how the system treats them'.
- Fair financing – whereby every member of society should pay the same share of their disposable income to cover health costs.

The elements of a health system are linked to the purpose and defined as

> *the people, institutions and resources, arranged together in accordance with established policies, to improve the health of the population they serve, while responding to people's*

legitimate expectations and protecting them against the cost of ill-health through a variety of activities whose primary intent is to improve health.

WHO, 2000

Mezzo-systems are subsets of healthcare systems, such as organisations or services that cross organisations. Whereas, micro-systems

are small functional, front-line units that provide most healthcare to most people. They are the essential building blocks of the health system. They are the place where patients and healthcare staff meet. The quality and value of care produced by a large health system can be no better than the services generated by the small systems of which it is composed.

Dartmouth Hitchcock Medical School, 2007

In complex healthcare systems, emphasis is placed on information, knowledge and personal reflexivity, meaning that individual accountability for practice is paramount and that to achieve this clinicians are required to interact with complex systems. Such complexity has been illustrated in 'high profile' cases such as the Bristol Hospital Enquiry (Kennedy, 2001) and The Queensland Public Hospital Commission of Inquiry (Davies, 2005). It is also reflected in the research utilisation/ implementation literature (e.g. Greenhalgh et al., 2004). These examples highlight the complexity of interactions between clinicians and their practice settings, illustrating that there are no simple solutions to complex healthcare problems/ issues.

In the United Kingdom, the Institute for Innovation and Improvement (2005) endorses the view that it is the micro-system level that has the biggest impact on the overall patient experience, proposing that it represents the most effective focus of action if widespread change is to be achieved. It is at the micro-systems level of front-line care that PD directs its activity (Manley & Webster, 2006), focusing on the development of an effective culture at the workplace (micro-systems) level rather than emphasising the organisational or corporate culture levels (Manley et al. in preparation). Workplace in this context mirrors micro-systems albeit from a cultural perspective and is defined as

the most immediate culture experienced and/or perceived by staff, patients, users and other key stakeholders. This is the culture that impacts directly on the delivery of care. It both influences and is influenced by the organisational and corporate culture as well as other idiocultures. Idioculture is used to imply that there are different cultures that exert an influence on each other rather than one organisational/corporate culture with sub-cultures within a hierarchical arrangement.

(RCN 2007)

Whilst micro-systems is the primary focus of PD, recognising the influence of mezzo- and macro-systems is essential if a coherent, systematic and strategic approach to PD is to be achieved within a whole systems approach. Previously, McCormack et al. (1999) referred to this as ensuring that there is a reflexive relationship between developments in patient care delivery, organisational systems and strategic planning. McCormack et al. proposed that a disconnection between these parts of the system results in ineffective development outcomes. As Nelson et al. (2002, p. 474) state, 'Ultimately the outcomes of the macro-systems can be no better than the micro-systems of which it is composed'. Health systems then include the resources, actors and institutions that relate to the financing, regulation and provision of health actions, where 'health actions' are defined as 'any set of activities whose primary intent is to improve or maintain health' (Murray & Frenk, 2000, p. 718). Systems approaches therefore provide a way of explaining, organising, delivering and modelling the complexity of healthcare provision at macro-, mezzo- and micro-levels.

Whole systems approaches

Whilst the discussion so far has illustrated systems principles in relation to healthcare, the exact qualities of effective systems have only been implied as being concerned with enabling flow and interaction within the broad purposes identified by the earlier WHO definition. This section explores the desirable features of whole systems approaches – approaches that are 'joined up'. It builds on the elements and properties described:

> *The Whole system is not simply a collection of organisations which need to work together, but a mix of different people, professions, services and buildings which have patients and users as their unifying concern, and deliver a range of services in a variety of settings to provide the right care, in the right place at the right time.*
>
> *Department of Health, 2003*

This understanding of whole systems as an integration of structures, processes, patterns and relationships identifies two key concepts central to a whole systems approach, namely relationships through person centredness and systems integration.

Person centredness: the pivotal concept in relationship patterns

One of the key flows and patterns within any system is that of the relationships that exist between and among people. In a study exploring the evidence underpinning whole systems working and its realisation in one healthcare system (McCormack et al., 2005) patients commented on the breakdown in relationships among staff in different parts of the system:

> *I have been referred to so many people here, a Mr A an orthopaedic surgeon, and my own consultant Mr B looks after all my other things. I am now apparently referred to a Mr C whoever he is, I don't know where I am in this place. I don't know who is going to treat who or what.*

The quote highlights the direct relationship between patients' experiences of daily care and their perceptions of service effectiveness. To this extent, healthcare policy places significant emphasis on the development of systems and processes in and among organisations that are 'person centred'. In the United Kingdom, person centredness is embedded in many policy initiatives (e.g. The National Service Framework for Older People; Department of Health, 2001). In a comprehensive review of the literature, McCormack (2004) identified 110 papers that were related to aspects of person-centred practice, the majority of which originated from the United Kingdom. Whilst it appears that developments in person-centred nursing theory and practice are predominantly taking place in a UK context, there appear to be commonalities with other international perspectives, such as the 'Quality Health Outcomes Model' (Mitchell et al., 1998; Radwin & Fawcett, 2002), the 'Synergy Model' (Curley, 1998) and 'family-centred care' (Wilson, 2005). There is growing emphasis on a person-centred approach to healthcare in general and nursing in particular (Mead & Bower, 2000; Carr & Higginson, 2001; Nestel & Betson, 1999; McConkey, 2000). It is of particular interest across the varied domains of nursing (McCormack, 2001, 2002, 2003, 2004; Nolan et al., 2004; Dewing, 2004; Wystanski, 2000; Binnie & Titchen, 1999).

Stewart (2001, p. 444) observes that whilst person centredness is a widely used concept, it is poorly understood. In fact she states, 'it may be most commonly understood for what it is not – technology centred, doctor centred, hospital centred, disease centred'. Kitwood's (1997, p. 8) definition of person centredness is widely cited and is indeed a well-established definition in healthcare. Kitwood defines person centredness as

> *a standing or status that is bestowed upon one human being, by others, in the context of relationship and social being. It implies recognition, respect and trust.*

In a review of the literature on person centredness in the field of gerontological nursing, McCormack (2004) suggested that Kitwood's definition leads to an understanding of person centredness that focuses on four modes of 'being': (1) being in relation; (2) being in a social context; (3) being in place; (4) being with self (see Table 2.3).

Table 2.3 Person-centred modes of being

Modes of being	
Being in relation	Persons exist in relationships with other persons
Being in a social world	Persons are social beings
Being in place	Persons have a context through which their personhood is articulated
Being with self	Being recognised, respected and trusted as a person impacts on a person's sense of self

These four modes of being represent the dynamic relationship that exists between persons, their social context and the relationships they have with others. This perspective of person centredness informs our understanding of the relationship patterns necessary to enable patient flow and continuity, but also this understanding has implications for the other patterns identified in Table 2.2, such as, learning and power, and the subsequent structures and processes necessary to achieve a whole systems approach. PD, with its focus on the development of sustainable cultures of effectiveness that are person centred and evidence informed, emphasises the importance of these four modes of being. Developing cultures that enable therapeutic relationships to flourish, helping persons become empowered to shape their social world of work and change contextual factors that might hinder effectiveness as well as developing modes of engagement that are respectful of persons are key foci in emancipatory PD. A number of studies highlighting the impact of developmental processes on shaping these cultures of effectiveness at a micro-level have been published (e.g. Harrison et al., 2005; Bellman et al., 2003; Ward & McCormack, 2000). However, there are fewer accounts in the PD literature of these micro-system developments being translated into developments at mezzo- and macro-levels (McCormack et al., 2006), i.e. systems integration.

Systems integration

From systems theory, the phenomenon 'organisation' (a system of humans, materials, machines and methods) is an entity made up of interlocking parts (the subsystems) (Baecker, 2001). In this respect an organisation is the whole and the parts are interdependent with each other, which implies that one part will influence all other parts through complex interlocking structural and procedural processes. This structure or architecture broadly defines what the organisation can and cannot do (Keating, 2001). These complex arrangements create a situation where one action may have many different results (Payne, 2000). Consider this example:

> In line with contemporary practice in the management of critical care patients and consistent with the evidence base supporting the need to reduce the time patients spend in critical care units, a regional hospital facility put forward a business case to develop a critical care outreach service. However, the health authority would only accept the business case if it was based on a reduction of existing in-patient critical care services, for the service cost to be transferred from an in-patient (bed based) to an ambulatory care model. The business case was accepted and a service redesign programme was set in motion. However, it soon became evident that there were a range of indirect impacts of the decision, including the knock-on effect on remote services who were dependent on the service, the lead-in time to establishing the service meant that there was in fact a service reduction for a period of 6-months, the staff development needs and the degree of 'marketing' needed to sell the new service to referring professional groups were extensive. These indirect impacts attracted a lot of unhelpful media attention and challenged the acceptability of the service among key stakeholders, with the overarching impact of slowing the pace of change.

This example demonstrates the way that healthcare organisations function both independently and as part of wider society. Haas and Kleingeld (1999) argue that the survival of an organisation is dependent on its ability to adapt to a changing social environment. Many of the tools of modernisation focus on helping health-care staff to cope with the changing demands of society (e.g. the demand for more information), the changing political world of healthcare (e.g. the shift from hospital led to community led care) and changing social boundaries (e.g. the changing demographic construction of local communities). Proponents of healthcare modernisation would argue that healthcare organisations have for too long coexisted alongside other social institutions without recognising that their resources were derived from these same societies. Modern healthcare organisations need to understand how their systems interface with other societal systems (such as housing, transport, etc.). For these reasons Silverman (1974) argues that organisations are best considered as open systems and must be able to see themselves as existing in a state of interdependence, or in other words, they must be able to achieve integration between their multiple constituencies.

One aspect of this is the integration of activity and the respective practices across the communities within a healthcare organisation. This is manifested by the dominance of initiatives to create interdisciplinary practice (Manley & Hardy, 2006), de-emphasise the monopoly of particular professions and create generic roles. According to Newhouse and Mills (1999) integrated systems should theoretically improve the coordination of services, reduce excess capacity, improve cost-effectiveness and quality. The economic benefits of integration have also been highlighted and these include economies of scale (such as reducing the duplication of services being purchased) and improvements in competitive position in the market. Features of successfully integrated healthcare systems include the following:

- Existence of a strong system-wide culture.
- Clarity of roles and responsibilities and sharing of responsibility between professionals and across the boundaries of healthcare subsystems.
- Strong channels of communication between and within healthcare organisations.
- Free-flowing information channels across the whole healthcare system.
- Centralised coordination systems for service users to access services.
- Effective healthcare team involvement at all levels of the system.
- Common and integrated clinical/financial management information systems and the development of incentives.
- Capacity to diversify through clarity of focus by each part of the subsystem.
- Integration of technology, strategy and service mix, taking into account the impact of new technology on both cost structure and the ability to differentiate services (McCormack et al., 2005; Handy, 1986; Hronek & Bleich, 2002).

These features can be difficult to achieve as the shared understanding of activity and the shared infrastructure of activity that make cooperation the norm within parts of the organisations, such as specialist teams, can act as a barrier to close collaboration with those working outside of that specialised activity. If this insight is coupled with the fact that (as discussed earlier) we have a tendency to attempt to reduce the complexity of large systems by thinking in reductionist ways, it is not surprising that large systems such as the health system tend to develop component parts that move into siloed ways of thinking and behaving. The system reaction to this phenomenon has been to emphasise the complexity of the system as a whole. This may actually work against integration as it may lead to a belief that the system is, at base, not understandable. Hence, this may reinforce partial and siloed views, which in turn work against integration. Such a cyclical situation can quickly lead individuals to believe that they are powerless in the face of such complexity.

Factors working against integration

In a review of the literature into whole systems working with older people and the challenges that arise to effective integration of services, McCormack et al. (2005) identified the factors that contribute to discontinuity in care provision for older people. These factors include the following:

- Demarcation of professional responsibilities and the 'turf wars' that exist in the boundaries between professionals.
- Reneging and shunting of responsibilities across the boundary of health and social care.
- Weak channels of communication between and within health and social care organisations.
- A lack of free-flowing information across the whole health and social care system.
- Existence of multiple points where older people access the health and social care system with no centralised systems to coordinate what/when older people access services.
- Routine and systematic assessment and reassessment of service user needs by multiple agencies and different professionals with minimal or no sharing of these data.
- Divisive budgetary controls that constrain the integration of services.

McCormack et al. mapped these key challenges that occur at every juncture in a care system with the way that these challenges play out in particular health and social care situations. These have been analysed form the perspective of systems structures, processes and patterns (Table 2.4).

From this accumulated knowledge about the difficulties that beset the care system, the idea has emerged that collaborative working and integration of the various parts of the care system will minimise the problems that service users and service providers encounter. There is general agreement that system integration is beneficial both to the service users and to service providers. For service users, strategies that reduce the complexity of accessing health and social care and enhance the provision of the services that they require are beneficial. For service providers, potential benefits exist of more cost-effective care provision, reduction in length of hospital stay, reduction in inappropriate hospitalisation and decrease in admission to long-term care. PD has much to offer the modernisation of health services and

Table 2.4 The interfaces where factors mitigate against the provision of coordinated and integrated care in services for older people (McCormack et al. 2005)

Interface between different systems negatively influenced	Examples of mitigating factors influencing different elements of the system		
	Structures	**Process**	**Pattern**
Service sectors	Information is shared within a service sector but not across sectors	Separate access routes to services	Gate keeping mechanisms inhibit the smooth transfer of patients from one care sector to another
Professionals	Discrete boundaries that define the function and responsibility of the professional group	Separate referral mechanisms and assessment processes	Variations in dominant values that drive decisions across professional groups
Professionals and clients	Strong adherence to professional identity and professional status	Value orientation, and attitude to disease management and risk differ – all perspectives may not be considered in decision-making processes	Unequal sharing of information between professionals and clients
Care settings	Subject to different targets, e.g. to reduce length of stay, to avoid inappropriate hospitalisations	Incompatible information systems for the transfer of patient data between care settings	Delayed/absent communication concerning patients, particularly during transition from one setting to another
Organisation types	Subject to different regulatory frameworks	Lack of/minimal knowledge of all the organisations that contribute to health and social care of older people	Suspicion concerning organisational aims and objectives
Types of care	Different types of care are subject to different forms of eligibility criteria	Bottlenecks occur at different points within various types of care	Suspicion that responsibilities are shunted from acute and primary care to long-term care without resources following patients

the integration of services. As will be highlighted later in this chapter, many of the tools of PD (such as values clarification, having a shared vision, mapping context, etc.) can contribute to breaking down many of these perceived barriers and contributing to collaborative working. Putnam (2000) refers to this as building 'social capital'.

Social capital: connections and relationships for integration

Social capital refers to connections among individuals – social networks and the norms of reciprocity and trustworthiness that arise from them (Putnam, 2000, p. 19). Social capital is located in the relationships between participants (Adler & Kwon, 2002) and refers to connections made among individuals, the social networks and the norms of reciprocity and trustworthiness that arise from these connections and networks (Putnam, 1993). Just like economic capital, Putnam argues that the more connected a citizen is to his/her social networks the more capital is accumulated for distribution among society at large. In other words, the more resource that exists in the 'social capital bank' the more resource there is for citizens to draw upon in order to improve the life of citizens. The extent to which social capital exists in a given context critically influences the success of collective and collaborative work. The examination of social capital in organisations is relatively new. However, there is increasing recognition that building such social capital in an organisation contributes to the integration of subsystems (Cohen & Prusak, 2001; Grant et al., 2002). In their study of social capital in organisations, Cohen and Prusak (2001, p. 10) suggest that the benefits of developing social capital include the following:

- Better knowledge sharing, due to established trust relationships, common frames of reference, and shared goals.
- Lower transaction costs, due to a high level of trust and a cooperative spirit (both within the organisation and between the organisation and its customers and partners).
- Low turnover rates, reducing severance costs and hiring and training expenses, avoiding discontinuities associated with frequent personnel changes, and maintaining valuable organisational knowledge.
- Greater coherence of action due to organisational stability and shared understanding.

Essentially, social capital creates workplace cultures where people are able to flourish through trust, shared values, mutual understanding and respect leading to greater potential for networking and commitment to cooperative action (Cohen & Prusak, 2001) – what Manley (2000, 2004) has referred to as effective workplace culture. A safe environment not only enables interpersonal risk-taking (Edmondson, 1999) but it also increases psychological safety, allowing team members to overcome constraints.

The social capital of an organisation is often an untapped resource. Whilst organisational change programs have emphasised human capital, the social nature of organisations, the social capital, has been ignored or even degraded; sometimes by the very change processes that were designed to lead to greater productivity and better quality (Prusak & Cohen, 2001).

According to Prusak and Cohen (2001) organisations will only thrive when there are dense social networks, norms of cooperation and high levels of trust. Management practices derived from management theory can destroy such social capital. Prusak and Cohen cite, for example, re-engineering practices, which value efficiency at the cost of human interaction and connectedness. Saul (2001) calls this the tyranny of the urgent. It may be seen in the unrealistic expectation that problems that have existed for many years must be solved in very short time frames; otherwise known as the 'let's just get it done' attitude (Saul, 2001, p. 36). How many times have we heard that the problem has existed for 30 years but we have 2 weeks to fix it? Hypocrisy and an emphasis on the charismatic leader rather than the power of the social group are other factors that mitigate against social capital. In addition to this, in healthcare organisations the emphasis has often been on knowledge generation and education in an effort to bring about modernisation and practice change. This can be seen most clearly in the rise of the evidence-based practice movement. As the knowledge base for effective healthcare practice has grown, the key question has moved from 'What is best practice?' to 'How can we implement best practice?' (Kitson et al., 1998; Walsh et al., 2005). Slowly we are coming to the realisation that solutions do not solve problems, people do. Even the best solution will not work if people do not embrace it and believe they have the capacity, skills, knowledge and support to put it in place (Walsh et al., 2006).

Parallels with the views of Putnam and Cohen and Prusak can be found in the work of other scholars. The research of Hodson (2001), for example, stresses the importance of dignity in the workplace. Understanding and supporting patient dignity has long been an important ingredient of high-quality healthcare. Patients want healthcare that values and preserves their dignity (Walsh & Kowanko, 2002). However, the notion of worker dignity and its place in healthcare reform and modernisation has been less well understood. Hodson (2001, p. 3) defines dignity as 'the ability to establish a sense of self-worth and self-respect and to appreciate the respect of others'. According to Marx (1992) dignity is lost when workers are alienated from *the products of their labour*, that is they no longer determine what is to be made or how it is to be used, *the process of work*, someone else controls the pace, techniques and processes of work and workers become emotionally separated from their work, *the ability to be creative*, when workers' capacity for self-directed creativity is denied, and finally when workers are alienated from *others*, when group interactions are dictated by rigid hierarchies, which determine who can relate to whom.

To a lesser or a greater extent these factors can be seen in the complex healthcare systems where patients and healthcare workers are turned into the object of 'worker' or 'patient'. According to Hodson (2001), successfully addressing these threats to dignity can result in the development of worker 'agency' that is the 'the active and creative performance of assigned roles in ways that give meaning and content to those roles beyond what is institutionally scripted (2001, p. 16)'. Hodson concludes that

The ultimate well-being of workers and the success of organisations are a result of a complex interaction of structure and agency, of organisations and employees engaged in a simultaneously collaborative and conflictual agenda of production.

2001, p. 20

Practices that support the well-being of workers and contribute to the development of social capital are available and when supported can make a difference both to the individual worker and to the organisation. Wilson (2005) studied the contribution of an action learning set (ALS) to the development of safety among a group of staff in a special care nursery (SCN). They found that the environment of the ALS created a safe space for risk-taking as they openly and honestly discussed problems, resulting in improved learning. The group developed a level of unconditional trust, which was based on mutual respect and shared values (Jones & George, 1998). Action learning designed to develop this 'level of trust' resulted in the formation of strong relationships and cognitive dimensions of social capital (Day, 2001). Wilson suggested that social capital is a useful concept to work with in the context of AL as the relationships formed serve as a way to influence processes and people, increase information flow, support reciprocity and facilitate effective action. Wilson et al. (2006) argue that the ALS created a safe space for building social capital among the team members as well as enabling growth to occur within the group. It also went some way towards forming a cohesive and positive working relationship as their journey continued.

Modernisation of healthcare then will benefit from a valuing of people (workers and patients), their social and individual capacity and their inherent dignity. The development of trust, safety, transparent ways of working, active engagement, dignity, social networking, self-esteem, self-efficacy and a sense of shared purpose will be needed if modernisation agendas are to be carried forward successfully. PD attempts to address these issues, not by forcing the embracing of complexity or by macro-solutions such as major structural reform of the system (such mechanistic and corporate orientated approaches to organisations' difficulties mask the deeply social nature of organisations [Cohen & Prusak, 2001]) but rather by working at the level of the individual patient and staff member and with individual teams. With its focus on person centredness, PD seeks to increase self-esteem and self-efficacy, both of which are key elements in developing individual responsiveness and motivation for change (Walsh et al., 2004). An emphasis on the development of individual agency and individual responsiveness and communication has the capacity to develop the social capital of the organisation and in turn assist coordination and integration of services.

The place of PD and what it has to offer the building of social capital

PD does what is often hard to do in large organisations and in large systems: it works with individuals and teams; it helps engage individuals with the larger vision, a shared vision; and helps to create links with their own aspirations. It has the potential to translate complex organisational and strategic agendas into practice reality. As can be surmised, when the vision of patients and healthcare workers and the greater organisation differ significantly conflictual agendas can develop. When this occurs, best practice is difficult or impossible to achieve. PD by working in respectful ways can help move healthcare staff and patients to a better alignment of what constitutes person-centred care. In so doing it moves the energy that would otherwise have been expended in conflictual agendas and resistance towards shared citizenship.

As has been discussed, rigid boundaries, work practices and polices that are overly prescriptive, controlling and based upon suspicion and a lack of trust in staff or patients will deplete the social capital available and undermine worker agency. What is necessary is for the system as a whole to re-engage with the untapped potential lying within the healthcare workforce and their patients.

Whole systems approaches and evaluation

Having considered whole systems approaches, the development of person cen-teredness and systems integration, the topics of health system performance and evaluation from a person-centred perspective will now be addressed.

Murray and Frenk (2000) identify weaknesses in the two common approaches taken to overall health system performance, namely, identifying the attributes of health systems and the indicators that are readily available. They argue that the first step in understanding overall health system (macro) performance is to identify its operational boundaries (so as to separate the system from elements outside of it) and to be clear what the health system's purpose is. Using the WHO's three intrinsic goals for health systems to reflect their purpose, Murray and Frenk derive key performance concepts (Table 2.5).

This example at the macro-system level illustrates the importance of a shared purpose for systems working as well as for guiding evaluation strategies. Because it reflects systems purpose, emphasis is on outcomes. Other frameworks for evaluat-ing whole system approaches at the mezzo-systems level include the development of a small number of 'whole systems measures' for providing feedback on pro-cesses and outcomes. For example, the toolkit developed by The US Institute for Healthcare Improvement (2006) influenced by the six dimensions of quality – safe, effective, patient centred, timely, efficient and equitable – is aimed to complement existing measures such as financial or human resource measures so at to provide feedback on overall organisation performance.

However, as noted throughout this chapter, relevant structures, processes and patterns need to be in place for achieving the systems purpose in a holistic, inte-grated and person-centred way. From a project using a whole systems approach to developing national critical care services (Manley & Hardy, 2006), a systems framework (Figure 2.1) is used to make sense of the indicators that reflect both mezzo (service) and micro (team) outcomes, processes and patterns in relation to critical care teams and services (Manley & Hardy, 2006).

Table 2.5 Key performance concepts related to three intrinsic health system goals (Murray & Frenk, 2000)*

WHO primary goals	Performance concepts related to primary goals
Health	• Increasing average health status • Reducing health inequality

Responsiveness	• Respect for persons:
	  ○ Respect for dignity
	  ○ Respect for individual autonomy
	  ○ Respect for confidentiality
	• Client orientation:
	  ○ Prompt attention to health needs
	  ○ Basic amenities, e.g. clean waiting rooms, adequate beds and food
	  ○ Access to social support networks during care
	  ○ Choice of institution and individual providing care

Fair financing	• Every household pays a fair share of the total health bill for a country ○ Very poor households pay nothing

* Intrinsic goals are goals of primary value in themselves as compared with instrumental goals that may contribute to the achievement of intrinsic goals; for example, improving access is an instrumental goal that will achieve increased health and responsiveness – the intrinsic goals.

The project used PD processes with 60 stakeholder groups in critical care, and as a result of wide consultation and collaborative working a number of organisational and team tools and frameworks have been developed to help critical care teams to measure their performance and continue to develop their effectiveness in providing

Different types of indicators

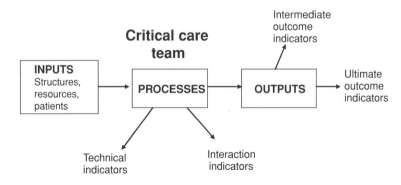

Figure 2.1 A systems-based framework for critical care indicators (Manley & Hardy 2006).

Table 2.6 Identifying the terms: team indicators of effectiveness (Manley & Hardy, 2006)

Type of indicator	Definition	Examples
Technical process indicators	The measures used to identify whether team actions are being performed and how the team works to achieve implementation of policy directives, clinical standards and protocols and context-related factors that effect the achievement of high-quality patient care	• The team consists of people relevant to provide effective healthcare to critical care patients • Percentage of cases judged to be managed appropriately on the most relevant quality dimensions
Interaction process indicators	The performance of care delivery (i.e. actions that the team have between them and with others) that relates to identifying, correcting and preventing health-related service provision	• The team recognise how engaging people who use the service in discussion and planning of care can improve and reduce anxiety, depression and PTSD symptoms in people who use their services
Intermediate outcome indicators	The impact of the teams' actions on healthcare practice and on people who use the service that leads towards achieving the ultimate outcome indicator	• Team regularly receive stakeholder feedback to promote and engage stakeholders in service developments
Ultimate outcome indicators	The achievement of the team goal/vision; for example, development of a team portfolio of robust evidence to demonstrate that recognised standards about person-centered, evidence-based care are met	• Evidence that the team works efficiently and effectively together to provide evidence-based, person-centred, high-quality healthcare

PTSD, post-traumatic stress disorder.

patient-centred services, as well as celebrating achievements (Manley & Hardy, 2006).

Different types of indicators will thus provide information on different aspects of micro-system function (see Table 2.6).

This project resulted in many of the requisites for a whole systems approach to providing critical care services at both the micro- and mezzo-systems level that reflect Benson's (1983) criteria in terms of partnership working:

- A common vision and purpose for critical care services shared by all stakeholder groups.
- Quality standards contributing to the development of national guidelines, namely, a single competency framework encompassing the full skill-set required for critical care services encompassing all professions contributions and stakeholders views.
- An assessment tool that is based on key principles for critical care team effectiveness using interactive process indicators (Table 2.7). These principles can be identified as 'enabling factors' and necessary prerequisites for professional and team development. A team, if accepting these key principles, would be able to establish a sustainable culture of team and workplace effectiveness that is evidence based and person centred.

Having explored some of the ways that whole systems approaches may be evaluated, the chapter will now conclude with a summary of the tools that are used in the methodology of PD to develop whole systems approaches to healthcare at the micro- and mezzo-levels. Many of these tools are used to both develop and evaluate services, as within a PD methodology, systematic and rigorous approaches to implementation, and evaluation are intertwined.

Tools and approaches to achieving integration and other criteria of systems

The Audit Commission (2002) in their report about building a whole systems approach to integrated services for older people identify a number of common steps that can offer a route map towards whole systems working. Table 2.8 identifies these

Table 2.7 Principles underpinning effective micro-systems at the team level (Manley & Hardy, 2006)

> - Learning can be used and translated into pathways, decisions and strategies that over time provide a 'road map' that enables a team to share a common definition of purpose and create an agreed direction towards achieving team goals
>
> - Work/practice-based learning promotes a partnership spirit within a framework of quality improvement
>
> - Ongoing evaluation, through critical inquiry, facilitates frequent and specific communication that fosters a culture of collaboration, person centredness and communication conducive to quality improvement
>
> - Sustainability in quality improvement work is significantly related to supportive leadership, facilitative human resources, increased activity in seeking new evidence and enhanced implementation of findings in clinical practice

Table 2.8 Steps towards whole systems approaches (after the Audit Commission, 2002) aligned to practice development tools and approaches that can support each step

Audit commission step	Processes	Practice development tools and processes
1. Start with the views and aspirations of users	Developing a shared vision starting with users and then involving other stakeholders and multiple perspectives	• Values clarification to develop a shared purpose and agreed mechanisms for achieving the purpose as well as ways of working with all key stakeholders • Visioning • Stakeholder analysis to identify the concerns, claims and issues of stakeholders • Patient stories/interviews
2. Understand your local whole system	Painting a picture using mapping services, flows and bottlenecks and existing data Defining the system boundaries Identification of barriers to flow	• Real-time tracking of patients journey (McCormack et al., 2006) • Patient stories and experience • Observation of care • Assessment of the workplace culture • Implementing systems that challenge barriers, contradictions and accepted norms
3. Invest in development capacity	Funding dedicated staff to carry out coordination/service development role across the system	• Developing a specific PD skill-set in practice-based facilitators • 360° analysis • Role clarification • Supervision systems
4. Encourage small-scale innovation	Assess impact and if it works roll it out	• Developing evidence-based care pathways • Implementing evidence-based guidelines • Work-based learning initiatives that feed into transformation • Participative practice based research approaches, e.g. action research
5. Ensure that there are well-placed enthusiasts at key points in the whole system	Identify key enthusiasts across system in different sites	• Role clarification • 360° analysis • Methods for achieving critical reflection

Table 2.8 *(cont.)*

Audit commission step	Processes	Practice development tools and processes
6. Exploit the opportunities for new organisational relationships and for rebalancing the system	Use policy initiatives to drive new ways of working	• Mapping and using key policy drivers • Enabling evidence-based and policy-based care
7. Create mechanisms to ensure that new approaches and ways of working penetrate mainstream services	Creating a culture that embeds the changes, e.g. rotating staff	• Workplace cultural assessment • Strategies for changing the culture • Developing transformational leaders • Developing work-based learning and cultural change facilitation expertise • Clinical supervision, active learning strategies • Implementing shared governance systems
8. Monitor progress	Involving users and other stakeholders	• Using stakeholder evaluation approaches • Developing evaluation criteria that reflect core purposes • Process and outcome evaluation • Participative practice based research approaches, e.g. action research

steps aligning them to common PD tools and processes. We would suggest that the alignment of these PD tools and processes with systems redesign enables those engaged in PD work to make a valuable contribution to the redesign of clinical services.

Summary and conclusions

This chapter has explored the relationships between healthcare systems and processes with an emphasis on person centredness. PD, with its emphasis on developing person-centred cultures and practices at the micro-level of healthcare systems, has much to offer the development of integrated care delivery. Person centredness emphasises the need for all persons to have the space and support to flourish. This flourishing enables creativity in practice and enhances the patterns embedded in systems. Person centredness enables expertise in practice to be realised, for dynamic interpersonal relationships to be embraced, for autonomy to be capitalised upon and for a culture of learning to be enhanced. All these factors contribute to the delivery of patient-centred care and ultimately to clinical effectiveness and improved patient outcome. We have argued that an integrated system that holds person centredness central to its integration builds social capital in an organisation and thus is essential to recruitment, retention and capacity building strategies. Systems that pay attention to the dignity and respect of staff ultimately make a difference to the social capital available to the organisation and consequently to the lives of patients and staff.

References

Adler, P. & Kwon, S. (2002) Social capital: Prospects for a new concept. *Academy of Management Review.* **27**(1), 17–40.

Audit Commission (2002) *Integrated Services for Older People: Building a Whole System Approach in England.* Audit Commission, London.

Baecker, D. (2001) Why systems? *Theory, Culture and Society.* **18**(1), 59–74.

Bellman, L., Bywood, C. & Dale, S. (2003) Advancing working and learning through critical action research: Creativity and constraints. *Nurse Education in Practice.* **3**(2), 186–194.

Benson, J.K. (1983) A framework for policy analysis. In: *Interorganizational Co-Ordination* (eds D.L. Rogers & O.A. Whetton). Iowa State University Press, Ames, IA.

Binnie, A. & Titchen, A. (1999) *Freedom to Practice: The Development of Patient-Centred Nursing.* Butterworth-Heinemann, Oxford.

Capra, F. (2002) *The Hidden Connection: Integrating the Biological, Cognitive, and Social Dimensions of Life into a Science of Sustainability.* Doubleday, New York.

Carr, A.J. & Higginson, J. (2001) Are quality of life measures patient centred? *British Medical Journal.* **322**(7298), 1357–1360.

Checkland, P. (2001) *Systems Thinking, Systems Practice.* John Wiley and Sons. 3rd Reprint.

Cohen, D. & Prusak, L. (2001) *In Good Company. How Social Capital makes Organizations Work.* Harvard Business School Press, Boston, MA.

Curley, M.A. (1998) Patient-nurse synergy: Optimizing patients' outcomes. *American Journal of Critical Care.* **7**(1), 64–72.

Dartmouth Hitchcock Medical School (22 June 2007) (www.clinicalmicrosystems.org)

Davies, G. (2005) *The Queensland Public Hospitals Commission of Inquiry.* The Health Quality and Complaints Commission. Brisbane, Queensland, Australia. Available from http://www.qphci.qld.gov.au/ [accessed 30/06/2007].

Day, D. (2001) Leadership development: A review in context. *The Leadership Quarterly.* **11**, 581–613.

Department of Health (2003) *Changing Places: Report on the Work of the Health and Social Care Change Agent Team 2002/3.* Department of Health, London.

Dewing, J. (2004) Concerns relating to the application of frameworks to promote person-centredness in nursing with older people. *International Journal of Older People Nursing.* **13**(3a), 39–44.

Edmondson, A. (1999) Psychological safety and learning behaviour in work teams. *Administrative Quarterly.* **44**(2), 350–383.

Grant, D., Wailes, N., Michelson, G., Brewer, A. & Hall, R. (2002) Re-conceptualizing organizational change: Strategies, processes, forms and discourses. *Strategic Change.* **11**(5), 237–242.

Greenhalgh, T., Robert, G., Bate, P., Kyriakidou, O., MacFarlane, F. & Peacock, R. (2004) How to spread good ideas: A systematic review of the literature on diffusion, dissemination and sustainability of innovation in health service delivery and organisation. *Report for the National Coordinating Centre for NHS Service Delivery and Organisation R&D (NCCSDO),* University College, London.

Grone, O. & Garcia-Barbero, M. (2002) *Trends in Integrated Care – Reflections on Conceptual Issues.* World Health Organization, Copenhagen. EUR/02/5037864.

Haas, M. & Kleingeld, A.D. (1999) Multilevel design of performance measurement systems: Enhancing strategic dialogue throughout the organization. *Management Accounting Research.* **10**, 233–261.

Handy, C. (1986) *Understanding Organizations.* Penguin Books, London.

Harrison, A., Hillier, D. & Redman, R. (2005) Utilizing practice development to implement an integrated care pathway for self-harm. *Practice Development in Health Care.* **4**(2), 77–85.

Hodson, R. (2001) *Dignity at Work.* Cambridge University Press, Cambridge.

Hronek, C. & Bleich, M. (2002) The less than perfect medication system: A systems approach to improvement. *Journal of Nursing Care Quality.* **16**(4), 17–22.

Institute for Innovation and Improvement (2005) *Working in Systems: Process and Systems Thinking,* Improvement Leaders Guides. NHS Institute for Innovation and Improvement, Coventry.

Institute for Innovation and Improvement (2006) *IHI's Whole System Measures Tool Kit: Version 2.0.* Institute of Health Care Improvement, Coventry. (www.ihi.org)

Jones, G. & George, J. (1998) The experience and evolution of trust: Implications for cooperation and teamwork. *Academy of Management Review.* **23**, 531–546.

Keating, C. (2001) An approach for systems analysis of patient care operations. *Journal of Nursing Administration.* **31**(7/8), 355–363.

Kennedy, I. (Chairman) (2001) *Learning from Bristol: The Report of the Public Inquiry into Children's Heart Surgery at the Bristol Royal Infirmary 1984–1995.* Department of Health, London.

Kitson, A., Harvey, G. & McCormack, B. (1998) Enabling the implementation of evidenced based practice: A conceptual framework. *Quality in Health Care.* **7**(3), 149–158.

Kitwood, T. (1997) On being a person. In: *Dementia Reconsidered: The Person Comes First* (ed T. Kitwood), pp. 7–19. Open University Press, Milton Keynes.

Manley, K. (2000) Organisational culture and consultant nurse outcomes: Part 1 organisational culture. *Nursing in Critical Care.* **5**(4), 179–184.

Manley, K. (2004) Workplace culture: Is your workplace culture effective? How would you know? *Nursing in Critical Care.* **9**(1), 1–3.

Manley, K. & Hardy, S. (2006) Improving services to patients through ongoing development of critical care teams. A project report commissioned by the Department of Health (England), London.

Manley, K. & Webster, J. (2006) Can we keep quality alive? *Nursing Standard.* **21**(3), 12–15.

Marx, K. (1992) Economic and philosophical manuscript of 1844. In: *Early Writings.* Penguin Classics, London.

McConkey, R. (2000) Community care and resettlement. *Currrent Opinion in Psychiatry.* **13**(5), 491–495.

McCormack, B. (2001) *Negotiating Partnerships with Older People – A Person-Centred Approach.* Ashgate, Basingstoke.

McCormack, B. (2002) The person of the voice: narrative identities in informed consent. *Nursing Philosophy.* **3**, 114–119.

McCormack, B. (2003) A conceptual framework for person-centred practice with older people. *International Journal of Nursing Practice.* **9**, 202–209.

McCormack, B. (2004) Person-centredness in gerontological nursing: An overview of the literature. *International Journal of Older People Nursing.* **13**(3a), 31–38.

McCormack, B., Dewar, B., Wright, J., Garbett, R., Harvey, G. & Ballantine, K. (2006) *A Realist Synthesis of Evidence Relating to Practice Development: Executive Summary.* NHS Quality Improvement. Scotland. (www.nes.scot.nhs.uk)

McCormack, B., Manley, K., Kitson, A., Titchen, A. & Harvey, G. (1999) Towards practice development – a vision in reality or a reality without vision? *Journal of Nursing Management.* **7**, 255–264.

McCormack, B., Reed. J., Cook. G., Childs, S., Hall, A. & Mitchell, E. (2005) *Whole Systems Working with Older People: A Critical Review and Case Study of the Evidence.* Research Report. Commissioned research from the DHSSPS R&D Office. Commissioned Research Programme.

McGuire, E. (1999) Chaos theory: Learning a new science. *Journal of Nursing Administration.* **29**(2), 8–9.

Mead, N. & Bower, P. (2000) Patient-centredness: A conceptual framework and review of the empirical literature. *Social Science and Medicine.* **51**(7), 1087–1110.

Mitchell, P.H., Ferketich, S. & Jennings, B.M. (1998) Quality health outcomes model. American academy of nursing expert panel on quality health care. *Image Journal of Nursing Scholarship.* **30**(1), 43–46.

Murray, C. & Frenk, J. (2000) A framework for assessing the performance of health systems. *Bulletin of WHO.* **78**(6), 718.

Nelson, E., Batalden, P., Huber, T., Mohr, J., Godfrey, M., Headrick, L. & Wasson, J. (2002) Microsystems in health care: Part 1. Learning from high-performing front-line clinical units. *Journal of Quality Improvement.* **28**(9), 472–493.

Nestel, D. & Betson, C. (1999) An evaluation of a communication skills workshop for dentists: Cultural and clinical relevance of the patient-centred interview. *British Dental Journal.* **187**(7), 385–388.

Newhouse, R. & Mills, M.E. (1999) Vertical systems integration. *Journal of Nursing Administration.* **29**(10), 22–29.

Nolan, M., Davies, S., Brown, J., Keady, J. & Nolan, J. (2004) Beyond 'person-centred' care: A new vision for gerontological nursing. *International Journal of Older People Nursing.* **13**(3a), 45–53.

Payne, M. (2000) *Teamwork in Multiprofessional Care.* Macmillan, London.

Plsek, P.E. (2001) Redesigning health care with insights from the science of complex adaptive systems. In: *Crossing the Chasm: A New Health System for the 21st Century.* National Academy Press, Washington, DC.

Prusak, L. & Cohen, D. (2001) How to invest in social capital. *Harvard Business Review.* **79**(6), 86–93.

Putnam, R.D. (1993) *Making Democracy Work. Civic Traditions in Modern Italy.* Princeton University Press, Princeton, NJ.

Putnam, R.D. (2000) *Bowling Alone. The Collapse and Revival of American Community*. Simon and Schuster, New York.

Radwin, L. & Fawcett, J. (2002) A conceptual model-based programme of nursing research: Retrospective and prospective applications. *Journal of Advanced Nursing.* **40**(3), 355–360.

Royal College of Nursing (2007) *Workplace Resources for Practice Development*. Royal College of Nursing, London.

Saul, J.R. (2001) *On Equilibrium*. Penguin, Toronto.

Schein, E.H. (2004) *Organizational Culture and Leadership*, 3rd edn. Jossey-Bass, San Francisco.

Silverman, D. (1974) *The Theory of Organizations*. Heineman, London.

Stewart, M. (2001) Towards a global definition of patient-centred care. *British Medical Journal.* **322**, 444–445.

Von Bertanlanffy, L. (1968) *General Systems Theory*. Braziller, New York.

Walsh, K. & Kowanko, I. (2002) Nurses' and patients' perceptions of dignity. *International Journal of Nursing Practice.* **8**(3), 143–151.

Walsh, K., Lawless, J., Moss, C. & Allbon, C. (2005) The development of an engagement tool for practice development. *Practice Development in Health Care.* **4**(3), 124–130.

Walsh, K., McAllister, M., Morgan, A. & Thornhill, J. (2004) Motivating change: Using motivational interviewing in practice development. *Practice Development in Health Care.* **3**(2), 92–100.

Walsh, K., Moss, C. & Fitzgerald, M. (2006) Solution focused approaches and their relevance to practice development. *Practice Development in Health Care.* **5**(3), 145–155.

Ward, C. & McCormack, B. (2000) Creating an adult learning culture through practice development. *Nurse Education Today.* **20**(4), 259–266.

Wilson, V. (2005) Developing a culture of family-centred care: An emancipatory practice development approach. Unpublished PhD Thesis, Monash University, Melbourne.

Wilson, V., McCormack, B. & Ives, G. (2006) Replacing the 'self' in learning. *Learning in Health and Social Care.* **5**(2), 90–105.

World Health Organization (2000) *Health Systems Performance Glossary*. Available from www.who.int/health-systems-performance/docs/glossary.htm [accessed 27/06/2007].

Wystanski, M. (2000) Patient-centred verses client-mental health care. *Canadian Journal of Psychiatry.* **45**(7), 670–671.

3. The Ever-Changing Discourse of Practice Development: Can We All Keep Afloat?

Lucienne Hoogwerf, Donna Frost and Tanya McCance

Introduction

In this chapter, we will attempt to make sense of the complex language underpinning and surrounding practice development (PD). In order to do this, attention will be given to developing an understanding of discourse, which is situated within the theoretical perspective provided by Habermas (1981). Using a nautical metaphor, we will argue that the language of practice developers reflects their understanding of PD and characterises where they are on their PD journey, thus leading to the emergence of multiple discourses. The implications of these multiple discourses for PD will be discussed in relation to the following: creating a safe environment and the importance of facilitation; different levels of expertise; learning within organisations; understanding organisational change; and the influence at strategic and political levels. These issues will be drawn out and illustrated through the presentation of two practice examples.

Raising awareness of discourse

When we were invited to write a chapter on the multiple discourses of PD, we used as our starting point the definition of PD provided by McCormack et al. (1999):

> *Practice development is a continuous process of improvement towards increased effectiveness in person-centred care, through the enabling of nurses and healthcare teams to transform the culture and context of care. It is enabled and supported by facilitators committed to a systematic, rigorous continuous process of emancipatory change.*
>
> *p. 256*

Garbett and McCormack (2002) developed this conceptualisation further, through the presentation of a model for PD, which draws out important relationships between key concepts that underpin PD work.

It can, however, be argued that at the most fundamental level, the discourse of PD focuses on developing practice with the ultimate aim of improving the quality of patient care. The continuous nature of PD and its focus on improvement places it within the context of quality improvement, modernisation and service development. This has been confirmed through a study conducted by Garbett and McCormack (2002), which involved focus group interviews with practice developers. These participants identified 'improvement' as a key reason for justifying the establishment of PD roles within organisations. This is also the context provided by McCormack et al. (2004):

> *developing practice (with its explicit focus on improving patients' experiences of healthcare) is everyone's responsibility . . . all nurses need to be aware of the processes of PD and to embrace a commitment to continuous improvement.*
>
> *p. 3*

At this level it can be argued that superficially there is a common discourse captured by the term 'PD' that is about *improving care*. Therefore, it is the commitment to improve practice that connects practitioners.

By working through issues that arise while engaged in this process of improving care, it is believed that language and discourse will change and develop. Language and discourse give meaning to actions. Understandings from actions give in turn meaning to language and discourse. All three – language, discourse and action – are vital to developing understandings and theories about PD, some of which we will explore in the next section.

Developing understandings of discourse

Discourse can be understood in a number of ways. *The Concise Oxford Dictionary of Current English* (1990) and Merriam-Webster (2005) give several closely related definitions of discourse. At its simplest, discourse is a synonym of 'conversation', denoting the verbal interchange of ideas. Discourse can also refer to the formal, orderly and extended expression of thought on a subject, such as a lecture, sermon or academic dissertation. At its most abstract level, discourse is defined by Merriam-Webster (2005) as a mode of organising knowledge, ideas, or experience that is rooted in language and its concrete contexts. In essence then, the same word can be used to describe both 'everyday talk' *and* the complex grouping of concepts and assumptions that arise from and impact on that 'everyday talk'.

Habermas' view of communication and discourse provides a theoretical base for our discussion. His work is located within the critical paradigm and is therefore appropriate since PD is informed by critical social science (Manley & McCormack, 2004). Habermas (1981) argued that communication between individuals is governed by basic, but required and implied, rules. These lead to conditions that create what Habermas called the ideal speech situation. These conditions are as follows:

- All people involved must have equal opportunity to start a discourse.
- All people involved must have equal opportunity to participate in the discourse.
- There may not be any difference in power between the participants.
- The participants must be truthful to each other.

Central throughout the whole process is the freedom of discourse (Habermas, 1974). Coercion and deception are sought to be overcome by a process of rational discussion and democratic political action. In other words, an environment needs to be created where democratic communication can occur. If neither democratic communication nor the development of a safe environment takes place then the understandings of the individuals involved will be based on distortion and so will be the resulting actions. The openness of expression that 'the ideal speech situation' demands can theoretically be created among members of any group or within any organisation. They reflect the emancipatory potential for individuals working in organisations. By providing every person with the same opportunity to participate in discourse, Habermas hopes to eradicate the prejudices that limit marginalised groups. Habermas (1990) has further developed and elaborated his theory of communicative action with his work *Moral Consciousness and Communicative Action*. In this work, he no longer speaks of a known ideal speech situation but instead of a new moral system ('Discourse ethics'). According to Habermas, discourse is the everyday practice of regulating conflict and reaching consensus; it is communication about communication (Outhwaite, 2005). Implicit in his work is the notion that discourse is at once shaping our experience and being shaped by the experience. Importantly, while 'taken-for-granted background assumptions and naively mastered skills' (Habermas, 1981, p. 335) remain unexamined, a discourse can function as a social boundary, defining what can be said – or thought – about a particular topic. Only by having the freedom to ask critical questions, and thereby expose and challenge underlying assumptions, can groups begin to change their actions – thereby broadening their discourse.

As pointed out by Elliott (2005), the work of Habermas has practical intent, but the concrete link from theory to practice is not explicit in his work and remains open to many interpretations. PD, with its intention to change practice based on common understandings, can provide a practical means to connect theory and practice. The starting point for practitioners in understanding the nature of a practice problem and the context in which practice occurs is to examine how the past has shaped their practice reality (Habermas, 1974). Social and political aspects are hereby taken into consideration. The language and discourses used by the practitioners in describing problems or issues reflect their knowledge and understandings of the problem at hand. Consequently, it is important that practitioners have an understanding of what knowledge is and how it is developed. To Habermas (1972) knowledge, rather than being a product of the pure, detached and intellectual act, is the outcome of human activity that is motivated by natural needs and interests. He describes three 'knowledge-constitutive interests': (1) technical interest focuses on explanation and is aligned with the natural sciences; (2) practical interest focuses on understanding and is aligned to hermeneutic or interpretive sciences; and (3) emancipatory interest using critical reflection to achieve freedom from restraints and sits within the critical sciences paradigm.

Whilst it is important to acknowledge the legitimacy of all types of knowledge, it is also important to understand what is achievable. Appling technical knowledge to developing practice relies on the assumption that evidence demonstrates effectiveness and will therefore be used. The way in which evidence is used to inform changes in practice and the nature of evidence sources that can be used are two important factors. It is fair to say that evidence does not drive the process within an emancipatory approach to PD, but rather informs the process in an ongoing way as the need arises. There is also wider recognition of the impact of other components in developing practice such as the importance of context and facilitation as well as evidence and the relationship between these elements in developing effective change strategies (Kitson et al., 1998; Rycroft-Malone et al., 2002). McCormack and Titchen (2006) would also argue that the practice understanding (practical interest) can inform and guide practice, but it may not result in a change in the ways nurses practice. They go on to clarify this: 'achieving understanding is necessary in order to identify possibilities for action, but it is only through the processes of taking action and the learning that results that true enlightenment can be achieved' (p. 244).

The processes described above are complex; skilled facilitation is almost essential for groups or individuals embarking on a PD project. Guided critical reflection enables practitioners to expose their existing knowledge and understanding of the context and critically evaluate it. Mezirow (1981) argues that critical reflection results in transformation of meaning and action and Johns (1995) suggests that learning through reflection is an emancipatory activity. In other words, it enables practitioners to seek the knowledge necessary to choose the most just course of action in a particular situation. When the agreed upon action is based on consensus, theoretically informed and with emancipatory intent, the process is described in critical social science language as 'the process of enlightenment'. Discourse becomes the vehicle for change as knowledge and action are informed by the language used by the practitioners. Knowledge is in turn informed by language and discourse and visa versa.

Habermas' notion on knowledge development has been influential within PD in terms of discourse, science and research arising from a practitioner's interests. Through knowledge, language and discourse practitioners are able to both reconstruct their practice and develop theories of practice.

We would like to share our understandings of discourse by means of a metaphor. While engaged in PD work we have found that many people describe – both in words and pictures – their PD journey as like being on a ship crossing the ocean, with all the turmoil of changing weather and heavy seas. We like this metaphor and will use it to examine the multiple discourses of PD.

A metaphorical exploration of discourse

Otto Neurath (1882–1945) used the image of floating in a boat on the open sea to illustrate a number of concepts, for example our linguistic situation (Cartwright et al., 1996). To remain afloat requires repairs, but with no dry dock we cannot inspect the boat from the outside. We can, however, examine and individually replace any rotten planks from inside the boat. So not only can we stay afloat, but gradually we are also able to repair or even refashion the entire boat (Quine, 1960, p. 3).

In PD we can also think of ourselves as sailors on a vessel, voyaging across the ocean. On our voyage the ocean represents the practice world, or the public sphere in which healthcare is organised and delivered. Like an ocean with varying winds and tides, the practice world is influenced by outside forces.

Organisations can be represented by the vessels that voyage the ocean. As well as differing destinations, each vessel has its own culture arising from the worldviews, wishes and competency levels of the people on the boat. How challenges are tackled depends in turn on the craftsmanship of the captain and crew, the resources available to them and the nature of the role of the passengers. While there are always captains and officers (managers), crew (employees) and passengers (patients), the interactions and relationships between these groups can vary widely.

In our metaphor, PD, with its tools and processes, is a particular way of sailing the ocean, or of navigating the practice world. More than the navigation systems and instruments, it encompasses the way in which the ocean is seen, described and interpreted, and the way in which the crew is organised, facilitated and interacts with others on the boat, including passengers. Within our metaphor, discourse enables understanding and problem-solving on the boat. It develops the understanding of how the vessel responds to the movement of the ocean and why; for example, certain planks in the hull become cracked or damaged. Through understanding on an individual and collective level the crew is able to take informed action based on consensus in order to make repairs. If a common discourse based on consensus[1] develops, it can enable effective maintenance or transformation of the entire vessel.

Within the overarching culture on the vessel there are of course various subcultures, for example, the sub-culture of the captain and officers, and the sub-cultures among the different groups in the crew and among the passengers. Discourses develop specific to the practice and shared assumptions of each sub-culture. This multiplicity of discourses enables the members of each sub-culture to develop their personal and professional knowledge – in other words, 'the prudent understanding of what should be done in practical situations' (Carr & Kemmis, 1986, p. 32). It can mean, however, that the different sub-cultures may have difficulty understanding each other's assumptions, reaching consensus or agreeing

---

[1] At this point it is important to note that full consensus cannot always be reached. The collaborative actions will then be based on the rule of the majority. Consensus can then be formed on process criteria.

on a course of action. These factors influence the ability of the crew to respond together to challenging situations and to reach the destination of the journey.

Sailing a PD vessel successfully is also dependent on the competency levels of the crew, not only in terms of their individual professions but also with respect to PD. Some crew members will focus on navigation systems and instruments, naive in the simple belief that these tools will enable them to safely sail their vessel to the chosen destination. Other crew members, however, will have an awareness of the unpredictable dangers of the ocean and the chance of stormy waters that can damage the integrity of their vessel. Some crew members, often veteran sailors, have developed an understanding of the ocean and its potential dangers and have learnt to read the weather seemingly effortlessly. They know intuitively what resources to use, bearing in mind the safety of their vessel, crew and passengers, enabling them to reach their final destination with developed insights and knowledge, which are transferable to new journeys.

The Dreyfus and Dreyfus model

The analogy represents differing levels of expertise, reflecting levels of proficiency not unlike those presented by Dreyfus and Dreyfus (1986). These authors present five stages of skill acquisition referred to as novice, advanced beginner, competent, proficient, and expert. Each stage reflects movement from what Dreyfus and Dreyfus (1986) refer to as rule-based 'knowing that' to experience-based 'know-how'. Applying this model to PD is useful in distinguishing the different levels of understanding/proficiency that are reflected in the multiple discourses of those engaged in this activity.

As a *novice* the individual learns to rely on objective facts and features and from this defines rules that determine action. At this stage rules are made clear and objective to the novice, which are applied without reference to what else may be happening in a given situation. Dreyfus and Dreyfus (1986) refer to such situations as 'context free' with the focus on processing information. The novice moves to the stage of an *advanced beginner* after gaining experience of coping with real situations. This enables the individual to consider more context-free situations and to use more sophisticated rules, while at the same time recognising additional elements that are not context free but are 'situational'. Performance at these two stages can reflect a technical approach to PD or indeed a focus on the isolated use of tools and techniques.

As the advanced beginner gains more experience the number of context-free and situational elements increases, thus requiring a level of performance that enables the processing of a situation as a set of facts. At this stage, the *competent* performer is able to determine the importance of some facts as dependent on the presence of other facts. Dreyfus and Dreyfus (1986) highlight the importance of choosing a plan with a particular goal or outcome in mind. At this stage, they identify a greater level of involvement in what occurs as a result. At this stage, the practice developer begins to demonstrate understanding of terms, the relationship between components, and how to make synergistic connections.

Proficient and expert are the two highest levels of skill, which are characterised by 'a rapid, fluid, involved kind of behaviour' (Dreyfus & Dreyfus, 1986, p. 27).

The *proficient* performer makes decisions after reflecting on various alternatives, informed by previous experience of similar situations and what worked in the past. At this stage, Dreyfus and Dreyfus (1986) describe an ability to 'intuitively respond to patterns without decomposing them into component features' (p. 28) and refer to this as practical 'know-how'. At the highest level, the *expert* arrives at decisions not as a result of detached deliberations, but based on 'mature and practiced understanding', with skills becoming so much part of the expert's way of working (Dreyfus & Dreyfus, 1986, p. 30). Practice developers working at these levels demonstrate both a philosophical and theoretical understanding of PD, enabling them to interpret complex situations and to decide on an appropriate course of action.

Applying this model to PD is useful in distinguishing the different levels of understanding and proficiency that are reflected in the multiple discourses of those engaged in this activity.

Aside from differing levels of proficiency, crew members and passengers may also be working with different understandings of the purpose of the journey depending on their worldview. Manley and McCormack (2003) articulate two main worldviews adopted by practice developers: emancipatory and technical PD. Emancipatory PD is located within a critical social science, with the focus on the social system, the assumptions held by individuals and groups about their own practice, and how reflection and self-understanding are influenced by these systems. According to Carr and Kemmis (1986) 'a critical social science will provide the kind of self-reflective understanding that will permit individuals to explain why the conditions under which they operate are frustrating and will suggest the sort of action that is required if the sources of these frustrations are to be eliminated' (p. 136). In contrast, McCormack et al. (2004) describe technical PD as 'a technical instrument for achieving the development of services to patients' (p. 36–37). It is thus logical that practitioners working from a technical perspective have a different worldview than those working from an emancipatory view. Their discourses, consequently, will differ.

In the preceding paragraphs, we have explored the theoretical underpinnings of discourse and presented beginning understandings through the use of a nautical metaphor and with reference to the Dreyfus and Dreyfus (1986) model. In order to deepen our understanding, we would like to share our lived experiences of multiple discourses within PD. The two practice examples (Examples 1 and 2) illustrate for us the ways in which the 'crews' from different 'vessels' were able to rebuild their boats while remaining afloat.

Example 1

Kauri ward

In an action research study that involved the introduction of patient participation (Hoogwerf, 2002), it became evident that the health professionals and manager in the study tended to work in consensus only while working mono-disciplinarily. Observations of multidisciplinary team meetings where patients' rehabilitation progress was discussed showed that all the team members used their own language. During

---

the meetings each participant attempted to convince the others of the rightness of their own view. The arguments used were at times meaningless to the other disciplines, at times resulting in inaction (although action plans were developed) and ineffective patient care. From Habermas' point of view on discourse, one can conclude that although the teams were starting to engage in discourse they had not yet reached consensus. Therefore they were not able to take transformative action.

During various research cycles the action research group (consisting of health professionals) worked together with the nurse consultant to develop participative care. This meant that a common understanding and language needed to be developed. The group started with developing their understanding and gathering evidence inspired by Habermas' (1974) notion on knowledge development.

The actions that resulted from the group were based on consensus. At the point that the group decided to work with goal setting (Locke & Latham, 1990), patients and their families became involved. It was at this point that a practice discourse developed. Returning to our metaphor, multidisciplinary team members were on board the vessel working from their own perspectives. They were each working with their own professional knowledge, which in turn created sub-cultures and language barriers. This influenced the course the boat took. The captain and navigator did not have the instruments at the time to set a common direction that would result in participative care based on consensus. In other words, a navigation system and instruments to repair the boat were missing. The nurse consultant was asked to facilitate the journey.

Example 2

Windmill Care

Windmill Care is a large nursing home. Over the last 7 years there have been varied attempts by several management teams to introduce change aimed at maintaining standards of care while improving efficiency. Although efficiency gains and better financial stability were realised, this was not the case with respect to quality of care and service delivery.

When the project described here began, members of all stakeholder groups (the chief executive board, the director of the organisation, residents and their families, and staff employed at Windmill Care) agreed that further action was necessary in order to improve resident care. Past experiences, however, had led to frustration, cynicism and mistrust. Groups and individuals in Windmill Care tended to locate the source of problems (and solutions) in the behaviour of other groups and individuals within the organisation. In discussions between these stakeholders conflict was not resolved and consensus was rarely achieved.

In mid-2005 the management team committed themselves, and thus the organisation, to a new approach to change management: PD. Two initial actions were taken to facilitate this process. An expert nurse was appointed who was also a competent practice developer, and two external facilitators were engaged.

The first steps taken by the PD facilitators were to open up a dialogue: they used creative workshops to enable people to share their experiences and feelings about working – and struggling – in Windmill Care. Different tools such as claims, concerns and issues and values clarification were used to examine the current situation and identify priorities for change and goals for the future. Such sessions occurred over time, daily work continued and some groups were better represented than others. There were regular evaluation moments, approaches were changed to meet the needs of those present or the circumstances, successes were shared and celebrated. Slowly, the climate of cynicism and frustration began to change into one of hope that new possibilities, a different future for Windmill Care, may be achievable.

There are currently a range of 'mini-projects' underway in Windmill Care. The projects tackle a number of priority areas identified collaboratively by stakeholders during the facilitated sessions described above. Members of all stakeholder groups are represented in the project teams (including clients and family members in some cases), and successes are celebrated through the whole organisation. The 'crew' of Windmill Care are beginning to rebuild their vessel.

Experiences from practice

In the given two examples, there are various issues that can be identified and which have a relationship to the multiple discourses of PD.

1. Creating a safe environment
2. Different levels of expertise
3. Learning within organisations
4. Understanding organisational change
5. Development of local theory

Although for the sake of clarity we will address each issue separately, in practice they are interlinked and developments in each area influence each other and often occur simultaneously. Important within them all is skilful facilitation, which is addressed in Chapter 8.

Creating a safe environment

As pointed out previously, freedom of discourse is vital if practice is to be transformed. An open democratic dialogue is necessary for the honest examination of a current situation and evaluation of learning that occurs.

The results of an *unsafe* environment were evident in Windmill Care when the PD project began. Metaphorically speaking, the early observations revealed an unseaworthy vessel, a seasick crew and passengers, with some members of both groups endlessly bailing water. The fact that the boat was both leaking and headed for the rocks was evident to many. Choosing an alternative to the rocks – a new destination ('better resident care') – could be seen as the easy part of the process. The challenging aspect lay in readying the crew (including the captain and officers), passengers and boat for the change in course that was required if the new destination was to be reached. The first step in 'getting ready' was the creation of a safe environment and the development of trust in each other and in the possibilities for positive change. One of the outside facilitators, for example, facilitated workshops with the crew, creating a safe environment for the free expression of lived experiences within the current culture of Windmill Care. The captain and officers were facilitated in participating in action learning sets and critical companionship (Titchen, 2001). These activities supported the development of collective project plans in which emancipatory principles and processes were explicitly used.

It was just as important on Kauri ward to create a safe environment for the action learning sets to enable the development of open democratic communication. In this example, an important tool was the consistent application of the group ground rules as formulated by Wheeler and Chin (1989). The development of trust allowed critical conversations to take place. This in turn aided understanding of each other's discipline-specific knowledge (procedural, practical, emancipatory and patients' knowledge). Here we saw the beginnings of critical conversations between disciplines.

Without skilled facilitation it is often difficult, when different disciplines, managers and practitioners work together, to achieve a safe environment. Habermas says that without being able to ask critical questions, a discourse can function as a social boundary. Such a boundary, in turn, prevents the asking of such questions as are necessary to begin the critical discussions that are the first step to understanding and learning to trust one another. Getting this process started was a crucial task of the facilitator(s) in both of the projects related here. The facilitator on Kauri ward described it as if she, one of the crew members on the boat, had several navigation instruments and tools with her in her duffel bag. With the help of these tools she was able to facilitate the crew in choosing their direction.

Different levels of expertise

The arrival of people with PD knowledge and skills was not – as some thought – the arrival of a life raft. It was the beginning of a process to rebuild the boats and equip those on them with skills they could use to continually look critically at their practice. This process would be experienced differently by everybody. At the start of the journeys described in our examples most of the people involved, except the nurse consultant and external facilitators, were novice practice developers, with differing levels of professional expertise.

In Windmill Care, many of those new to a PD approach to change could have been described as frightened. Their 'boat' was, after all, in danger of sinking. The decision to turn the boat around and aim for 'better resident care' seemed irrelevant and almost impossible to those focusing on survival. Their situation can be contrasted with that on Kauri ward. Here a number of 'crew members' were professionally expert. Their knowledge and craftsmanship meant that they agreed with the decision of the captain and navigator to take the boat out of heavy seas, which were damaging the hull. The similarity between the two situations is that both crews were novices with respect to PD. This new navigation system needed to be proven before the crews would trust that it worked. People were worried, for example, about the negative emotions and experiences that would be shared. The refusal of some people to actively participate with the new method was viewed by others as proof that such an approach would never work.

In Windmill Care an expert nurse had 'come aboard' at about the same time as the expert facilitators. With some experience of PD she felt at ease with its tools and work methods. Not surprised by the scepticism of some crew members, the presence of the waves or leaks in the boat, she possessed the skills necessary to hear the perspectives of other stakeholders and involve them in planning and evaluating actions. She struggled, however, with being so close to the rocks. She struggled, in other words, to apply the PD approach when confronted with serious shortcomings in practice that required immediate action. The sharing of experiences among staff, for example, felt like a luxury when residents and families were being short-changed.

The nurse consultant (on Kauri ward) and the external facilitators (in Windmill Care) were proficient practice developers. They were not overawed by the situations they encountered on arrival in the organisations nor by the emotions and stories that emerged during the beginning stages of the projects. In contrast, the reactions from various stakeholders and the struggles and triumphs experienced by people within the organisation were recognisable, to the more experienced practice developer, as belonging to and necessary for the process. Metaphorically speaking, the expert practice developer can respond intuitively to the weather and water surrounding the boat. Recognition of patterns not only enables anticipation of waves, but also anticipation of group processes that are taking place among the crew. Through critical conversations and reflection on previous experiences they are able to consciously choose from a range of integrated strategies with which to face the sailing conditions and facilitate the crew.

It can be seen that although all present on the boat are experiencing the same events, their perceptions, opinions and descriptions of those events are different from each other. Different individuals and professional groups will vary with respect to the meaning they assign, the language they use and the strategies they will use in particular situations. Their discourses, in other words, will vary. Just as importantly within PD is the realisation that discourses will also vary depending on practice developer's level of expertise with PD.

Skilled facilitation is therefore crucial. Critical conversations are needed to connect the multiple discourses that exist even within the same project. The goal is a local discourse understood by and useful to all stakeholders within a particular project. For this to occur, a safe environment and skilled facilitation will not be enough. The different stakeholders must be able and willing to learn from their practice and from each other.

Learning within organisations

By engaging in the process of action learning, health professionals can learn, among other things, each other's language and develop an insight into each other's professional knowledge. By doing so they can come to a course of action that is based on consensus, multiple evidence and which truly solves the problems they are faced with in an emancipatory fashion. The process of action learning, therefore, can be recognised as discourse.

Formal critical learning strategies, such as action learning and critical reflection, sit within a reflective model that places emphasis on learning in and from practice.

Different models of reflection are advocated within PD, with Johns' (1995) and Mezirow's (1981) being two commonly used frameworks. Deliberate reflection allows professionals to practice thoughtfully, intelligently and carefully. This kind of reflection involves higher order processes of thought such as planning, preparing, analysing, synthesising, predicting and evaluating. Practitioners must draw not only on their professional knowledge but also on their knowledge of the context in which they work. The outcome is professional judgement and such judgement takes place before, during and after practice (Clarke et al., 1996).

Reflection forms a large component of the process of action learning where we are asked, or ask ourselves, questions (Weinstein, 1999; McGill & Beaty, 1992). Weinstein (1999) describes action learning as a process that is 'a way of learning in and from our actions, and from what happens to us, by taking time to question, understand and reflect, to gain insights and consider how to act in future' (p. 3). Importantly, the goal of action learning, according to Revans (1982), is to enable individuals to move from talking about action to taking action and herein lies the biggest challenge. Transferring the learning that takes place through formal strategies such as action learning into concrete actions that can change practice is one aspect that distinguishes a proficient practice developer from a novice practice developer.

To return to the example of Kauri ward, one could speak in the beginning stages of a language gap among the different practitioners and their patients, based on different professional or lay backgrounds, worldviews and experiences (Hoogwerf, 2002). The varied stakeholders did not understand each other's perspectives or language. Necessary to the process of change was the setting up of action research cycles and their skilled facilitation. Group members began to support each other to take different viewpoints and try out new approaches in their work. The action research progressed to a point where practitioners and patients were learning together and consequently developing a common language. The involvement of clients in the process was the crucial step, which enabled practitioners on Kauri ward to effectively solve some of the problems they were facing. This would not have been possible if the practitioners had not been able to make the transition from learning theoretically to applying what they had learnt and changing their practice. They were no longer fully reliant on the formal protocols of collaborative goal setting but could apply the principles of this process to other areas of their practice. They were therefore moving from being novice practice developers towards being competent practice developers.

Understanding organisational change

Professionals and practitioners with differing levels of professional expertise and at every level of an organisation can be practice developers. The practice developers who go on to become expert will not always come from high up in the hierarchy, just as those in traditional leadership roles may well be novice practice developers. However, vital to the success of a PD project is the effective discourse between different stakeholders regardless of their hierarchical level within the organisation. It is necessary that they develop a common language about the issue of interest or difficulty they are facing. Although the principles of PD would support a grassroots development of practice in a situation where the impetus, direction and energy originated from the practitioners, it is, in reality, almost vital that a team has the support of its manager when engaging in PD.

In our experience, a PD project will struggle and probably flounder without the support of managers, preferably those who are willing and able to engage in transformational leadership. This is important to recognise because it often means that as certain stakeholders become empowered others become disempowered. This has implications for practice, especially for traditional leadership roles. Careful facilitation is therefore needed to enable all stakeholders to feel safe, valued and supported while transforming towards their new role. These changes are political and occur throughout the entire journey. The skilful facilitator must be able to engage in political discourse while ensuring that it does not dominate the whole process.

On reflection, healthcare organisations, like any other, are subject to political processes associated with change. Critical conversations and reflection expose these and enable practitioners to find strategies to deal with them. A challenge for practice developers is to be able to facilitate critical conversations at every level within the organisation. The practice developer needs, therefore, to be comfortable in the various discourses present in a given context, and be able to 'translate' the necessary information to a language understandable to other stakeholders; in other words, be able to function as a linking pin (Hoogwerf, 2002).

At the beginning stage of the journey the navigators, in Kauri ward an experienced practitioner and a proficient practice developer, carefully brought the issues to the practitioners. In the case of Windmill Care outside facilitators facilitated this process. It involved examining systems and processes, the effect of legislation, the logistics and finances. By doing so it became evident that change brought about uncertainty. Although it brought excitement for some there was anxiety for others, irrespective of level within the organisation. However, because a safe environment was created in which the participants were able to trust the process they were better able to cope with the certainties brought about by the letting go of everyday practice and routines. On Kauri ward we saw beginnings of critical conversations between disciplines. They explored the organisational structure, knew who the opinion leaders were and the political processes in the organisation.

Development of local theory

McCormack et al. (2006) identify three dimensions that comprise the 'how' of PD:

- How learning happens, focusing on a reflective model using tools such as action learning and critical reflection.
- How change happens, focusing on the emancipatory approach, which raises awareness of culture and context through the use of values clarification, developing a shared vision, workplace culture analysis, developing shared ownership, and working through methods that are collaborative and participative.
- How knowledge is used and generated, focusing on the use of both deductive and inductive knowledge with the important emphasis on developing new knowledge and theory through processes that are rigorous and systematic.

Those involved in PD at Windmill Care are in the beginning phases of all three of these dimensions, with the current focus on the second dimension. Kauri ward, as described, saw active engagement in all three dimensions, including the last – to do with knowledge use and generation. Critical conversations among all stakeholders in Kauri ward led to a local practice discourse. Patients and nurses in the study began to use the same language. This enabled the team members, over time, to both implement and evaluate strategies of participative care. The practitioners most closely involved developed a local theory about their practice and made connections between theory and practice based on consensus. Moreover, it enabled them to reflect in and on action (Schon, 1983), thereby testing and further developing their local theories. This local discourse about practice was in turn shared with a broader community (through conferences and publication), thereby contributing to the discourse of practitioner research, which feeds into the discourse of PD.

In both Windmill Care and Kauri ward the organisations collaboratively agreed to rebuild their 'boats' to make it possible to reach a new destination. Because the direction and the design are based upon consensus, the organisations are engaged in a local discourse that can lead to the development of local theory. This in turn feeds into the wider discourse of PD. Metaphorically speaking, the boats these organisations aim to build will look like artisans have built them, and not as if they have come off an assembly line. As a result of being built for local conditions all such boats look different, but their crews would be able to effectively communicate with other boats where PD is also used.

Coming into the harbour

Every journey has an ending. The journey we have taken as authors has been both exciting and challenging. When beginning to write this chapter, we asked ourselves if the question about multiple discourses in PD was not purely academic. Along the way, however, we have developed insights into the relevance and importance of discourse with respect to deepening understandings and coming to consensus – in part through the discourses we ourselves have engaged in while writing the chapter.

As we have seen in our journey each discipline or stakeholder group tends to have their own language, culture and knowledge base from which a specific discourse evolves. Members of each group are usually able to engage in monodisciplinary or group-specific discourse without much difficulty. Their assumptions and constraints, however, tend to remain invisible and unexamined. This can also occur among groups of people who are engaged in PD (both within and across projects). The challenge is to examine and expose group-specific discourse and render it understandable and useful to all stakeholders involved. Conversation about conversation, or examining our everyday talk and discovering what we really mean and what we actually bring into effect with our words, is therefore crucial to reaching consensus. These processes are necessary at many different levels – between health professional and patient, at an organisational level and in academic circles – if we hope to engage in transformative action that improves quality in healthcare organisations.

In our title, we pose the question of whether or not we can all keep afloat within the multiple discourses of PD. We assert that it is the multiple discourses of PD that are in fact keeping us afloat. Without being able to reach consensus and solve problems our vessels will fall into disrepair and might even sink. In contrast, effectively reaching consensus and taking transformative action means that the multiple discourses of PD can be likened to many artisan built vessels all sailing together in one flotilla.

Future journeys

Given that the process of discourse is vital to the ongoing development and quality of care and service delivery, it is crucial that practice developers can skillfully engage in discourse across the different settings and within different groups. The current PD literature reports on various collaborations between practitioners, patients, scholars and educators. Outside healthcare there are examples of successful collaborations between all stakeholders where the role of chief executives is also made explicit (see, e.g., Senge, 1990; Senge et al., 1999). Future journeys within PD should also seek active collaboration with people in traditional positions of power. Only when those with influence actively participate in PD will the resulting discourse be one that actually examines empowerment and disempowerment. The real challenge would be to come to consensus while avoiding coercion and distortion. In this way, we would continue our journey, being more explicit about the existence of distorted realities and developing instruments and skills with which to counter them. We remain hopeful that the evolving discourse will enable the achievement of transformative action and changes that are embedded in practice at all levels of healthcare organisations.

Acknowledgements

We would like to thank all our critical friends who gave valuable feedback, enabling us to finish the chapter. Particular thanks are due to Theo Niessen, Teatske van der Zijpp, Shaun Cardiff and Brendan McCormack.

References

Carr, W. & Kemmis, S. (1986) *Becoming Critical: Knowing Through Action Research*. Deakin University Press, Melbourne.

Cartwright, N., Cat, J., Fleck, L. & Uebel, T.E. (1996) *Otto Neurath: Philosophy Between Science and Politics*. Cambridge University Press, Cambridge.

Clarke, B., James, C. & Kelly, J. (1996) Reflective practice: Reviewing the issues and refocusing the debate. *International Journal of Nursing Studies*. 33(2), 171–180.

Dreyfus, H.L. & Dreyfus, S.E. (1986) *Mind over Machine: The Power of Human Intuition and Expertise in the Era of the Computer*. The Free Press, New York.

Elliott, J. (2005) Becoming critical: The failure to connect. *Educational Action Research.* **13**(3), 359–374.

Garbett, R. & McCormack, B. (2002) The qualities and skills of practice developers. *Nursing Standard.* **16**(50), 3–36.

Habermas, J. (1972) *Knowledge and Human Interests.* Beacon, Boston.

Habermas, J. (1974) *Theory and Practice.* Heinemann Educational Books, London.

Habermas, J. (1981) *The Theory of Communicative Action.* Beacon, London.

Habermas, J. (1990) *Moral Consciousness and Communicative Action.* MIT Press, Cambridge.

Hoogwerf, L.J.R. (2002) *Innovation and Change in a Rehabilitation Unit for the Elderly Through Action Research*. Wetenschappelijke Uitgeverij Academia Press, Gent.

Johns, C. (1995) Framing learning through reflection with Carper's fundamental ways of knowing. *Journal of Advanced Nursing.* **22**(2), 226–234.

Kitson, A., Harvey, G. & McCormack, B. (1998) Enabling the implementation of evidence based practice: A conceptual framework. *Quality in Health Care.* **7**, 149–158.

Locke, E.A. & Latham, G.P. (1990) *A Theory of Goal Setting and Task Performance*. Prentice-Hall, Englewood Cliffs, NJ.

Manley, K. & McCormack, B. (2003) Practice development: Purpose, methodology, facilitation and evaluation. *Nursing in Critical Care.* **8**(1), 22–29.

Manley, K. & McCormack, B. (2004) Practice development: Purpose, methodology, facilitation and evaluation. In: *PD in Nursing* (eds B. McCormack, K. Manley & R. Garbett), pp. 33–50. Blackwell, Oxford.

McCormack, B., Dewar, B., Wright, J., Garbett, R., Harvey, G. & Ballantine, K. (2006) *A Realist Synthesis of Evidence Relating to Practice Development*. NHS Quality Improvement Scotland, Scotland.

McCormack, B., Manley, K. & Garbett, R. (2004) *Practice Development in Nursing*. Blackwell, Oxford.

McCormack, B., Manley, K., Kitson, A., Titchen, A. & Harvey, G. (1999) Towards practice development: A vision in reality or a reality without vision? *Journal of Nursing Management.* **7**(5), 255–264.

McCormack, B. & Titchen, A. (2006) Critical creativity: Melding, exploding, blending. *Educational Action Research.* **14**(2), 239–266.

McGill, I. & Beaty, L. (1992) *Action Learning A Practitioner's Guide*. Kogan Page, London.

Merriam-Webster (2005) Merriam-Webster, Inc. Available from www.Merriam-Webster.com [accessed 23/09/2006].

Mezirow, J. (1981) A critical theory of adult learning and education. *Adult Education.* **32**(1), 3–24.

Outhwaite, W. (ed) (2005) *The Habermas Reader.* Polity, Cambridge.

Revans, R.W. (1982) What is Action Learning? *Journal of Management Development.* **1**(3), 64–75.

Rycroft-Malone, J., Harvey, G., Kitson, A., McCormack, B., Seers, K. & Titchen, A. (2002) Getting evidence into practice: ingredients for change. Factors influencing implementation and facilitation, and presentation of Promoting Action on Research Implementation in Health Services (PARIHS) framework. *Nursing Standard.* **16**(37), 38–43.

Quine, W.V.O. (1960) *Word and Object (Studies in Communication)*. MIT Press, Boston.

Schon, D.A. (1983) *The Reflective Practitioner: How Professionals Think in Action.* Basic Books, Cambridge, MA.

Senge, P. (1990) *The Fifth Discipline: The Art and Practice of the Learning Organization.* Double Day, New York.

Senge, P., Kleine, A., Roberts, C., Ross, R., Roth, G. & Smith, B. (1999) *The Dance of Change: The Challenge of Sustaining Momentum in Learning Organisations.* Double Day, New York.

The Concise Oxford Dictionary of Current English (1990) 8th edn. Clarendon Press, Oxford.

Titchen, A. (2001) Critical companionship: A conceptual framework for developing expertise. In: *Practice Knowledge and Expertise in the Health Professionals* (eds J. Higgs & A. Titchen), pp. 80–90. Butterworth-Heinemann, Oxford.

Weinstein, K. (1999) *Action Learning A Practical Guide.* Gower, Hampshire.

Wheeler, C.E. & Chin, P.L. (1989) *Peace and Power: A Handbook of Feminist Process.* National League for Nursing, New York.

4. *A Methodological Walk in the Forest: Critical Creativity and Human Flourishing*

Angie Titchen and Brendan McCormack

Forest energy
Regenerating forces
Transformation walk

Welcome to our story in which we take you on a journey to help you experience critical creativity in your practice development (PD) work. Critical creativity is a new framework for PD that blends being critical (e.g. challenging assumptions, pointing out contradictions, paradoxes and dilemmas, reflecting in and on practice) with using creative imagination. We, therefore, invite you to begin your experience of this chapter through the use of your own creative imagination.

We suggest that, *in a moment when you have read this paragraph and the next two*, you make yourself comfortable (maybe lie on the floor). Close your eyes and when you feel yourself beginning to relax, listen to the sounds of the world outside the space you are in. Observe them . . . and then let them go. Move your attention then to the sounds of the space you are in. Listen, note them . . . and then let them go. Then listen to your breath, relaxing deeply as you breathe out, in and out, the sounds of your body.

When you are ready, imagine you are entering a forest. This forest symbolises your PD project, practice or research. We invite you to explore your forest landscape with all your senses. What does your PD smell like, look like? What do you see, notice? What is the quality of the light and the dark? What do you hear, taste, feel? What is the texture, the density of the different parts of your PD forest? What emotions does it evoke in you? How does it make you feel?

Try not to rationalise whatever comes to your imagination, however bizarre. Go with it, trust the wisdom of your body, some important hidden knowing or insight might rest there for you. When you are ready to leave your forest, listen to your breath, to your body, to the sounds in your space and then gently open your eyes.

Point of departure: spiralling through the forest

A group of stakeholders, including those who provide and receive healthcare, are at a forest retreat (Figure 4.1) to plan their organisation's PD journey together. Two of the stakeholders, Rory and Anna, have offered to facilitate. They are reasonably experienced in facilitating and developing practice within an emancipatory framework (see Manley & McCormack, 2004). They have recently read a paper by McCormack and Titchen (2006) and want to experiment, for the first time, with moving their emancipatory PD into a critical creativity frame. It says in the paper that working in nature is often found to be energising, inspirational and uplifting. As morale is low and there is a lot of confusion and uncertainty at this time of change in their organisation, they have chosen, for the two away days, a place of great beauty to uplift colleagues and enable creative, as well as critical working together. However, having arranged the natural venue, Anna and Rory think no further about how to promote energy, inspiration and uplift and leave these things to chance. Instead, they pay attention to structure, for example, providing a detailed programme with no time or space for blue-skies thinking or contemplation. Having previously created a shared vision for the PD project with all stakeholders, they focus on achieving the task set out for the day, that is, for small groups of stakeholders to talk about what they think needs to be done to improve the service that their organisation delivers. The first day is hot and most participants choose to sit for their discussions in the gardens immediately surrounding their conference chalet or in the chalet itself.

At the end of the day, Rory and Anna invite participants to evaluate the day's work using objects that they are attracted to or to engage in a piece of reflective writing. Whilst some participants remain indoors writing, most go outside and pick up from the edge of the forest, pieces of wood, water, soil, fir cones, for instance. They return indoors to express their evaluations using these artefacts. The facilitators then invite people to share the meaning of their creations or writing. Whilst new potential for growth and connections has been experienced, there is a pervading, palpable feeling of disconnectedness and flatness. A few participants are more explicit. Holding up a hollow chestnut case, Dave says:

> *There is structure around to protect us, but there has been a feeling of emptiness in the day. Our project vision didn't get enough attention.*
>
> Dave

Maria points at her piece of rotting wood covered by a tiny fern and some moss:

> *There has been lots of potential coming up today, but I don't feel that it has been capitalized upon. There is new growth, but I want to be more expansive, more flowing, more creative. I have been too much in my head today and I have not made the most of our glorious surroundings.*
>
> Maria

Lucy shares her poem:

> *Early morning feet firmly grounded on the grass.*
> *Deep breath in feel the air, smell the forest, sun is embracing*
> *There is energy!*
>
> *As the day passes my mind and body become disconnected*
> *Away flows my energy*
>
> *I feel empty, sad and out of place*
>
> Lucy

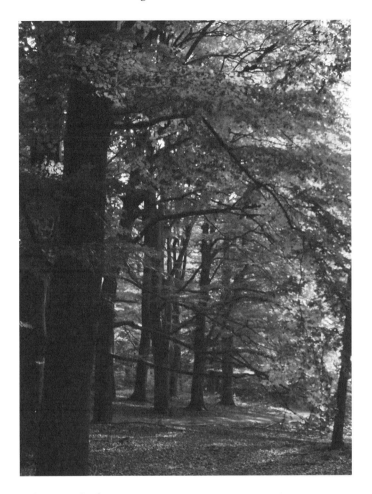

Figure 4.1   Entering the forest.

Rory and Anna hear what people are saying; they recognise that they haven't got the balance right between providing programme structure and pacing for the day and providing open space and creativity, so as to enable everyone and the work to flourish. They decide to go for a walk in the woods with their two colleagues, Lucy and Elsa, before dinner and agree to begin walking, in pairs, in silence.

The purpose of this chapter is to show how human flourishing (i.e. the outcome for individuals who achieve their maximum potential for growth and development) can be nurtured in those who co-create and implement critical and creative methodologies to develop practice and research that development. Our story, *Spiralling through the Forest* will show, at face value, how this nurturing can occur whilst developing practice, but at a deeper level, through the use of *resting points*, we will reveal how parallel processes have been used in our International Practice Development Colloquium (IPDC) cooperative inquiry. This study is a part of a movement that values and enables human flourishing for both actors and beneficiaries, as both the *ends* and *means* of research and development (see Lincoln & Denzin, 2000). In our case, the movement is building on emancipatory PD, as described by Bellman (2003), Manley and McCormack (2004), Titchen and Manley (2006). Human flourishing is seen as both ends and means in the development of, and investigation into, person-centred, evidence-based healthcare. The chapter is a performance text in the sense that we portray, through the story, imagery and resting places, how the *conditions* for human flourishing can be enabled through praxis (practice wisdom/mindful action with a moral intent) that is critical and creative. Such praxis is achieved through creative thinking, 'thinking about thinking' (metacognition) and critique *blended* with creative imagination and expression. We show how this blending occurs through the professional artistry of two facilitators, Anna and Rory, who pay attention to creating nourishing conditions, much as the gardener or forester might do to provide conditions for plants, trees, insects, birds and animals to grow, transform and flourish. Professional artistry, as described by Titchen and Higgs (2001), is the blending of practitioner qualities, different types of knowledge and ways of knowing, intelligences, practice skills and creative imagination processes all with the therapeutic or, in this case, facilitative use of self.

So above we have identified three key concepts: praxis, professional artistry and human flourishing. Their reciprocal relationship to each other is at the heart of a new paradigmatic (worldview) synthesis that we have called *critical creativity*. This work forms some of the products of the cooperative inquiry undertaken by the IPDC.

It is bold to confront an established worldview (paradigm) and propose additions to it, but this is what the IPDC inquiry is striving to do. Recently, we have exposed, for public scrutiny, our challenge to the critical worldview as an adequate location for the transformational PD and research approaches that we are developing in healthcare (McCormack & Titchen, 2006). Whilst we accept the fundamental assumptions of the critical worldview (i.e. understanding of power relationships that may cause oppression is fundamental to enabling empowerment to take meaningful action), as described by Fay (1987) for example, it does not, from our perspective, recognise the creativity required in our approaches. Neither does it explicitly acknowledge that creativity often involves moral and spiritual dimensions as people push out the boundaries of the known within their own practices. In particular, these gaps within Fay's (1987) eight critical theories for practice (Table 4.1) have informed our PD practice thus far (McCormack & Titchen, 2006).

Over the last decade, we have addressed these gaps, by combining the assumptions[1] of the critical worldview with our experiences of using creative imagination

---

[1] In this chapter, the term 'assumptions', when used in connection with philosophy, theory and methodology, means accepted positions that are made explicit.

Table 4.1 Fay's (1987) eight critical theories for practice

Theory	Description
1. False consciousness	Shows how our understandings are false, how these came about and potential alternatives
2. Crisis	Spells out what a 'crisis' is and why it exists
3. Education	Learning processes to help us become enlightened
4. Transformative action	Identifies those 'crisis elements' that need to be changed and a plan of action for doing so
5. The body	Understanding of how we inherit roles and how these limit our freedom
6. Tradition	Identifies which parts of a particular tradition are changeable/not changeable
7. Power	The nature and limits of power in a given context
8. Reflexivity	Explains the past, accounts for the present and plans for liberation whilst paying attention to context and limits

and expression in our emancipatory PD work. Then through a critical review of our work, we have created a new synthesis for action-focused development and research to add to the critical worldview. As stated above, we call this synthesis 'critical creativity'. In our previous paper (McCormack & Titchen, 2006), we described our reflexive journey that led to the articulation of critical creativity. We critiqued current assumptions underpinning the critical worldview and articulated the unique philosophical, theoretical and methodological assumptions of critical creativity. As a result, we proposed a substantial elaboration of Fay's sub-theory 10 (a sub-theory of his theory 4 – *transformative action* (see Table 4.1 for Fay's theories, and McCormack & Titchen [2006] for the associated sub-theories). We have called this elaboration of sub-theory 10, *creativity* (see McCormack & Titchen, 2006).

We recognise that increasing numbers of people engaged in PD and PD research use creative arts media in their work and that a few are positioning themselves with the notion of human flourishing as ends and means. We are also aware that the term 'critical creativity' has been used by others. However, it appears that they draw on very different sets of assumptions and frame creativity and criticality in distinctly different ways to those we present here. According to Ragsdell (1998), for instance, critical creativity is a critical approach to cognitive and creative thinking leading, through understanding or enlightenment, to empowerment. Her theoretical base flows from creative problem-solving, organisational, critical systems thinking and total systems intervention. Others justify their work through a variety of other traditions, such as indigenous knowledge, humanities and embodied knowing (perceiving through the senses). Whilst we frame our journey through a Westernised critical tradition, we also draw upon a variety of other sources of wisdom and knowledge (ancient, spiritual and indigenous).

We present, in this chapter, the first refinement of our theoretical framework for human flourishing within a critical creativity worldview (see McCormack & Titchen, 2006). We describe the methodology and methods that we have co-constructed within the IPDC cooperative inquiry and show how they have been shaped through critical creativity's unique philosophical, theoretical and methodological assumptions. Throughout the chapter, we offer a *faction* growing from walks that members of the IPDC have taken together (both metaphorically and metaphysically) in a forest near Utrecht in The Netherlands. A faction is fiction based on empirical fact. The faction itself is indicated by the use of a different font, but it contains quotes in italics. These quotes are from real IPDC co-inquirers to whom pseudonyms have been given. The quotes enable the reader to get a sense of the empirical IPDC data upon which the faction was created. The photographs in Figures 4.3, 4.5 and 4.6 are further sources of empirical evidence. The faction is also rooted in our experience of many years of PD, researching PD and researching ourselves. It provides an example of how our inquiry methodology is also a methodology for developing practice. Resting and meeting points, symbolised by a spiral, offer our commentary on the story.

At the end of the chapter, we set out the methodological walk we have undertaken so far and where we are planning to go next.

Melding, exploding, blending: a refinement

In silence, Rory and Anna hold the frustrations of the day. Their own and others' flourishing has been absent: 'Oh why did we sit in our heads all day and not venture out into the woods? What was stopping us?' Gradually, they notice the points of light on the forest path and their hearts begin to lift on birdsong wings. The earth is fragrant with the scent of pine and, within minutes, the forest soothes their frustrations and heals their sense of failure. Rory stops and folds his arms around the rough bark of an ancient tree. Anna hangs back until he beckons her and they link arms, without words, bodies pressed on the massive trunk. Continuing along the dappled path, they gently begin to share their experiences of the last few moments, framing them, using their senses, in the landscape:

> *Human flourishing is points of light on trees*
> *Light transforms, enables light and death*
> *Young saplings and ancient canopy must both flourish*
> *To maintain the balance of the forest*
> *Anna*

At a meeting point, they join up with Lucy and Elsa and comment on the devastation of beauty; a patch of felled trees. Lucy invites them to re-frame the scene; logs to keep us warm in winter, creating space and light for saplings to grow:

As we walk on, we step off the path and stop in a pile of dead leaves.
You can regard them in two ways – as having done their job or as a new beginning given that we need them for new development. The youngsters (meaning the trees) need the oldies (meaning the rotting leaves) to nurture and support them (i.e. provide them with nourishing compost for growth). The forest's ecosystem is a wonderful metaphor for practice development – we all have a place and value in our practice world with our own understandings that inform our actions. But we need the light fall (critique) and life juice (common language) in order to grow.

That is the way it is.

We stop at an open space which at the first glance looks awful, destruction! But then at a second glance, there it is a beautiful spot for deer to graze.
Being here, standing here breathing deeply, I feel my blood streaming and feel connected to the system again!

Lucy

The four decide that human flourishing is an ecosystem of balancing life–death–life, creating conditions for interdependency and the losses and gains of each position. Fragility and strength. Strength and fragility. Dynamic balance.

In the IPDC inquiry, we are a group of people with varying degrees of experience of research and facilitating research that is collaborative, participative and inclusive. Those of us who are more experienced are concerned with enabling others' capacity to co-construct the inquiry methodology and methods. However, this places considerable tension in the group: on those who are enjoying a rare opportunity to work with experienced, creative others; to fly, to be creative and innovative. The tension is between flying and bringing less experienced others along at a pace comfortable for them. There is a tension also for some who do not want to hold others back. How can we all, in a transparent, nurturing way, ensure that there is a commitment to exploring tensions, so that the forest canopy can flourish without taking away the light that will enable the saplings to flourish and grow?

Talking, reasoning,
Power of programme silently pervades,
Loss of interest and energy drain

Invitation to walk,
Framing reflection in landscape experience,
Feeling ground, layered with richness,
Microcosm beneath our feet
Pine smell of living air
As light dances through leafy filters

In stillness, beauty absorbed
Adds relish to being.

> *Privileged few*
> *Travelling paths worn by others*
> *And seeking new*
>
> *Freedom within form*
> *Green openness midst trees erect*
> *Living reminders to ages past*
> *Rendering us in perspective*
> *Like wisdom sought*
> *In nature revelation*
>
> *Much more than talk*
> *This living, feeling, knowing*
> *Rich integration point of infinite reference*
> *And in appreciation learn*
>
> *Elsa*

This last poem within the faction captures the essence of the transformative engagement that the group experienced in the wood. *'Much more than talk; living, feeling, knowing'*, as the poem expresses, reflects the feelings we had about the theories and frameworks we used in our emancipatory PD and research. In our critique of critical social science (McCormack & Titchen, 2006), we identified limits to its usefulness as a framework to enable transformative and creative action. More specifically, in our critique of Fay's (1987) eight practice theories of being critical, we concluded that the creative nature of the work in which we are engaged is omitted within these theories. The critical approach, as elaborated by Fay, does not sufficiently explain or direct attention to the issue of how a critical theory can be turned into actual practice. We identified that even within *transformative action* (theory 4 in Table 4.1), sub-theory 10 of Fay's model (a plan of action that indicates how people are to carry out a social transformation) leaves the impression that the movement from the level of abstract theory to the level of practice is nothing more than application. But this is misguided; practical activity involves skills, sensitivities, and capacities that require an artistry that involves far more than knowing the contents of a theory. This is why we elaborated sub-theory 10 and named it *creativity*, as introduced above.

Practical activity involves praxis through which practitioners learn how to pick out significant features of their environment, develop insightful responses to these features, and adjust and adapt themselves to the particularities of a given situation. Of course, praxis can be informed by theory, but genuine praxis requires that practitioners go far beyond learning this theory in order to be effective practitioners, i.e. we need to place ourselves in the context of theory by how we live, feel and know the environment/landscape of practice. In particular, in trying to implement a critical theory, practitioners need to employ a kind of creative activity whereby they enable themselves to perform in particular situations. Practising this creative activity and developing practical knowing will enable practitioners to develop a professional artistry without which their interventions or transformative actions in the practical world would be clumsy, routine or unresponsive. We identified that what was needed to augment Fay's critical model, then, was a *praxis spiral* that focuses attention on the important creative work in which practitioners must engage if they are to be effective in taking or facilitating transformative action.

We suggest therefore that creativity enables holistic engagement of mind, heart, body and spirit at the heart of critical social science, which has, traditionally, centred on using the mind for critiquing historical, social, political and cultural contexts of practice. Thus the sub-theory of *creativity* blends and melds all the other sub-theories as set out by Fay (see Table 4.1 for Fay's theories and McCormack & Titchen [2006] for the associated sub-theories). Without such creativity, the knowing that is at the heart of transformative action cannot be fully realised through the professional artistry of practice. We set out the sub-theory of *creativity* as

> *the blending and weaving of art forms and reflexivity (critical consciousness) located in the critical [worldview]. Blending and weaving occur through professional artistry in order to achieve the ultimate outcome of human flourishing. Thus this theory has critical, moral and sacred dimensions.*
>
> McCormack & Titchen, 2006, p. 259

This sub-theory has a critical dimension because it builds on critical theory, a moral dimension because it encompasses praxis and a spiritual dimension because we use our spiritual intelligence to make meaning, uplift ourselves and to take or facilitate transformative action at the edge of the unknown.

We have come to see that whilst Fay sets out his theories as a typology (Table 4.1), he does not discuss the relationships between them. Thus, we are exploring, inductively, what these relationships might be.

As the four talk in the forest, they realise that Fay's typology of eight critical practice theories does not show the relationships between the theories. Their experience this evening is that they have been able to spell out to themselves what the *crisis* (theory 2), revealed in the evaluations of the first away day, was and why it existed. They have been able, through their bodies first, to know that something was wrong, rather than through reflecting on their practice, which is what practitioners and managers are urged to do when they go about improving people's experiences of healthcare. Rather, it is centrally and significantly through *the body* and then through *reflexivity* (theory 8) that Anna and Rory have overcome the *crisis* (as it related to themselves). They learn that they must pay attention to *the body* (theory 5 – understanding of how we inherit roles and how these limit our freedom), in this context to work within a critical creativity worldview, if they are to enable the conditions for human flourishing and transformation the next day. This has suddenly assumed huge significance for them as facilitators of the PD planning process. They are also beginning to sense that theory 5 needs to be supplemented to capture how they are using, in this work, the wisdom and pre-reflective knowing that their bodies hold. They realise that this knowing is often hidden and overshadowed by their cognitive knowing and thus by *reflexivity*.

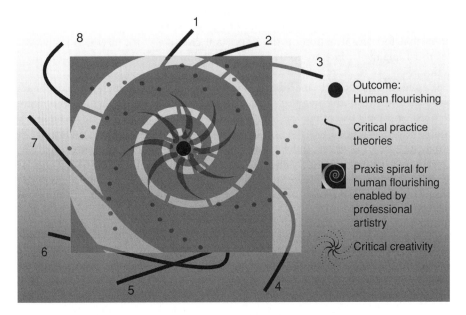

Figure 4.2 A theoretical framework for human flourishing located in the critical creativity worldview (McCormack & Titchen, 2006).

After dinner, Rory and Anna, decide to use their experience of the evening walk to create conditions that could re-energise the group and enable stakeholders to create a shared vision, common purpose and methodology for the PD project. They want to do this within the theoretical framework for human flourishing (see Figure 4.2), not only to achieve the shared vision that everyone can sign up to, but also to introduce and model ways of critical, creative working that the stakeholders might decide to build on in the project. They also want to explore the *praxis spiral* idea and how this may help them to be more effective in working creatively with stakeholders and to become more aware of the relationships between Fay's theories in their own practice.

 The facilitators in our faction realise that they could shape their facilitation, developed within an emancipatory PD (EPD) tradition by combining it with more ancient ways that honour and work with nature, energy, spirituality and creativity. Here we see Fay's (1987) critical practice theory of *tradition* (theory 6 – identifies which parts of a particular tradition are changeable/not changeable) at work. They can see, for example, that they could combine the cognitive processes and tools of EPD, such as the claims, concerns and issues tool (RCN, 2007), with the use of creative imagination and expression. They are aware that there is a tension between the cognitive and the imaginative in that they require the use of different aspects of ourselves and thus facilitation approaches and indeed helping people to overcome a resistance to using creative methods; an 'I can't' resistance often stemming from negative school experiences. Our facilitators are also aware that some traditions are worth keeping, in this case the cognitive tradition of many EPD tools and processes, and that bandwagon-jumping should be avoided, for example, using paint and clay as media for engaging creatively with such activities as 'values clarification' without integrating these media with rigorous thematic analysis of the data emerging. The best of different traditions, ancient, contemporary and new fusions, can be used in complementary ways to engage the whole of ourselves authentically in PD work.

Framing action in landscape experience: cooperative inquiry methodology

The next morning, still slightly bleary-eyed and heavy-headed from midnight revelry in the bar, Anna invites the group to get a sheet of folded A4 paper and a pencil and then gather in a circle on the grass outside the chalet. She offers to teach them a T'ai Chi exercise. The group agrees, some of them thinking it might help to wake them up:

Place your feet hip-width apart and feel and connect with the earth ... Imagine now that there is a silver thread suspending you from the crown of your head to the sky. Lengthening in the back and neck ... Soften your knees. Let the sky energy pour through you to the earth. Suspended between the heavens and the earth ... Now, I am going to show you an exercise with movement and breath that will help us to draw in the wonderful energy from the trees surrounding us.

Gently, breaking the silence, Rory invites the group to play, to have some fun, an adventure into the unknown. He gets agreement on some ground rules for their adventure. Everyone will be responsible for their own safety (emotional, physical, spiritual) and they will choose to follow or to find their own way. Rory points out that if they are to feel their way to a shared vision and common purpose and cooperative ways of working, then they need to stay attuned, engaged and connected to each other, through their senses, each in their own way. They also agree that they would dare to step out of their comfort zone.

Anna and Rory run off into the wood, shouting, 'Follow us!' 'Trust the process' – running, jumping, whooping; intentionally, to release residual energies and feelings associated with participants' expressions of 'flatness' yesterday. Such energies inhibit the embodiment of experience and the engagement with creative spaces. They are working on the idea that a fundamental way of accessing creativity is through taking risks, leaping into the unknown, being the playful child.

At a meeting point, in the forest, Rory invites everyone to pair up and for each pair to find a tree and link arms around it. 'Look up to the sky', he says (Figure 4.3). After still moments, Anna and Rory run on. Some follow, some stay behind and talk about what they have experienced. Connecting with nature and with another person, they rooted/grounded in the earth and connected with the sky. They say that this helped them to

- *Take a risk*
- *Let go of inhibitions*
- *Ground ourselves in nature*
- *Connect with the 'here and now'*
- *Make a physical connection with another and nature*
- *Feel belonging*

- Prepare for stepping into something new, and
- Move into metaphorical & metaphysical spaces.

We discover a tall tree in an open space. On the left side there is a beautiful light fall. We see re-growth of young plants on this side, but not on the right. We wonder although the left and right are connected with the trunk and enjoy the same life juice they differ! What is the language that connects them? Is that how we are at the moment, disconnected?

Lucy

Anna and Rory are aware that not everyone is following. Feeling a slight anxiety that some may lose connection with the activity, they remind themselves of the necessity to feel the interpretations of a situation in order to engage with Fay's theory 2 (*crisis*). This felt effortless to them and enabled the crisis to become a risk that was grounded in their mutuality as co-facilitators:

The trust that the group would stay together was realistic. My concern was the feeling (be it limited) of disconnection – running, jumping and following was a complex moment that raised issues such as: Do I want to do this (emotionally)? Can I do this (physically)? Why am I doing this (rationally)? I remember being critical of 'not blindly following the leader(s)'. Me and my 'partner' were conscious of keeping the rest of the group in view, and felt comfortable taking up the invitation to use our senses – but then in our own time, way, and route. Upon reflection, this works better as each member is able to participate within/at the edge of their own comfort zone.

Pieter

When everyone catches up, Anna suggests that people walk in their pairs in meditative silence, using their senses to really experience the forest world. Her intention here is that by emptying the mind through awareness, we free ourselves up for criticality and creativity.

Fay's *false consciousness* (theory 1) may explain why some stakeholders held back and questioned themselves when invited to play and to go on 'an adventure into the unknown'. Being playful is not usually seen by many as part of healthcare work. Moreover, jumping into the dark abyss of the unknown is likely to be avoided as certainty in contemporary healthcare interventions and outcomes is increasingly sought. However, the facilitators are encouraging the stakeholders to take a leap of faith into a new consciousness to enable creative visioning. This consciousness-raising is a PD process within the critical social science tradition, but it is usually achieved through cognitive means. Here the facilitators are doing it through the body, for example, through inviting a physical embodiment with the tree and hands clasped, using the senses to embody the forest and using the imagination to go on an adventure.

Working within the critical creativity theoretical framework, the facilitators are able to turn the *crisis* (theory 2) of confidence into potential for *transformative action* (theory 4) by identifying those crisis elements that need to be changed and devel-

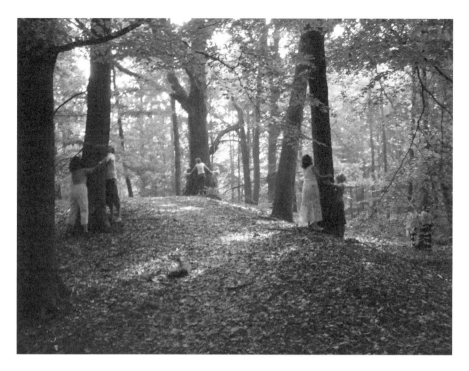

Figure 4.3 Sensing the forest world: consciousness-raising through the body and imagination.

oping a plan of action for doing so. As often happens, this plan is created in very short space of time. This is the effortless magic, the shape-shifting of this way of working.

In the IPDC inquiry, we accept the philosophical assumption of spiritual intelligence as the capacity and quickness to address and solve problems of meaning and value and place our transformative actions, lives and pathways in wider, richer meaning-giving contexts (Zohar & Marshall, 2000). Thus, as Wright (2007) says, spirituality is a call to action. As we are ultimately concerned, in PD and its facilitation with human flourishing (in its myriads of ways), we believe that it is likely to involve the human spirit and being in tune with nature (see Lincoln & Denzin, 2000). Moreover, spiritual intelligence gives us our moral sense and allows us to discriminate, to aspire, to dream and to uplift ourselves. Spiritual intelligence lets us work *with* the boundaries of the known and shape and transform the situation. We, therefore, honour all forms of spirituality that encompass a moral concern for others and recognise that particular spiritual beliefs imbue and shape knowing, doing, being and becoming within our inquiry. People in our inquiry hold a variety of spiritual beliefs or none at all, but through a long, deep, critical and creative exploration we have found a point of connection by searching for commonalities. We have found that the three commonalities of significance are as follows: spiritual intelligence; helping relationships imbued with a professional love within clear boundaries (the moderated love described by Campbell (1984); a respectful relationship with, and sense of awe emanating from, beauty and nature.

Praxis and professional artistry

The concept of praxis has been around for millennia (Aristotle created the term). It takes a key place as the central spiral of the critical creativity framework (Figure 4.2). It represents the spiralling journey from wherever we are now towards human flourishing. The journey spirals as we deepen and extend our capacity for praxis, constantly returning near to, but never at, the same place, always moving on. Movement is facilitated through the processes of blending, connecting, energising, reflecting, practising, learning and becoming. As we are concerned with overcoming internal and external barriers and transformation, the *praxis spiral* in our framework is influenced by a blending of approaches to reflexive action that free us from obstacles to effective action, with a facilitated understanding of the learning from these processes. We propose that it is the practice developer's professional artistry that enables this blending and creates the dynamic energy of the spiral. This artistry is the meaningful expression of a uniquely individual view within a shared tradition and involves the blending of practitioner qualities, practice skills and creative imagination processes (Titchen & Higgs, 2007). It is the hallmark of expertise (Titchen, 2000), in this case, of a practice developer/facilitator. According to Titchen and Higgs (2001), the qualities, skills and processes of professional artistry and their blending are built up through extensive introspective and critical reflection upon, and review of, practice. This view supports our notion of reflecting, practising, learning and becoming within the *praxis spiral*. Through a blend of cognitive and artistic critique, practice developers and facilitators are able to turn Fay's eight critical practice theories (Figure 4.2) into informed, transformed and transforming action with the moral intent of social justice, equity and human flourishing for all stakeholders, including themselves. We argue that professional artistry, within the practice of any discipline, enables the continual re-construction of theory in and on practice.

After experiencing the forest, in silence, through the *body*, Anna and Rory begin to talk. They realise, to their amazement, that they have now entered the praxis spiral because they are re-constructing Fay's theory in and from their practice in the here and now. They realise that it was through the body that they were able to be *reflexive* in a creative way (relationship between theories 5 and 8). To facilitate reflexivity in the others, they invite pairs of participants to talk to each other about what they noticed. The pairs follow Rory and Anna down another forest path, talking softly.

Further on, Anna suggests that the pairs re-frame their vision and purpose for their PD project through the forest sights, smells, textures and so on. She bases this suggestion on her experience that such re-framing not only seems to elicit new and deepening insights, but also provides a frame for remembering them. She reminds people, however, of the folded A4 paper and points out that they might like to record or draw insights, images, analogies or metaphors that emerge (theory 3 – *education*).

Anna and Rory now step off the road well travelled, drawn by a veil of mist and light towards the unknown (Figure 4.4). They are surprised immediately to see devastation, decaying wood like carcasses, old bones. They sense that this devastation represents the things they must let go of; the things they must let die in themselves, like the fear of uncertainty and the unknown. Stepping through the mystic veil, they spiral through the pathless forest. The others follow, some close, others at a distance. Knowing the stakeholders as persons, Rory and Anna are confident that everyone will stay attuned to and connected with each other once they step into the tremulous dark of the ancient wood. Rory realises that the 'tremulous dark' is like some of the fear he is experiencing right now having decided to engage with Anna in critically creative PD, rather than EPD with which they are both familiar. His previous understanding of Fay's theory of the *body* (theory 5) helps with framing this fear, i.e. the need to understand where this fear comes from and why he becomes fearful. It has been through his critical companionship relationship (see Titchen, 2004) with Anna over many years that he has come to learn how to free himself from such fears and do what is asked of us by Fay's theory of *education* (theory 3) – to develop an account of the conditions necessary for transformation to occur.

This section of the story is informed by Titchen and Higgs (2001) critical and creative model of becoming. The felled trees and decaying wood represent what we have to let die in ourselves before we can make room for creativity, new life, growth. Whilst this letting go is often painful for us, it is necessary. Just as the forester, in a seemingly brutal way, thins dense woodland to enable everything in it to flourish. Stepping through the mystic veil symbolises the act of 'becoming' a transformational practice developer and facilitator. This act is sometimes almost mystical or magical for those we have worked with and very often for ourselves. What is astonishing is that this act often occurs very quickly when working with critical creativity. The dark wood represents an abyss; a fertile void of uncertainty into which we have to leap if we are to engage in critical, creative, ethical and spiritual becoming. The points of light coming through the trees symbolise the light or the transformation or new life and direction that we attain through practice development/facilitation/professional artistry and creativity.

Rory and Anna spiral, feeling their way towards the place in the woods where they want to invite the pairs to join up to engage in a critical dialogue; prickles under foot, spongy ground, earthy fragrance of rotting leaves, ferns unfurling. They pass a huge tree that has fallen between two straight-trunked pines standing close together. Magically, no branches of either standing tree have been broken. They discuss how this symbolises something of the culture that they want to work towards in their PD project:

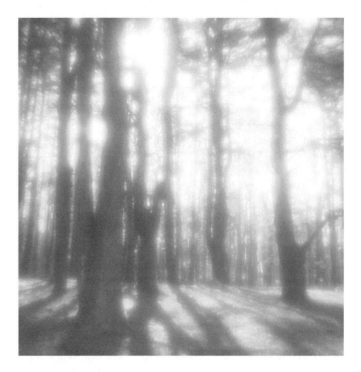

Figure 4.4   Stepping through the mystic veil.

> *Slip through the wall crack*
> *Of blockage and resistance*
> *Hands clasped, effortless*
> *To new synergy*
> *Different stories, knowings*
> *Re-creation*
> *Sharing action*
> *Transformation!*
> *Anna*

Spiralling, they see their conference chalet through the trees. Rory resists the desire to return and frames this desire in words to Anna that reflect a bodily reaction to the surroundings and an embodiment of emotion over rationality. Anna gently leads on like the confident critical companion that she is. Rory and Anna continue to discuss the power of the tree to be so precise, even in its falling, and realise that from a critical perspective, *power* (theory 7) is often considered a negative force or a power over, rather than a power to enable (see Hokanson Hawks, 1991). But as reflected in Anna's poem, power as 'hands clasped' can be sensitive, careful, deliberate and well intentioned. They reflect on the relevance of this metaphor to much of their own PD work.

IPDC co-inquirers intentionally resist the desire to return to the known pathways of EPD research. We aspire to having no formal leader roles and all co-inquirers having an equal power in decision-making about the research and responsibility for organising, designing and facilitating our six monthly gatherings. And we are making some progress towards that aspiration. But in the meantime, there are amongst us more experienced researchers and practice developers who express critical creativity as a way of living, being, learning, becoming, practising. As might be expected, they have become sapiential leaders, that is, leaders leading through their wisdom and depth of knowledge and experience, rather than through their role or position. In our forest metaphor, the sapiential leaders are the forest canopy who can sense the way forward towards a fuller understanding of critical creativity, whilst others, at ground level, are, in a well-worn phrase, just beginning to see the woods for the trees. The metaphor of the fallen tree symbolises how the sapiential leaders are managing the tension between flying and bringing others along in ways that promote human flourishing. We, for example, are trying to make space and light for others to grow by sharing our craft knowledge of using a critical creativity framework in PD and PD research. This faction is based on one such sharing.

> At last Rory and Anna find the meeting point, and when everyone arrives, they invite the pairs to join up with other pairs to engage in a critical dialogue about what they have learned about the vision, purpose and ways of working for their PD project. The groups engage in animated conversation, sharing metaphorical and metaphysical insights. Anna and Rory record what people are saying. Energy levels are very high. People are excited.

Our proposed new sub-theory of *creativity* (McCormack & Titchen, 2006) illustrates how the emotional engagement experienced through metaphorical and metaphysical dialogue moves beyond rational reflection and is felt instead through the body and the bringing together of all our senses in order to bring about new learning and understanding that impacts on our actions (i.e. trans-formation).

> After a while, another invitation to walk alone with others, this time in contemplative silence. 'Notice what you notice (Figure 4.5) and pick up, either physically or imaginatively, anything that you are attracted to and bring it with you – you don't have to have a reason for it. What we are attracted to is often symbolic of something that we haven't yet recognised cognitively, raised to our consciousness and/or articulated'.
> At last, they reach a special meeting point, experienced as a sacred place of transfor-mation. Without words or instructions, Rory and Anna begin to create a piece of landscape art with the artefacts they have gathered (Figure 4.6). They were intentionally modelling artistic expression using nature, silence, attunement and sensitivity to others and their creations. The others join in spontaneously, in silence. Some are quickly finished and stand back and watch in a respectful, reverential way. Rory and Anna are aware of some

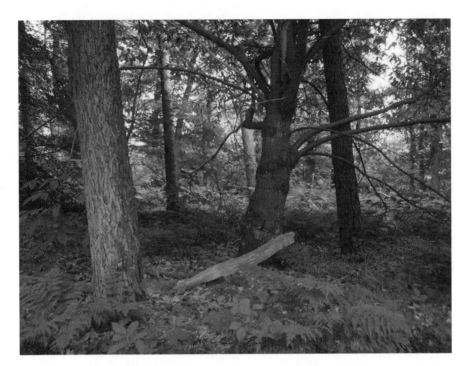

Figure 4.5   Mariolijn noticed this.

finishing quickly and others taking longer. So they deliberately hold the space open for those who need longer by continuing to contribute to the artwork:

I remember this point clearly – and was very aware of being authentic and true to myself – I didn't want to 'reproduce' or 'imitate.

Pieter

 Transformative action is a nexus of *power* to enable, *the body*, consciousness-raising, creative facilitation (*education*) embedded in ancient *tradition* and nature, ritual, and *reflexivity*. In the IPDC inquiry, as facilitators of *transformative action*, we often enable ourselves and others to use silence and inner listening to self as key to accessing professional artistry (i.e. a blending of different kinds of knowing, intelligences, cognition, metacognition, practice wisdom and creativity). We also use artefacts to capture the essence of experience and any intuitions, bodily, emotional, artistic or spiritual intelligences that may come into our consciousness during such work, which can be turned into words with other activities. Working with artefacts and other creative expressions, we have found that people gather large amounts of synthesised data in a seemingly effortless way that is yet systematic and rigorous.

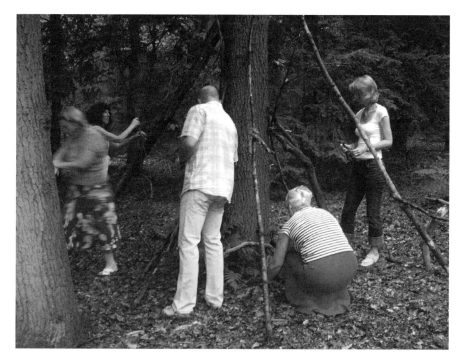

Figure 4.6   Creating the vision as a piece of landscape art.

Creating landscape art is one example of how IPDC co-inquirers express artistically and with others their inner wisdom and new ideas. Silence is absolutely central. Words or verbal sounds tend to break the magic of such moments. Working together in this way bonds people at a deep level. Sometimes, it creates a metaphorical or a metaphysical space (sacred space – in whatever tradition or not people choose, each for own self). Such co-expression often enhances the human flourishing of individuals and the group. It creates a holistic expression of individual experience. Facilitators using a critical creativity approach will draw on many different traditions of facilitation; for example, Brendan is strongly influenced by John Heron's (1989) work and Angie by Carl Rogers' (1983) and by indigenous wisdom expressed by Angeles Arrien (1993) in her synthesis, 'the four-fold way'.

The artwork complete, Rory invites each person to share the meaning of their part of the creation. After each sharing, he invites the rest of us, with the permission of the creator, to express what that part of the artwork evokes in us. He says, 'Express what it brings up in you by saying, "I see, I feel, I imagine". Using these words helps each person to own their own interpretation/response to the artwork'. He encourages us not to interpret others' work because the philosophical position of critical creativity is that multiple realities are honoured and included at the same time as identifying shared meanings.

Anna captures what people say to ensure that the critically creative process is translated into 'data' that those who do not engage with critical creativity can still recognise as evidence for rigorous and systematic analysis. She will use these notes later in the processing session to ensure that shared meanings are made explicit for the creation of the project vision.

To reaffirm the group bonding, a sense of belonging and closure of the experiential part of the activity, Rory asks us to stretch a circle around the creation. We stand in silence for a moment or two and then share one word, a sound or movement to get at the essence of the creation and/or experience of creating it. Anna captures words, energies and movement on her paper. As processing is essential with this kind of activity, Rory suggests that we move out of our metaphorical/metaphysical place and space and go back to the 'real world' where there are chairs!

A whisper away lies the 'real' world of kitchens, workmen and conference groups. We are amazed that we created such a beautiful space so near the 'real' concrete world. Magically, a circle of chairs appears! Sound of water. Now we are ready to move into cognitive critique of our sensory, aesthetic experiences through critical, creative conversations, contemplations, receiving the observation notes and drawings. After the processing is over, Anna invites one word or short phrase evaluations of the walk in the woods.

This processing stage is when the critical and artistic juxtapose or collide and potentially something new is created or the previously inexpressible or unknown is articulated. It uses particularly the PD processes of graceful care, sympathetic presence, learning in and from practice, intentionality, saliency, temporality, consciousness-raising, problematisation, self-reflection and critique (Titchen, 2004; McCormack, 2001). These processes are facilitated by, for example, the strategies of observing, listening and reflective questioning, story-telling, high challenge/high support, facilitating theorisation of practice, engaging multiple discourses or cultural analysis. The analysis of the processing in our real walk in the forest led us to a new understanding of our original theoretical framework for human flourishing. As highlighted earlier, the relationships between Fay's (1987) theories appear to be unarticulated. The new understanding that emerged for us is that central to our theoretical framework must be Fay's theory of the *body*, as it is through our bodies that we integrate a *reflexive* analysis of our engagement with our creativity and our framing of that, through theoretical and methodological perspectives. Thus we have refined the original framework and now place *the body* and *reflexivity* at the centre, with *the body* being the entry point into the framework (Figure 4.7).

Blending and weaving: underpinning assumptions

The story has shown how critical creativity informs the IPDC inquiry strategy. The inquiry is shaped by the philosophical, theoretical and methodological assumptions described by McCormack and Titchen (2006). We want to point out two of the philosophical assumptions here. The first is that we use creative expression

78

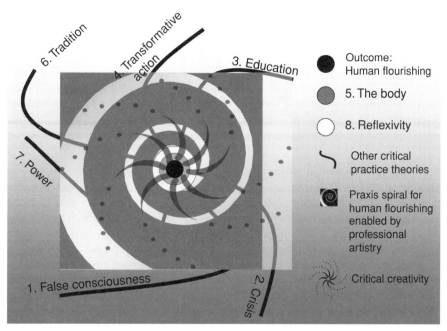

Figure 4.7 A theoretical framework for human flourishing located in the critical creativity worldview (revision 1).

to create synergy between cognitive and artistic approaches to critique. A movement between creative expression, critical dialogue and contestation is enabled to develop and understand the key concepts of human flourishing, transformation, praxis and professional artistry. Each stage combines cognitive with artistic critique, creating a synergy through a reiterative, reciprocal dialogue between words and art forms. The second assumption is that our work is person centred. Being person centred is linked to beliefs and values about the intrinsic moral good of personhood and to a universal moral principle that extends beyond politics, religion, wealth, privilege, cognition, rationality, ethnicity or sexuality. Three main characteristics of person centredness shape our inquiry: (i) the uniqueness of the human individual, (ii) a concern with the meaning and purpose of human life and (iii) the individual's freedom to choose. We have blended the moral intent of the critical worldview with its focus on improvement and transformation within the social world, with the moral intent of creating conditions that will enable improvement and transformation of the individual life worlds of persons.

What we have shown in the story is how skilled facilitators are co-inquirers, observing, questioning, experiencing and engaging with the concept being investigated, all at the same time. They are immersed in the world, connected to it in all their roles. They are epistemologically and ontologically authentic, that is, their ways of creating new knowledge about human flourishing are congruent with the way they are as human beings, connecting with others in the world and fostering conditions for the human flourishing of co-inquirers:

> *Green is so green and blue is vivid,*
> *Yes, the energy is flowing*
> *Thank you, critical companions,*
> *For walking, jumping and running across this beautiful forest.*
> *Lucy*

An important theoretical assumption that we make is that critique of assumptions in our inquiry begins consciously through individual and group processes in order to link new ideas with what people already know and also to blend different worldviews (epistemological concerns). This work begins as a conscious blending process, but as we begin to genuinely live the assumptions in our inquiry practices, there appears to be a move from conscious to unconscious blending. In other words, the blending becomes embodied and part of human being in the world (ontological concern). Another theoretical assumption is that we see human becoming as the development of mind, heart, body and spirit through approaches to learning and facilitation that draw upon a variety of perspectives and traditions. So we use these theoretical assumptions to work with Fay's eight critical practice theories through our newly proposed sub-theory 10, that is, *creativity*.

Our key methodological assumption is that we assume a critically creative approach to reflexive action. Professional artistry provides the synergy and positive/enabling power to blend the philosophical and theoretical assumptions above and convert them into such action. We use this blend to mediate Fay's critical theories in our investigation of ourselves as co-inquirers developing an international theory for PD. In other words, we are particularising Fay's propositional knowledge to make it useful to our particular situation and selves. Blending and particularisation seem to involve artistic processes, such as appreciation, attunement, harmonisation, synthesis, being able to see the whole and the parts of some aspect of professional practice or experience and moving between them and getting the balance and form right.

Whilst accepting the central assumptions of EPD and research (see Manley & McCormack, 2004; Titchen & Manley, 2006), we have now set out through story and resting places the features of our practice epistemology (knowing) and ontology (being), as co-inquirers and enablers, that are unique to critical creativity.

 ## Resting after walking (for now)

In this chapter, we have re-articulated a new paradigmatic synthesis called critical creativity through a physical walk in a wood, capturing metaphorical and metaphysical meaning in order to engage in body-situated, reflexive analysis of PD. We have embraced EPD processes, tools and outcomes in order to illustrate the strength and wisdom of the energy that flows from critically creative dialogical action. Critical creativity is not merely a method using creative arts media and critical dialogue. Rather it is a way of learning, practising and living PD that shares philosophical and methodological assumptions with EPD, but also having distinct sounds, fragrances, hues, textures and flavours of its own. This is not to say that using creative arts media and critical dialogue, debate and contestation is not good, because for many practice developers and facilitators embracing the overt tools of critical creativity provides a medium for experimentation and initial stepping into the unknown[2]. We have started in this and other writings to unravel the rubric that is critical creativity in order to articulate and make explicit the links between philosophy, theory, methodology and method. We intend for these articulations to enable the canopy of the tall trees to flourish and through such flourishing and forestry work create the conditions for others to grow and flourish too. As we have articulated throughout the chapter, the concept of *human flourishing* is a central methodological focus as both the means and the end of critical creativity and one in which we continue to develop conceptual understanding through creative concept analysis. The articulation of human flourishing and a methodological framework will be the focus of future publications.

Two more final points. Firstly, an IPDC inquirer on reading a draft of this chapter pointed out that our image is so strong that she wondered if readers might be left thinking that critical creativity is only about walking in the woods or that it only happens when we are in nature. We have used the metaphor of 'a walk in the woods' to frame our exploration of critical creativity in this chapter. The metaphor is real, as in this particular case critical creativity was further refined by a walk in the woods. So in this way, the real became metaphorical, as a means of shaping concepts and theories that are complex and difficult to grasp. The embodiment of the concepts and theories through the walk and their articulation through metaphor, we hope, enables you to actively engage in an experience of critical creativity rather than be a passive recipient of concepts and theories. Critically, creative PD takes on many shapes and forms and this 'walk' is just one such example (see Coats et al., 2006 and Titchen & Horsfall for others). Secondly, we have shown how Fay's (1987) critical theories can be articulated within a critical creativity worldview, but we do not wish you to be left with the impression that they are the only theories that are used within critical creativity. Many theories that are likely to inform your PD work can be positioned within this worldview, so whilst the theories might change, the constants would be the praxis spiral, professional artistry and human flourishing.

And so to conclude your journey and rest your tired feet, we ask you, *after reading these final words*, to make yourself comfortable (maybe lie on the floor again). Close your eyes and think about the journey you have been on. Record in your

---

[2] Possible starting points for novice facilitators who want to work in this worldview include using a free, downloadable learning resource, entitled *Opening Doors on Creativity* (Coats et al., 2006) or attendance at an IPDC Practice Development School. These are held in the four countries: United Kingdom, The Netherlands, Australia and New Zealand. Details are available on http://www.rcn.org.uk/resources/practicedevelopment/news/

mind significant images, dialogues, metaphors and meanings that fly around your imagination, carried on the wings of the birds of the forest. Note the sounds, feelings, smells and tastes that you connect with.

Let your mind move towards the end of your journey and leave the woods behind you. Acknowledge the sacred space you have been in and the privilege you have been given of sharing this beautiful and engaging surrounding. When you have said goodbye to the forest, listen to your breath, to your body, to the sounds in your space and then gently open your eyes.

Acknowledgments

We would like to honour those IPDC co-inquirers who accepted with us the challenge of walking in the woods and engaging in critical creativity, namely, Christine Boomer, Bob Brown, Karen Cox, Margaret Devlin, Marja Legius, Famke van Lieshout, Kim Manley, Kate Sanders, Theresa Shaw, Annette Solman, Val Wilson, Roz Young, and especially and in addition, Shaun Cardiff, Liz Henderson and Lucienne Hoogwerf for their written contributions to this chapter. Finally, we would like to thank Jan Dewing, a newcomer in the IPDC, for her critique of this chapter.

References

Arrien, A. (1993). *The Four-Fold Way*. Harper, San Francisco.

Bellman, L. (2003) *Nurse-Led Change and Development in Clinical Practice*. Whurr, London.

Campbell, A.V. (1984) *Moderated Love*. SPCK, London.

Coats, E., Dewing, J. & Titchen, A. (2006) *Opening Doors on Creativity: Resources to Awaken Creative Working*. A learning resource. Royal College of Nursing, London. Available from http://www.rcn.org.uk/resources/practicedevelopment/about-pd/processes/creative/ [accessed 20/01/07].

Fay, B. (1987) *Critical Social Science*. Polity, Cambridge.

Heron, J. (1989) *The Facilitator's Handbook*. Kogan Page, London.

Hokanson Hawks, J. (1991) Power: A concept analysis. *Journal of Advanced Nursing*. **16**, 754–762.

Lincoln, Y.S. & Denzin, N. (2000) Paradigmatic controversies, contradictions, and emerging confluences. In: *Handbook of Qualitative Research* (eds N. Denzin & Y.S. Lincoln), 2nd edn, pp. 163–188. Sage, London.

Manley, K. & McCormack, B. (2004) Practice development: Purpose, methodology, facilitation and evaluation. In: *Practice Development in Nursing* (eds B. McCormack, K. Manley & R. Garbett), pp. 33–50. Blackwell, Oxford.

McCormack, B. (2001) *Negotiating Partnerships with Older People: A Person-Centred Approach*. Ashgate, Aldershot.

McCormack, B. & Titchen, A. (2006) Critical creativity: Melding, exploding, blending. *Educational Action Research: An International Journal*. **14**(2), 239–266. Available from http://www.tandf.co.uk/journals.

Ragsdell, G. (1998) Participatory action research and the development of critical creativity: A natural combination? *Systematic Practice and Action Research.* **11**(5), 503–515.

RCN (2007) *Workplace Resources for Practice Development.* Royal College of Nursing, London.

Rogers, C. (1983) *Freedom to Learn for the 80s.* Charles E. Merrill, London.

Titchen, A. (2000) *Professional Craft Knowledge in Patient-Centred Nursing and the Facilitation of Its Development.* Ashdale Press Tackley, Oxfordshire.

Titchen, A. (2004) Helping relationships for practice development: Critical companionship. In: *Practice Development in Nursing* (eds B. McCormack, K. Manley & R. Garbett), pp. 148–174. Blackwell, Oxford.

Titchen, A. & Higgs, J. (2001) Towards professional artistry and creativity in practice. In: *Professional Practice in Health, Education and the Creative Arts* (eds J. Higgs & A. Titchen), pp. 273–290. Blackwell Science, Oxford.

Titchen, A. & Manley, K. (2006) Spiralling towards transformational action research: Philosophical and practical journeys. *Educational Action Research: An International Journal.* **14**(3), 333–356.

Titchen, A. & Higgs, J. (2007) Research artistry: Dancing the praxis spiral in critical-creative qualitative research. In: *Being Critical and Creative in Qualitative Research* (eds J. Higgs, A. Titchen, D. Horsfall & H.B. Armstrong), pp. 282–297. Hampden Press, Sydney.

Titchen, A. & Horsfall, D. (2007) Reimaging research using creative imagination and expression. In: *Being Critical and Creative in Qualitative Research* (eds J. Higgs, A. Titchen, D. Horsfall & H.B. Armstrong), pp. 215–229. Hampden Press, Sydeny.

Wright, S. (2007) There is nothing soft about spirituality. *Nursing Standard.* **21**(19), 26–27.

Zohar, D. & Marshall, I. (2000) *SQ: Spiritual Intelligence the Ultimate Intelligence.* Bloomsbury, London.

5. *Evidence Use and Evidence Generation in Practice Development*

Tracey Bucknall, Bridie Kent and Kim Manley

Introduction

Accessibility, availability and use of the best available evidence on which to decide the most appropriate healthcare interventions to benefit the patient are key concerns for practitioners. Yet the debate on what is evidence, let alone determining the best available evidence, remains controversial. The evidence based practice movement strongly advocates that, wherever possible, research should be the primary determinant for clinical decisions. Although practitioners need to know the latest research, this is only one element of the decision-making process in clinical practice. In practice development (PD), evidence use and its development are derived from an array of different knowledge sources (Manley, 1997). Arguably all evidence needs to be considered for relevance and appraised for quality. The use of evidence is dependent on the practitioner's ability to reflect on, question and research their own practice to make the best decisions with and for their patients.

This chapter begins with a discussion about the importance of decisions made in practice, under varying conditions, that are influenced by individuals and organisational culture. Next, we examine the nature of evidence for use in practice and the challenges associated with its implementation in PD. Finally, to assist practice developers create a strategy for using evidence in practice, some starting points for practitioners and clinical teams are suggested. Approaches such as critical reflection, action learning and participatory action research are considered and illustrated with examples from practice or research.

Making decisions in a clinical context

Decision-making involves comparing and evaluating information to form an opinion or judgement about future behaviour. It is a critical activity in supporting practice-related decisions. The attributes of an effective nurse include having *sound clinical judgement* (Bucknall, 1996). All patients wish to be reassured that the nurses working with them are both smart and caring, that is, strong of mind and a kind heart. A common view is that knowledge of the correct treatment options should lead to the correct treatment of an individual. Yet, to what extent is a clinical encounter between the nurse and patient simply a matter of scientific application? Downie and Macnaughton (2000) argue that the scientific facts only become evidence when the practitioner decides the information is pertinent to a particular patient. Indeed, many clinical decisions are not supported by clear robust evidence. Clinical decisions are frequently a jumble of factual information and value judgments. In the real world, decisions often have to be made with limited relevant or incomplete information, from a variety of sources and with significant uncertainty attached to the decision. Added to this complex mix is the interaction that occurs between the nurse and patient, with potential differences in values and beliefs surrounding healthcare issues and the resource implications related to selected treatments (Tavakoli et al., 2000).

Consequently, for facts or information to become evidence a practitioner needs to judge the information to be relevant and important enough to use before determining treatment (Downie & Macnaughton, 2000). Unfortunately there is no single, best method to assess the importance of evidence. The type of question being asked will determine the evidence being sought and its relevance to the practice issue. Reflection on practice requires considerable effort and may, in fact, alter over time with changes to the environment.

Individual characteristics, such as personal attributes, values and capabilities, as well as the complexity of the task and the external environment, all shape the behaviour of the practitioner (Bucknall, 1996). In relation to PD, the individual is also influenced by theoretical (domain), practical (tacit), and situational knowledge. Table 5.1 illustrates the influences that impact on an individual's decisions in practice.

Table 5.1   Influences on nurses' decisions in practice (Bucknall, 1996, 2003, 2006)

Theoretical (domain) knowledge combines theory, research findings, facts and information that are necessary to understand patient changes and perform technical skills. Knowledge comes from within the discipline and from other fields.
Practical (tacit) knowledge is gained from nursing experience in the clinical setting. It is the knowing 'how' after learning 'why'. Clinical experiences develop the nurses' perception and identification of cues, as well as the ability to discriminate and prioritise them.
Situational knowledge arises from a nurse's repeated exposures to particular clinical situations and settings. Frequent experiences with individual patients, families, staff, equipment, policies and procedures influence a nurse's decision-making through constant data comparison with earlier encounters.
A nurse's personal attributes, values and capabilities will influence the decision-making process. A critical event may leave an imprint on the nurses' memory, just as their state of health and emotions may also.

Table 5.2   Contextual influences on decisions made in practice (Bucknall, 2003, 2006)

Type of patient problem: determines the types of decisions, the speed of decisions and the complexity of the decisions made. Unusual patients will slow decisions down; patients with similar diagnoses, frequently encountered will lead to speedier decisions. Shared decision-making between nurses and patients may require nurses to accommodate different preferences for treatment.

Resource availability: determines the types, speed and processing of decisions. These include the physical layout, equipment and the staffing within that context. Technology can be a time saving adjunct to the practitioners' clinical assessments interventions and communication with team members. It may improve accuracy, speed, use of evidence, patient safety and comfort or alternatively be a stressor because of information overload. The staffing mix of experienced and inexperienced nurses and the number of nurses may alter the balance from quality nursing care to unsafe practice.

Relationships in organisations: based on work area, discipline, teamwork, appointment levels and experiential hierarchies. Hierarchies provide informal checking processes on decisions such as during the handover and ward rounds. Increased communication and collaboration between staff, patient and families facilitates knowledge sharing to be patient centred.

The context of practice and the organisational culture exert significant influences on PD (McCormack et al., 2002). When the environmental effects on an individual's practice decisions have been explored, it is clear that the type of patient or their situation, the human and physical resources of the setting, and the communication and relationships between individual practitioners and team members all influence the use of evidence in practice (see Table 5.2).

By being aware of the factors that influence decisions in practice, practice developers step closer to both enabling and providing effective care. Effective care is both person centred and evidence based and will be embedded in the culture of the workplace through leadership and critical dialogue between peers. The next section will review the concept of evidence and discuss the types of evidence available to practitioners as sources of information to improve decisions in practice.

What is evidence?

Evidence for practice has grown in complexity over the past decade. Levels or types of evidence initially reflected the needs of medical practice. Evidence was generated by quantitative methods and focused on effectiveness of interventions. Today other evidence is sought to answer questions that arise from the diversity of health professions engaged in patient care, and the patients themselves. All health professions need to use a wide range of available evidence to assist their decision-making and achieve the goals of effective and efficient care delivery. The nature of evidence for decision-making in practice has been classified into four types: research; clinical experience; patients, clients and carers; local context and environment (Rycroft-Malone et al., 2004a).

Types of evidence

In PD, it is common for all four types of evidence to be used but the emphasis placed on each may vary when working with different stakeholder groups or different situations.

Research evidence

Ever since the first definition of 'evidence' for evidence-based medicine was based on quantitative research such as randomised controlled trials, there have been calls for a broader definition (Pearson, 2002). Within nursing and midwifery, the past decade has seen a growing acceptance that research evidence should also include qualitative research, to the extent that traditionally quantitatively focused organisations such as the Cochrane Collaboration have developed qualitative research groups. Later in this chapter, the evidence generated by action research is explored further.

All the research evidence rating tools reflect the principle that a higher value is placed on research that is objective and systematically developed; however, practice developers need to be aware that all forms of research can be subjectively interpreted and the findings analysed to determine the applicability for a particular setting (Rycroft-Malone et al., 2004b; Downie & Macnaughton, 2000).

Levels and quality of research evidence

In recognising the interdisciplinary differences and growing debate on the question of evidence, research evidence has been classified on the basis of type and scientific rigour. The Scottish Intercollegiate Guideline Network (SIGN) developed a grading system that has been adopted by the Guidelines International Network (GIN) members and can be located on the web (http://www.bmj.com/cgi/content/full/323/7308/334). This grading system is a useful way to appraise research evidence and identify the level of research evidence supporting PD initiatives. In particular, it is important in convincing practitioners of the advantages to the patient. Another grading system was developed by the National Health and Medical Research Council (NHMRC) (1999) in Australia. The NHMRC have moved away from solely considering the empirical nature of the evidence to a more comprehensive assessment that includes the following:

- Volume of evidence
- Consistency of the study results
- Potential clinical impact
- Generalisability of the evidence to the population being targeted by the guideline
- The applicability of the body of evidence to the local, regional or national context

Each of these variables is rated on a scale from A (excellent) to D (poor) and a matrix has been developed to explain this further; http://www.nhmrc.gov.au/publications.

Since qualitative research requires different modalities for critical appraisal to those used for quantitative research, the terms rigour, credibility, trustworthiness and believability are widely used as measures of quality, rather than validity of data (Russell & Gregory, 2003). There is a useful web-based resource to assist with the evaluation of qualitative studies:

- Evidence Based Nursing users' guide: http://ebn.bmj.com/cgi/content/full/6/2/36

Clinical practice guidelines are another form of research evidence that are used to assist both practitioners' and patients' decisions about specific aspects of healthcare (Newhouse et al., 2005). However, not all guidelines have been developed using rigorous processes as advocated, for example, by SIGN, and on appraisal, are found to be poorly developed and lack clarity. Practice developers may also find useful a tool developed for assessing the quality of guidelines: AGREE (Appraisal of Guidelines Research and Evaluation), http://www.agreecollaboration.org/instrument. It is a generic instrument that guides the assessment of quality and application to practice using six different components of guideline development:

- Scope and purpose
- Stakeholder involvement
- Rigour of development
- Clarity and presentation
- Applicability
- Editorial independence

Evidence in the form of practitioners' experiences

Not surprisingly, research evidence cannot provide all the answers to practitioners who need assistance with their decision-making (Bucknall, 2003). Practitioners, therefore, need to consider alternative sources to provide the knowledge needed for practice. Practical knowledge and experiential knowledge are terms that have been used to describe the knowledge that is gained from experience built up over time. In PD, practitioners' experiences are crucial for determining the relevance and importance of patients' signs, symptoms and personal experiences. Rolfe (1997) argues that it is the acquisition of know-how or personal, experiential knowledge that separates the novice from the expert. The origins of this type of knowledge are unclear because there are a number of possible sources. It may have come from previous experiences of caring for particular patients in certain settings, or it may arise from others informing practitioners of their own experiences. Either way, it is important that such knowledge is made explicit so that it is open for others to critically appraise and debate (Rycroft-Malone et al., 2004b).

Evidence from patients/clients and carers

Today, patients' and carers' experiences and views are becoming increasingly important in EBP; particularly, as they become more informed about their conditions or problems through greater access to information technology. This has led to the growing realisation that models used by practitioners to guide evidence utilisation need to incorporate the patients' perspectives (Davis et al., 2003). In PD, providing patient-centred care is a core purpose; integral to this is the ability of practitioners to engage with patients to elicit their preferences and opinions on treatment and care plans. Therefore, practitioners need to be able to seek out information about patient's or carer's past experiences or views about intervention options, and integrate these into the decision-making process.

Evidence from the local context and environment

Contextual evidence is derived from local factors that influence PD. It includes micro- or macro-factors related to the physical location, the people who use or work within a setting and timing. Contextual evidence may be physical, psychological or sociological; it includes underlying or associated factors that affect the interactions that need to take place. An example of contextual evidence is an organisation's readiness to change. Assessment of this as part of the PD process is crucial because it may impact on the effectiveness of practice changes. Local data are often underestimated or unrecognised by practitioners. Contextual factors impacting on practice within any setting are complex and multiple in nature, and yet need to be understood if practice change is to be achieved (McCormack et al., 2002). Van Driel et al. (2005) cite examples of cultural preferences that may impact on practice and prevent change occurring such as reducing female circumcision among refugees who still want to continue with the practice.

Manley (2004) identified the specific indicators of an effective workplace culture with regard to evidence within the context of PD, as follows:

- Evidence use to inform decision-making is drawn from policy (local to global), propositional knowledge, personal knowledge, craft knowledge, local theory (contextual knowledge) and patients' own personal knowledge.
- Evidence is also generated from practice through systematic and rigorous approaches at individual and collective levels.

PD may fail if sufficient attention is not paid to the specific characteristics of the practice setting, the problem being addressed or the macro-issues such as politics, policy and funding. By understanding more fully the context in which PD is taking place, or the patient/clinical encounter, practitioners are better equipped 'to bridge the gap between efficacy—what works in isolation in an ideal setting— and effectiveness (what works in everyday practice)' (De Maeseneer et al., 2003, p. 1316). Since culture and contexts have such an impact on what can be achieved, transforming them is one of the main purposes of PD (Manley, 2004; Garbett & McCormack, 2004).

Using evidence in practice

The discussion so far has focused on the nature of evidence in PD. The next section will outline the challenges to using the different types of evidence in practice. It is a complex interplay between practice developers, practitioners, the patients requiring care and the practice setting. We will also introduce examples of implementation models and frameworks identified in the literature for readers as a starting place for developing a PD strategy.

Challenges to using evidence in practice

Knowledge transfer in healthcare organisations is often a complex and protracted process, with numerous publications identifying the difficulties encountered in using evidence in practice (Greenhalgh et al., 2004). There are five main challenges faced when using evidence in practice:

1. Type and availability of evidence.
2. Characteristics of the person using the knowledge.
3. Communication channels for transferring the evidence.
4. Healthcare system or context where PD occurs.
5. The incorporation of patient's preferences and their involvement in healthcare decisions to increase patient-centred care (Bucknall, 2006).

Tables 5.3–5.7 present each challenge and associated attributes derived from the literature. Questions to consider when planning a strategy for implementing new evidence into practice are also suggested.

Table 5.3   Challenge 1: The type and availability of evidence

Characteristics	Questions for practice
Evidence	What is the quality and accessibility of the evidence?
Relative advantage	Will it be an advantage to use it? Will patients benefit? Will anyone else benefit?
Compatibility	How compatible is the evidence with current practice? Will it fit with our practice and resources?
Complexity	How complex are the interventions? Are different levels of practitioners involved? Are different disciplines involved? What do we need to change?
Trialability	Can we trial different approaches? Can we adapt what we have or do we need a new approach?
Observability	Can we watch others before we implement?
Reinvention	Do we need to adapt the evidence before using it locally? How can we do this?

Table 5.4   Challenge 2: Characteristics of those adapting the knowledge

Characteristics	Questions for practice
Practitioner/learner	What practitioner attributes determine the use of evidence in practice?
Personality	What motivates the practitioner? What learning styles will be required? What approach will suit the practitioner(s)?
Meaning	How important is the problem to the practitioner(s)?
Cognitive competence	Will the practitioner(s) be able to understand the evidence?
Independence	Can the practitioner(s) make the decision or is permission needed?

The types, quality and availability of evidence have been shown to influence the rate, extent and adherence to practice changes by different individuals (Rogers, 1995; Greenhalgh et al., 2004). Evidence is more likely to be used in practice when there are perceived benefits to patients and to those using the evidence (see Table 5.3). Evidence needs to be reflected upon and adapted before being integrated with the local context. Not surprising, this requires considerable time; a frequent barrier identified by Hutchinson and Johnston (2005).

The ability of each practitioner to process information varies and may, in part, be determined by personal factors such as motivation, learning style and capability (Greenhalgh et al., 2004). These may vary as their concerns change over time. Given evidence may take significant time to implement, motivation is critical in sustaining the enthusiasm of team members (see Table 5.4).

Table 5.5   Challenge 3: Communicating and facilitating the evidence in practice

Characteristics	Questions for practice
Communication and facilitation	What approaches will promote evidence transfer and uptake?
Homophily	What are the staff demographics of the organisation?
Change champions	Who is a likely change champion in the organisation?
Opinion leaders	What types of opinion leaders are contained within the organisation? Are external opinion leaders required?
Boundary spanners	Who is a likely boundary spanner? Does the organisation have links with external boundary spanners? What professional groups need to be accessed?
Social networks	How might these be established or enhanced? Do different professions have different types of social networks?

Table 5.6   Challenge 4: The practice context

Characteristics	Questions for practice
Context	What is the context of practice?
Structural determinants	What type of management structure is in place? Does it have clinical governance?
Absorptive capacity	Who is responsible within the organisation for analysing and reframing the evidence for the local context? Is it a learning culture that fosters widespread interdisciplinary sharing of evidence? Is leadership in place?
Receptive to change	Who is monitoring the change? What audit and feedback system is in place? What quality indicators are measured? Do practitioners receive the results?
Organisational networks	What organisation networks support practice development? Do these need to be fostered?

A significant challenge to getting evidence used in practice is communicating the evidence. Different approaches may be useful at different times depending on the purpose of the communication (Greenhalgh et al., 2004) (see Table 5.5). Networking with others in similar circumstances is one useful approach since this can provide friendship, support and advice in informal settings, learning from each other and developing communities of practice (Wenger, 2000).

Another approach to communicating new evidence is through change champions; informal and passionate clinical peers, who are able to motivate their colleagues through enthusiasm and 'can do' attitudes (Greenhalgh et al., 2004). Similar success has been shown with opinion leaders who may be internal or

Table 5.7   Challenge 5: Incorporating patients' preferences in practice

Characteristics	Questions for practice
Patients	To what extent can the patient participate in shared decision-making?
Level of involvement	Does the patient wish to be involved? How could the patient be involved?
Competence	Is the patient competent and able to be involved?
Meaning	How important is the problem to the patient?
Personality	What motivates the patient to participate in care? What approach should be taken to engage the patient in care?

external to the organisation. They are highly respected, able to evaluate new information, adapt it for the local context, and achieve success by modelling, peer influence, and altering group norms (Rogers, 1995). Practice developers may be both change champions and opinion leaders, as they are able to influence the actions and beliefs of their peers in promoting practice change.

In PD, a key method is facilitation (Manley, 2001; Garbett & McCormack, 2004; Titchen, 2004). This enables others to understand the process they need to go through in order to change behaviour of practitioners. It is also required to assist others in generating evidence from practice, as lack of support in changing practice is a frequently cited barrier to EBP (Hutchinson & Johnston, 2005).

Strong leadership and a culture of ongoing learning and experimentation also facilitate interdisciplinary knowledge sharing. These attributes are dependent on the ability of the organisation to monitor the changes and feedback to those involved for further refining of the process (Greenhalgh et al., 2004). Contextual factors, such as those identified in Table 5.6, need to be examined because of their impact on PD.

A further challenge central to PD is enabling person-centred care and the involvement of the patient in treatment decisions. Practitioners need to take account of the patient's condition, their values and circumstances when making decisions about healthcare treatments (Sackett et al., 1996). Shared decision-making is preferred by patients who have the capacity to comprehend the treatment information (Degner et al., 1997). However, practitioners should ask the questions identified in Table 5.7 to determine the level of involvement that is right for that patient. While support for patient involvement in healthcare decisions is increasing, there is little research that has focused on the role of the patient in promoting the rate of adoption of this activity amongst practitioners (Bucknall et al., 2004). Indeed, designing care around patients' concerns and needs is a key component of PD (Manley, 2004).

The challenges faced by practitioners using evidence in practice are complex in nature. In recognising the difficulties associated with implementation, practice developers need to systematically plan their practice changes to influence the behaviour of other practitioners since successful implementation is highly dependent upon changes being made to organisational and individual behaviour. Historically practitioners have lacked drive and action: 'Much of what passes as research dissemination is in fact passive diffusion focused on expanding individual awareness to promote behaviour change' (Kerner et al., 2005, p. 2). Greater understanding of team development, systems change, professional decision-making and clinical effectiveness has been accompanied by the realisation that a more active approach is needed to effect change.

Over the past 20 years, numerous models to facilitate the uptake of evidence in practice have been developed or refined. The main problem faced by practitioners is that of excessive choice, although many of the North American EBP implementation models are similar, particularly when assessed for clarity, conciseness, comprehensiveness and ease of use by direct care nurses (Mohide & King, 2003).

A wealth of models exists from disciplines outside of healthcare including psychology, management and sociology. Models being used effectively today reflect the complexity of contemporary healthcare in that they are multifaceted. One of these, Promoting Action on Research Implementation in Health Services (PARIHS) (Rycroft-Malone, 2004) appears to have resonated with practitioners, particularly those engaged in PD, and has led others to develop tools based on the concepts in this framework (Walsh et al., 2005).

The PARIHS framework is founded on the principle that implementation of evidence into practice, by practitioners, is more likely to be successful if undertaken using a systematic, context-specific approach to facilitation. This tool guides practitioners to explore aspects of evidence, context and facilitation, which influence the success of evidence implementation.

Growing international interest in model and framework development in evidence based practice implementation is increasingly evident. Yet there seems a shift towards implementation or utilisation measurement (Wallin et al., 2006). The changes to practice, particularly those involving information technology, that have occurred in recent times have prompted further research such as that by Gerrish et al. (2007). They developed a comprehensive tool to measure the extent to which practice is evidence based, and tested it in acute and community settings in England. The findings suggest that this could also be used as an outcome measure for PD.

Developing evidence from practice

The discussion so far has focused on understanding different types of evidence that may inform decision-making in practice and the models that guide evidence use in PD. However, PD is also concerned with developing evidence from practice (McCormack et al., 2006). In PD, evidence generation influences patient care by informing the transformation of individuals and teams integrating work-based learning with being a practitioner–researcher of one's own practice. 'Practitioner–researcher' is a term used to describe a practitioner who is systematically and rigorously researching some aspect of his/her own everyday practice. Such practitioners can generate evidence from practice about, for example, how to provide patient-centred interventions, how to enable a team culture of effectiveness, or how to use evidence from research in their work with patients. Practitioner–researchers therefore explore *how* they work with each other and key stakeholders, as well as *what* they do.

The practitioner as researcher of their own practice

The development of evidence from practice is associated with the practitioner–researcher movement, the concepts of reflexivity and reflection, and the recognition that practitioners work with the realities of practice, in varied contexts, with

Table 5.8 The aims of consultant nurses (CNs) and aspiring consultant nurses (ACNs) co-researchers within a study where they were supported to become researchers of their own practice (Manley et al. in preparation)

- CNs were researching and investigating their own practice as practitioner–researchers, aiming to become more effective and demonstrate their impact
- ACNs were researching and investigating their own practice as practitioner–researchers, wanting to develop evidence of their increased effectiveness and readiness for CN roles

colleagues and users who are individuals, and often unpredictable situations. Practitioners can generate evidence by working individually or in critical communities with intent to develop their practice, effectiveness and expertise, or some element of it, through rigorous investigation of their own practice (Titchen & Manley, 2006). Table 5.8 illustrates the intentions of 'practitioner–researchers' who were consultant nurses and aspiring consultant nurses and the evidence they intended to develop in relation to their own practice.

Reflexivity is the concept used to describe how practice changes in response to alterations in knowledge and thinking that have arisen from participating in critical, reflective inquiry. The word 'critical' is key as it highlights the association between the practitioner–researcher movement and critical theory. Critical theory is concerned with uncovering and overcoming taken-for-granted aspects and barriers in practice, work contexts and cultures, so that action follows from increased self-knowledge and understanding of practitioners (Fay, 1987; Freire, 1972). Understanding alone does not guarantee action, but critical science enables the barriers to action to be identified, challenged and dismantled through critique and reflection (Carr & Kemmis, 1986).

Reflection in and on practice is the process that enables individuals to systematically and creatively think about and evaluate their practice in order to reach new insights and understandings (Mezirow, 1981; Schon, 1983; Boud et al., 1985). These new insights and understandings source evidence derived from practice that can be captured and verified. When such understandings are experienced by other practitioner–researchers within critical communities then this evidence can contribute to practice theories that can be shared, transferred, tested and refined by others in different contexts.

Table 5.9 illustrates the experience of becoming a practitioner–researcher within a critical community where participants were researching their own expertise and compiling a portfolio of evidence.

Just as facilitation has been identified as important in achieving evidence use, it is also required to help practitioners investigate their own practice, transform their learning into action, and generate evidence from practice (Manley et al., 2005; Dewar & Sharp, 2006; Wilson et al., 2006). Supporting practitioners in this approach to evidence development has a number of benefits (see Table 5.10).

Table 5.9   Experience of being a practitioner–researcher within a project that explored expertise in the practice of nursing (Manley et al., 2005)

> Practitioner–researcher: *Participating in this project has helped me develop as a practitioner. Analysing and reflecting on what I do, and how and why I do it, in a systematic way has helped me recognise my own skills and knowledge. Prior to this project, I did not recognise a lot of what I do, articulating them [i.e., skills and knowledge] has made them visible to me. I feel this portfolio can make them visible to others. At the beginning of the project I found it difficult to pick out concise and specific evidence relating to expert practice, and immensely difficult to write down. I would sit at my computer for hours and produce what felt like a pathetically small amount of work. The writing flows now, and that feels like a gift to me.*

Nature of evidence that can emerge from practice

The evidence emerging from investigating one's own practice provides insights into new ways of thinking and acting, as well as contributing to theory about how and what is practiced, the impact of practice, and how practice can be transformed. In the context of PD, these insights relate to the individual and/or collective action necessary for developing effective workplace cultures characterised by person-centred and evidence-based care. McCormack and Titchen (2006) identify several methods practitioners and practice teams can use to generate evidence and achieve transformation in practice (see Table 5.11).

However, these methods do not provide guidance about where to start or what to do with the evidence resulting. The following section will do so.

Table 5.10   Benefits of supporting practitioners as researchers of their own practice

- Learning from the inquiry process is immediately incorporated into everyday action so inquiry and implementation are integrated (Manley, 2001; Titchen & Manley, 2006; Titchen & Manley, 2006)
- Individuals and teams become self-empowered and take ownership for developing their own practice (Manley, 2001, 2004; Wilson et al., 2006)
- Individuals become truly accountable for their actions in that they are able to articulate the rationale informing their action (Manley, 2001)
- Individuals develop the skill-set necessary for becoming self-sufficient in their own learning and development within the context of lifelong learning (Manley & Webster, 2006; Wilson et al., 2006)
- This way of working fosters the development and maintenance of a 'culture of effectiveness' where critique, work-based learning and the giving and receiving of feedback becomes the norm (Manley, 2001, 2004; Wilson et al., 2006)
- It enables the potential of all to develop and flourish (McCormack & Titchen, 2006; Titchen & Manley, 2006)

Table 5.11 Methods for developing evidence from practice (adapted from McCormack & Titchen, 2006)

Activities for providing evidence of intent, outputs and outcomes	
Action planning	
Objective setting	
Taking action	
Implementing practice change	
Evaluation	
Role-modelling	
Methods that can be used by individual practitioners or teams	**Methods that can be used by practice dyads, groups or teams**
Observing	Reflective conversations
Listening	Critical dialogue
Questioning	Critical reflection
Critiquing	Providing and receiving high
Self-reflection	challenge and high support
Creative expression and analysis	Feedback
	Feedback on performance
	Focused conversations
	Storytelling
	Appreciative inquiry
	Engaging multiple discourses
	Analysing, interpreting and
	evaluating shared experiences
Methods requiring facilitation by others	**Specific tools that can be used to generate evidence from practice**
Action learning	Values clarification
Problem-based learning	Role clarification
Clinical supervision	360° feedback
Facilitation of theorisation of practice	Cultural analysis
Facilitating the articulation of craft knowledge	Audit
Reflective questioning	
Development of transformational leaders	
Identifying how craft knowledge is developed	

Starting points for developing evidence from practice

Developing evidence from practice may start with

- the motivation and natural curiosity of the practitioner about her/his practice;
- the next steps required to achieve a team's shared vision;
- the need to implement and evaluate a practice initiative, policy or strategy;
- internal or external feedback received about individual or team performance;
- participation in an action research study, cooperative inquiry or action learning.

At the individual level a practitioner–researcher may be interested in

- refining a technical skill,
- improving their skills in providing feedback,
- developing their effectiveness across a number of areas,
- demonstrating their impact,
- developing their leadership potential,
- actioning feedback from users' experiences,
- developing their expertise,
- facilitating others, and
- clarifying their role.

These interests need to be translated into questions that the practitioner uses to guide action cycles or objectives that can be evaluated through an action plan or learning contract. Questions are action orientated because they are about how practitioners work, what they do and when, and the knowledge and evidence from different sources that inform their actions, for example

- How can I demonstrate my effectiveness?
- How can I enable others to develop expertise?
- When is it appropriate to use a specific intervention with patients?

Support from a facilitator who acts as a critical companion (Titchen, 2000) will help the practitioner explore these questions and identify practical strategies that need to be tried, tested, reflected on, and evaluated. Evidence will be generated from implementing these practical strategies and from this arises new insights that can be shared with others or that guide ongoing inquiry.

Whilst the methods identified in Table 5.11 may be used by practitioner–researchers to obtain feedback and evidence about her/his own practice, one approach, qualitative 360° feedback, may be useful to start the ball rolling. This method involves gathering feedback (evidence) from one's peers about how a role or some aspect of it is experienced by others. This helps to identify areas for development and refinement or to deconstruct and explain outstanding practice. This method has been used by practitioner–researchers to develop evidence of their expertise (Manley et al., 2005; Garbett et al., 2007).

At a critical community level, the generation of evidence may use similar approaches to that for the individual. Alternatively, once a common vision has been agreed with regards to a strategy, vision or project focus, then a tool termed *claims, concerns, and issues* can be used as a starting point (Titchen & Manley, 2006, 2007). This tool derived from fourth generation evaluation (Guba & Lincoln, 1989) enables stakeholders to be identified, valued and engaged, and starting points identified in relation to different purposes (Titchen & Manley, 2006) (See Table 5.12), as well as, strengthening stakeholder involvement in participatory action research approaches (Titchen & Manley, 2007).

Table 5.12 Using *claims, concerns and issues* for different purposes associated with getting started as a critical community in developing evidence from practice (Titchen & Manley, 2006)

- Helping critical communities decide what to focus on and when
- Developing action research questions
- Informing collaborative action planning and action strategies
- Developing a consensus about what is important to the critical community
- Providing a source of data for analysis about the journey
- Showing that all views and experiences are listened to and contribute to formulating questions that stimulate the formulation of action plans and their evaluation
- Using claims to develop action hypothesis requiring testing

Approaches to systematically and rigorously developing evidence from practice

PD is arguably a systematic rather than ad hoc activity (Garbett & McCormack, 2002; McCormack et al., 2006). The frameworks for guiding systematic approaches to developing evidence from practice are structured around action cycles, or more accurately action spirals, as we never return to the same place again but always move forward in our learning and development. Each action spiral has stages including planning, acting, observing and reflecting that are systematically and self-critically implemented (Grundy & Kemmis, 1981). An action spiral may start at the individual level by asking action-orientated questions or using feedback about how others perceive our role. At the critical community level it can begin by focusing on claims, concerns and issues.

Critique and reflection are active and necessary processes that enable evidence, developed from practice about practice, and the conditions under which practice takes place, to be exposed to rigorous and open scrutiny, therefore minimising the unquestioning acceptance of inherited modes of thinking. Assumptions can constrain our ways of thinking and actions. Critical science assists the critique of, and reflection upon, our assumptions as a starting point for developing evidence and ultimately critical theory. Carr and Kemmis (1986) identify the role of reflection in relation to the critique of barriers to practical action that exist within ourselves and the systems in which we work. They provide examples of how the practitioner–researcher may reflect at different levels and how this may be used as data for analysis.

Action research exists on a continuum of approaches as wide-ranging as research itself, from technical through to emancipatory (Grundy, 1982). Emancipatory action research is an approach for developing evidence from practice that integrates all the above: processes of reflection and critique; action spirals; strategic intent and collaboration with stakeholders into a sophisticated research approach characterised by participation, collaboration and inclusion – principles that characterise PD as well as action research (McCormack et al., 2006).

Emancipatory action research is consistent philosophically with emancipatory PD (Manley & McCormack, 2004) since it integrates both development of practitioners with changing practice encompassing evidence generation as well as evaluation (McCormack & Manley, 2004). Specific criteria are used to judge the quality of an action research study and therefore the evidence generated from it (McCormack & Manley, 2004).

Action research is an approach that locates research in practice and it provides a systematic framework for assisting practitioner–researchers, as either individual or critical communities, to generate evidence from practice at the same time as changing practice. Action learning, in contrast, is similarly systematic but is located in learning from practice. PD draws on research and learning to inform action (McCormack et al., 2006).

Action learning is a structured and disciplined approach that supports practitioners, through facilitation, as individuals and groups explore issues from their own practice, implement learning, and use and generate evidence to enable change to occur in practice (McGill & Brockbank, 2004; Wilson & McCormack, 2006; McCormack et al., 2006). It is frequently a key method within action research, providing data that can contribute to and corroborate outcomes (Dewar & Sharp, 2006; Manley et al., 2005; Meyer et al., 2003; Charlotte et al., 2004). Dewar and Sharp (2006) illustrate case studies using action learning as a collaborative mechanism for developing communities of inquiry as part of an action research study aimed at helping practitioners use evidence in end of life care. Dewar and Sharp recognise that evidence is available to inform practitioners about *what* to do, but not *how* to implement it in practice. Through action learning, Dewar and Sharp were able to support key change agents in implementing best practice guidelines, and developed new evidence from practice that would enable others to implement similar changes.

Conclusion

Using and generating knowledge is a central tenet of PD. A practice developer must have the ability to be both an astute observer and critical thinker. They must be able to analyse a situation, compare the best available alternatives for treatment or intervention, and engage with the patient to incorporate their preferences in the selection of the best option. Yet, as straightforward as this sounds, practitioners work in very complex and chaotic environments where information is either incomplete or in oversupply, often uncertain, received from multiple sources, both subjective and objective, and shrouded in value judgements. As a consequence, practitioners need to be detectives, piecing together information to reach a suitable conclusion.

As researchers of their own practice, practice developers must draw upon a range of approaches that have been systematically developed using rigorous and transparent processes. Practitioners must be able to appraise and evaluate evidence used in practice not just to determine quality but also for applicability or relevance to the practice setting. Evidence generated by practice developers must be achieved using a systematic, transparent, rigorous process so that it can also be used by other practitioners.

When making a clinical decision, restricting evidence used to that of research imposes significant limitations on the suitability or applicability of the choice for practice. In PD, there is widespread recognition that different types of evidence can and should contribute to practice decisions. Similarly, these decisions are influenced by individuals and the context in which the decisions are being made. Just like a kaleidoscope, where each small turn changes the picture, the practice environment is influenced by different things occurring on any given day, including the patients. Consequently, practice developers need to question and challenge existing practices. This requires significant reflection by individual practitioners and teams, focusing specifically on practice behaviours, to generate the understanding and insight needed to provide the best care for that patient. Every interaction with the patient is unique and if due consideration is not given to different types of evidence, wrong decisions can be made. Practitioners need to embrace evidence-based practice as a key principle of PD; this can lead to new insights that can be shared with others or guide ongoing inquiry. As Maria Robinson stated: 'Nobody can go back and start a new beginning, but anyone can start today and make a new ending'.

References

Boud, D., Keogh, R. & Walker, D. (1985) *Reflection: Turning Experience Into Learning.* Kogan Page, London.

Bucknall, T.K. (1996) Clinical decision making in critical care nursing practice: Decisions, processes and influences. Unpublished Thesis, La Trobe University, Australia.

Bucknall, T.K. (2003) The clinical landscape of critical care: Nurses' decision making. *Journal of Advanced Nursing.* **43**(3), 310–319.

Bucknall, T.K. (2006) Knowledge transfer and utilization: Implications for home health care pain management. *Journal of Healthcare Quality.* **28**(1), 12–19.

Bucknall, T.K., Rycroft-Malone, J. & Mazurek Melnek, B. (2004) Integrating patient involvement in decision making. *Worldviews on Evidence Based Nursing.* **1**(3), 151–153.

Carr, W. & Kemmis, S. (1986) *Becoming Critical: Education, Knowledge and Action Research.* Falmer, London.

Charlotte, A., Meyer, J., Johnson, B. & Smith, C. (2004) Using action research to address loss of personhood in a continuing care setting. *Illness, Crisis, & Loss.* **12**(1), 23–37.

Davis, D., Evans, M., Jadad, A., Perrier, L., Rath, D., Ryan, D., Sibbald, G., Straus, S., Rappolt, S., Wowk, M. & Zwarenstein, M. (2003) The case for knowledge translation: Shortening the journey from evidence to effect. *BMJ.* **327**(7405), 33–35.

Degner, L.F., Kristjanson, L.J., Bowman, D., Sloan, J.A., Carriere, K.C., O'Neil, J. et al. (1997) Information needs and decision preferences in women with breast cancer. *JAMA.* **277**(18), 1485–1492.

De Maeseneer, J.M., van Driel, M.L., Green, L.A. & van Weel, C. (2003) The need for research in primary care. *The Lancet.* **362**(9392), 1314–1319. (http://www.sciencedirect.com/science/article/B6T1B-49SW3C7-10/2/d8eb1449 98681525f1fae8e744b15541).

Dewar, B. & Sharp, C. (2006) Using evidence: How action learning can support individual and organisational learning through action research. *Educational Action Research.* **14**(2), 219–237.

Downie, R.S. & Macnaughton, J. (2000) Judgement and science. In: *Clinical Judgement: Evidence in Practice* (eds R.S. Downie, J. Macnaughton & F. Randall). Oxford University Press, Oxford.

Fay, B. (1987) Critical Social Science: Liberation & Its Limits. Polity, Cambridge.

Freire, P. (1972) *Pedagogy of the Oppressed*. Herder & Herder, New York.

Garbett, R. & McCormack, B. (2002) A concept analysis of practice development. *Nursing Times Research.* **7**(2), 87–100.

Garbett, R. & McCormack, B. (2004) A concept analysis of practice development. In: *Practice Development in Nursing* (eds B. McCormack, K. Manley & R. Garbett). Blackwell, Oxford.

Gerrish, K., Ashworth, P., Lacey, A., Bailey, J., Cooke, J., Kendall, S. & McNeilly, E. (2007) Factors influencing the development of evidence-based practice: A research tool. *Journal of Advanced Nursing.* **57**(3), 328–338.

Greenhalgh, T., Robert, G., Bate, P., Kyriakidou., O., Macfarlane, F. & Peacock, R. (2004) How to spread good ideas. A systematic review of the literature on diffusion, dissemination and sustainability of innovations in health service delivery and organization. *Report for the National Coordinating Center for NHS Service Delivery and Organization R & D*, University College, London.

Grundy, S. (1982) Three modes of action research. *Curriculum Perspectives.* **2**(3), 23–34.

Grundy, S. & Kemmis, S. (1981) Educational action research in Australia: The state of the art. Paper presented at the *Annual Meeting of the Australian Association for Research in Adelaide.*

Guba, E.G. & Lincoln, Y.S. (1989) *Fourth Generation Evaluation*. Sage, Newbury Park, CA.

Hutchinson, A.M. & Johnston, L. (2005) Bridging the divide: A survey of nurses' opinions regarding the barriers to and facilitators of, research utilization in the practice setting. *Journal of Clinical Nursing.* **13**(3), 304–315.

Kerner, J., Rimer, B. & Emmons, K. (2005) Introduction to the special section on dissemination. Dissemination research and research dissemination: How can we close the gap? *Health Psychology.* **24**(5), 443–446.

Manley, K. (1997) Operationalising an advanced practice/consultant nurse role: An action research study. *Journal of Clinical Nursing.* **6**(3), 179–190.

Manley, K. (2001) Consultant nurse: Concept, processes, outcomes. Unpublished PhD Thesis, Manchester University/RCN Institute, London.

Manley, K. (2004) Transformational culture: A culture of effectiveness. In: *Practice Development in Nursing* (eds B. McCormack, K. Manley & R. Garbett), pp. 51–82. Blackwell, Oxford.

Manley, K., Hardy, S., Titchen, A., Garbett, R. & McCormack, B. (2005) Changing patients' worlds through nursing practice expertise. Exploring nursing practice expertise through emancipatory action research and fourth generation evaluation. *A Royal College of Nursing Research Report 1998–2004*. RCN, London.

Manley, K. & McCormack, B. (2004) Practice development: Purpose, methodology, facilitation and evaluation. In: *Practice Development in Nursing* (eds B. McCormack, K. Manley & R. Garbett). Blackwell, Oxford.

Manley, K., Titchen, A. & Rowe, R. (in preparation) *Being and Becoming a Consultant Nurse*. Research Report. RCN, London.

Manley, K. & Webster, J. (2006) Can we keep quality alive? *Nursing Standard*. **21**(3), 12–15.

McCormack, B., Dewar, B., Wright, J., Garbett, R., Harvey, G. & Ballantine, K. (2006) *Realist Synthesis of Evidence Relating to Practice Development: Executive Summary*. NHS Quality Improvement, Scotland. (www.nes.scot.nhs.uk/)

McCormack, B., Kitson, A., Harvey, G., Rycroft-Malone, J., Tichen, A. & Seers, K. (2002) Getting evidence into practice: The meaning of 'context'. *Journal of Advanced Nursing*. **38**(1), 94–104.

McCormack, B. & Manley, K. (2004) Evaluating practice developments. In: *Practice Development in Nursing* (eds B. McCormack, K. Manley & R. Garbett), pp. 83–117. Blackwell, Oxford.

McCormack, B. & Titchen, A. (2006) Critical creativity: Melding, exploding, blending. *Educational Action Research*. **14**(2), 239–266.

McGill, I. & Brockbank, A. (2004) *The Action Learning Handbook*. Routledge Falmer, London.

Meyer, J., Johnson, B., Proctor, S., Bryer, R. & Rozmovits, L. (2003) Practitioner research: Exploring issues in relation to research capacity building. *Nursing Times Research*. **8**(6), 407–417.

Mezirow, J. (1981) A critical theory of adult learning and education. *Adult Education*. **32**(1), 3–24.

Mohide, E.A. & King, B. (2003) Building a foundation for evidence-based practice: Experiences in a tertiary hospital. *Evidence-Based Nursing*. **6**, 100–103.

National Health and Medical Research Council (1999) *A Guide to the Development, Implementation and Evaluation of Clinical Practice Guidelines*. Commonwealth of Australia, Canberra.

Newhouse, R., Dearholt, S., Poe, S., Pugh, L.C. & White, K.M. (2005) Evidence-based practice: A practical approach to implementation. *Journal of Nursing Administration*. **35**(1), 35–40.

Pearson, A. (2002) Nursing takes the lead: Redefining what counts as evidence in Australian health care. *Reflections on Nursing Leadership*. **28**(4), 18–21.

Rogers, E. (1995) *Diffusion of Innovations*. The Free Press, New York.

Rolfe, G. (1997) Beyond expertise: Theory, practice and the reflexive practitioner. *Journal of Clinical Nursing*. **6**(2), 93–97.

Russell, C.K. & Gregory, D.M. (2003) EBN users' guide. Evaluation of qualitative research studies. *Evidence Based Nursing*. **6**(2), 36–40.

Rycroft-Malone, J. (2004) The PARIHS framework – a framework for guiding the implementation of evidence-based practice. Promoting action on research implementation in health services. *Journal of Nursing Care Quality*. **19**(4), 297–304.

Rycroft-Malone, J., Harvey, G., Seers, K., Kitson, A., McCormack, B. & Titchen, A. (2004a) An exploration of the factors that influence the implementation of evidence into practice. *Journal of Clinical Nursing*. **13**(8), 913–924.

Rycroft-Malone, J., Seers, K., Titchen, A., Harvey, G., Kitson, A. & McCormack, B. (2004b) What counts as evidence in evidence-based practice? *Journal of Advanced Nursing*. **47**(1), 81–90.

Sackett, D.L., Rosenberg, W., Haynes, R.B. & Richardson, W.S. (1996) Evidence-based medicine: What it is and what it isn't. *BMJ*. **312**, 71–72.

Schon, D.A. (1983) The Reflective Practitioner. How Professionals Think in Action. Basic Books, New York.

Tavakoli, M., Davis, H.T.O. & Thomson, R. (2000) Decision analysis in evidence-based decision making. *Journal of Evaluation in Clinical Practice*. **6**(2), 111–120.

Titchen, A. (2000) Professional Craft Knowledge in Patient-Centred Nursing and the Facilitation of Its Development. Ashdale Press Tackley, Oxfordshire.

Titchen, A. (2004) Helping relationships for practice development: Critical companionship. In: *Practice Development in Nursing* (eds B. McCormack, K. Manley & R. Garbett), pp. 148–174. Blackwell, Oxford.

Titchen, A. & Manley, K. (2006) Spiralling towards transformational action research: Philosophical and practical journeys. *Educational Action Research*. **14**(3), 333–356.

Titchen, A. & Manley, K. (2007) Facilitating research as shared action and transformation. In: *Being Critical and Creative in Qualitative Research* (eds J. Higgs, A. Titchen, H. Byrne Armstrong & D. Horsfall). Hampden, Sydney.

Van Driel, M.L., De Sutter, A.I., Christiaens, T. & De Maeseneer, J.M. (2005) Quality of care: The need for medical, contextual and policy evidence in primary care. *Journal of Evaluation in Clinical Practice*. **11**(5), 417–429.

Wallin, L., Estabrooks, C.A., Midodzi, W.K. & Cummings, G.G. (2006) Development and validation of a derived measure of research utilization by nurses. *Nursing Research*. **55**(3), 149–160.

Walsh, K., Lawless, J., Moss, C. & Allbon, C. (2005) The development of an engagement tool for practice development. *Practice Development in Health Care*. **4**(3), 124–130.

Wenger, E. (2000) Communities of practice and social learning systems. *Organization*. **7**, 225–246.

Wilson, V. & McCormack, B. (2006) Re-generating the self in learning: Developing a culture of supportive learning in practice. *Learning in Health and Social Care*. **5**(2), 90–105.

6. Learning – The Heart of Practice Development

Charlotte L. Clarke and Val Wilson

Introduction

Practice development (PD) implies that there is a development in practice. This requires two aspects to be explored further – does 'practice' mean what is done and/or what is thought? Does 'development' mean a change and/or an improvement? These questions are consistent with the principles underpinning PD as articulated in Chapter 1. In particular, they relate to principles 3 (learning) and 4 (evidence use and development). For PD to be effective, it needs to impact first and foremost on what is thought (the doing will follow naturally) and to seek to achieve an improvement in patient care. This places learning by individuals and by organisations at the heart of PD activity. This chapter explores the role of learning theory and processes in developing healthcare practice.

Learning theories in professional and practice development

For professionals to advance their practice requires them, in part, to engage in a process of learning through reflection and learning of their current practice. However, the fragmented approach to contemporary practice in healthcare results in discontinuities of experience and the individual practitioner is frequently shielded, or buffered, from the consequences of their actions. As a result, they lose the opportunity to evaluate, reflect and be reflexive in their practice.

There are a number of examples of healthcare delivery that are vulnerable to this process. For example, midwives' support of breastfeeding in the immediate post-natal period and pharmaceutical management of patients in Emergency Department where staff are buffered from the longer term implications of their administrations. For example, someone may fall after admission to a ward following administration of a sedative in Emergency Department.

One of the major learning theories that promotes as essential, observation and reflection of concrete experiences is Kolb's experiential learning model (1995) (see Figure 6.1).

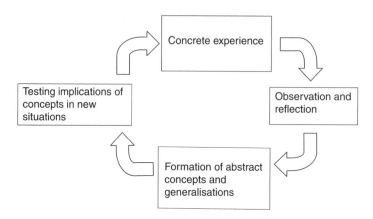

Figure 6.1 Kolb's experiential learning cycle.

It is the disruption to this cycle caused by lack of exposure to the consequences of one's actions that may fragment the reflective learning. For example, midwives who do not have more than a few days continuity of caring for a woman may be unable to have 'concrete experiences' about the duration of breastfeeding for the woman and any associated problems – for example, poor positioning may result in trauma to breast tissues that are not evident for some days after the trauma has occurred. Without these concrete experiences, there can be no observation and no reflection to inform future practice.

However, there are critics of models of reflection that they concern solely the individual practitioner (e.g. Quinn, 1998; Eby, 2000) and certainly models of reflection offer no solutions for situations in which there are structural and organisational disruptions to the reflective cycle as described above in relation to breastfeeding support in midwifery. The literature about professional learning focuses on the way in which professionals think. Polanyi (1962) coined the expression 'know-how' and used it in his description of two kinds of knowledge, 'knowing-that' and 'knowing-how' (Easen & Wilcockson, 1996). The expert knowledge that professionals use, but find difficult to articulate, is known as tacit knowledge (Meerabeau, 1992; Meyer & Batehup, 1997). Boreham (1994), arguing for a dual cognitive architecture as a means of explaining professional thinking, says that thinking involves moving between the two processes of explicit and implicit thinking. Both systems are used at the same time and interact with each other. Novice and expert professionals are believed to think in different ways. Expert professionals have the ability to organise knowledge in a more sophisticated way that highlights the important relationships between different concepts (Roehler et al., 1988) and their performance responds to a 'deep understanding of the total situation' (Benner, 1984).

Schon (1992) offers an important distinction between 'problem-solving' and 'problem-setting', the latter requiring a learning process that is more collegial than the rather individualistic process described by Kolb. The process of identifying and analysing problems (problem-setting) rather than solving problems that build on assumptions (problem solving) requires a process of reflection that is advanced

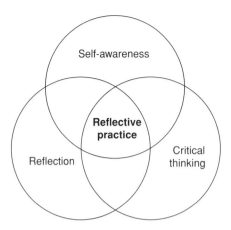

Figure 6.2 Reflective practice.

through not only experience but also feeding in new ideas and knowledge and exploring the implications of these with colleagues. Indeed, the primary driver for developing practice is problem-setting that results in an awareness of lack of fit between the services provided and the needs of the service users (Clarke et al., 1998; Wilson-Barnett et al., 2000). Eby (2000) describes this as critical reflection, and a key component of critical practice. Eby (2000) outlines the components of such a process (see Figure 6.2).

Hammond and Collins (1991) describe such an approach to critical practice as being underpinned by a certain set of beliefs and values concerning professional development.

These include

- promoting self-awareness and social awareness and social action;
- supporting the principles of lifelong learning;
- stimulating self-expressions and peer expressions or dialogue;
- improving self-expression, learning and cooperation;
- linking theory and practice.

All of these values derive from a set of philosophical origins that include phenomenology and critical theory. It is these philosophies that similarly underpin the model of critical practice that is promoted by Barnett (1997) and Brechin (2000). Critical practice is described as having three components that intersect to create critical practice, each component having an associated set of actions and skills.

1. Critical action:
   - Sound skill based, used with awareness of context.
   - Operating to challenge structural disadvantage.
   - Working with difference towards empowerment.

2. Critical reflexivity:
   - Engaged self.
   - Negotiated understanding and intervention.
   - Questioning personal assumptions and values.
3. Critical analysis:
   - Evaluation of knowledge, theories, policies and practice.
   - Recognition of multiple perspectives.
   - Different levels of analysis.
   - Ongoing enquiry.

These debates are critical in the current healthcare environment that promotes evidence-based practice and clinical governance. Where once the learning during a pre-registration training was considered to contain sufficient knowledge for a professional's work, thereafter requiring the skill of application of that knowledge base, the emphasis now is on lifelong learning and a recognition that professional decision-making is 'too complex to take the form of simply applying general rules to specific situations' (Winter & Munn-Giddings, 2001). Schon (1983) was critical of the application of knowledge model (technical rationality), recognising the need for professions to construct a situation through the experimentation and learning associated with reflective practice. Similarly, others argue that in attempting to comply with a technical–rational evidence base, the artistry and reflexivity of context-specific practitioner knowledge is compromised (Eraut, 1994; Meyer & Barehup, 1997; Fish, 1998). Indeed, one of the more major concerns about evidence-based practice is that the dominance of positivist science may devalue, or even exclude, other sources of knowledge known to the professional such as the wishes of the service user (Trinder, 2000). Stewart (2001), in studying midwives' perceptions of evidence-based practice, emphasises the difficulty of implementing evidence that challenges cultural norms.

Professional practice is a development process characterised by ongoing learning (Eby, 2000). Clearly, professional learning that depends on a sustained opportunity to witness consequences of actions and reflect on these cannot develop independently of service systems. Cowley (1995) argues that organisations need to be places of learning to support professional developments. Increasingly, organisations are seen as a collective that can learn as well as the individuals within it. Argyris and Schon (1996) describe how an organisation can hold knowledge through its individual members and through developing strategies for completing complicated activities. They refer to knowledge such as routines and practices that can be 'inspected' as 'theories of action'. For example, in midwifery these may be protocols or guidelines. Fish (1998) argues that such theories of action are creatively adapted by practitioners to local circumstances and individual problems.

There are two distinct effects of each kind of learning. Single-loop learning increases the effectiveness of actions to achieve the values and norms previously decided. Single-loop learning may not bring about a desired change and it is then that the need to change the organisational values and norms may be recognised (Davies et al., 2000). This then is called double-loop learning. 'It is through double-loop learning alone that individuals or organisations can address the desirability of the values and norms that govern their theories-in-use' (Argyris & Schon, 1996, p. 22). It is this form of learning that practitioners active in PD are harnessing in order to reconceptualise patient care and move forward services that match patient need.

The importance of double-loop learning depends on the extent to which the organisation's essential values and norms are involved. Learning is affected by the size of the organisation and the number of layers within the organisation and the extent to which changes may have repercussions in other areas. In this way, the pervasiveness of an individual development, and the impact of any individual practitioner, is necessarily linked to the mode of organisational learning. Where the organisation favours the process of an inquiry that is to take place, Argyris and Schon (1996) refer to them as 'enablers'. Important to double-loop learning is the questioning of 'assumptions and behaviour' (Argyris & Schon, 1996). The nature of the organisation's 'behavioural world' is key to the process of inquiry. In an atmosphere where individuals are friendly, 'open' and 'cooperative', organisational inquiry is facilitated. If individuals in the organisation are, for example, 'hostile' and 'competitive', then the opposite effect is achieved. Although the midwives interviewed did not identify such overtly hostile activity, they did describe several situations in which their attempts to support breastfeeding had been undermined by colleagues. The theories-in-use, which guide the behaviour of individual members are interdependent with the organisation's learning system (Argyris & Schon, 1996).

The close integration of learning with practice, the development of practice and the advancement of knowledge for the individual professional and for the organisation was identified in a soft systems study of PD by Clarke and Wilcockson (2001):

One clear message from the study is the importance of a close integration of learning, practice and knowledge development (or research). Indeed, disaggregating these elements will result in dissonance between knowledge, practitioners and the organisation – rather like a car's gearbox, if all the cogs do not move simultaneously the whole will seize.

Clarke & Wilcockson, 2001

Clinical decision-making is located, or 'situated', in the context of local service, professional and service user knowledge, changing as that contextual knowledge fluctuates in time and between place and person (Clarke & Gardner, 2002a). It is in the area of bringing together local contextual knowledge with more remote technical knowledge that there is most concern expressed within the literature (Greenhalgh, 1999; Trinder, 2000) with some arguing that most desirable is a synthesis of scientific, theoretical, experiential and personal knowledge (Schon, 1987; Eraut, 1994; Rolfe, 1998). Where there have been many advocates for services that promote continuity of the carer as a means of improving the quality of midwifery care, Green et al. (2000) suggest that more important is to have continuity of care. Perhaps promoting continuity in both aspects of care and carer needs to be attended to, the explanatory framework being the need to promote the simultaneous development of professional and organisational learning. In this way, the reflective cycle of professional practice is respected and services are structured to maximise consistent care through a shared value base and approach.

Strategies for engaging in professional learning in practice development

Within a PD framework there is the opportunity for practitioners to engage in a variety of learning strategies that focus on critical reflection. Reflective learning processes are central to an emancipatory PD (EPD) approach. Reflective processes are integrated with other developmental processes and thus achieving PD is enabled through the changes in the perspectives of individual practitioners to recognise the need for change. Thus, unlike technical approaches to PD where learning is a consequence of the work, in EPD learning is integrated with development activities and is a primary intended outcome of development activities (Manley & McCormack, 2003). In this chapter, we will explore a number of strategies that may be used for this common purpose with individuals or groups. An outline of the strategy will be offered together with an example of how it works in practice.

High challenge with high support

High challenge is a process used to raise participants' awareness about what is happening around them, the role they play in what is happening and to foster a reflexive mode of inquiry. This is undertaken in a supportive way, where challenge is balanced with support to ensure that the participant does not feel threatened or judged by the challenger, and is therefore more prone to act on their findings (Manley & McCormack, 2003; Johns & Freshwater, 1998; Johns & McCormack, 1998). A facilitator or practitioner uses guided reflection to challenge another's normative attitudes, assumptions and actions. High challenge is used to confront contradictions and high support to sustain commitment and effort to resolve contradictions as well as to transform self (Johns, 1996). These skills are often first learned within the context of an action learning set and then used very effectively in day-to-day clinical practice. Practitioners use these skills to challenge the 'taken-for-granted' decisions about patient care.

High challenge/high support (HC/HS) was one strategy used within a PD study carried out in a special care nursery (Wilson et al., 2007). One of the issues identified early on in the study was the fact that the nurses referred to the babies only by their surname. The facilitator (researcher) used HC/HS techniques to challenge the use of language and the impact it may hold for families in the unit. This also enabled the nurses and the facilitator to explore the underpinning assumptions about the ritualistic component of behaviour. Figure 6.3 indicates how this experience impacted on practice for Jane, one of the nurses.

We can therefore see from Jane's journey that the use of HC/HS not only enabled her to review and change her own practice but also encouraged her to adopt the strategy in working with others. The use of HC/HS enabled Jane to

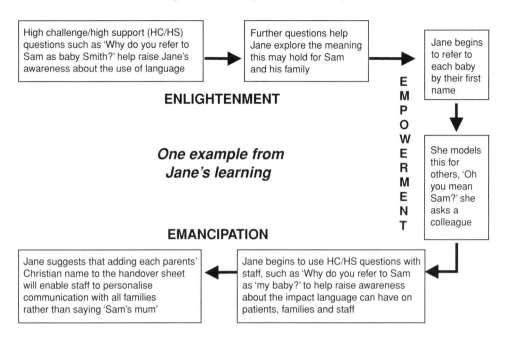

Figure 6.3 Jane's Journey.

move through the stages of enlightenment, as she began to see the significance that her practice held for families. The next phase was where Jane began to incorporate changes in her own behaviour to reflect new understandings of the importance of language. The facilitator provided ongoing support and encouragement of the changes Jane was making. The final stage of emancipation occurred when Jane herself began to use the HC/HS techniques with staff as she questioned them about their practice. Jane also offered further suggestions for change, which highlighted the significant growth for Jane in undertaking this journey.

Critical companionship

Critical companionship is a relationship in which an experienced practitioner helps another, for example in becoming increasingly person centred. This is achieved through critical reflection and dialogue, which helps the learning practitioner to understand what they need to change and how they can make those changes in order to transform practice. A critical companion is a facilitator who helps the learning practitioner to grow personally and professionally, to generate knowledge and become empowered to transform the culture within which they work (Titchen, 2003; McCormack, 1999). Critical companionship as developed by Titchen (2000) incorporates the following elements:

brings mind, heart, body, and creative imagination into helping relationships for practice development. It offers a metaphor and framework for an experienced facilitator (often, but not necessarily a colleague) who accompanies another on an experiential learning. . . Creating trust and using 'high challenge' and 'high support', critical companions enable individuals, teams and organisations to transform their roles, relationships, cultures and ways of thinking, being, doing and feeling

Titchen, 2004, p. 149

This definition by Titchen highlights the important aspects of creating meaningful learning partnerships for facilitation development.

When establishing a critical companionship relationship a carefully negotiated process has to be considered, which requires the facilitator and participant to be clear about their relationship, how they will work with one another, and where and when they will meet. The brief story given in Box 6.1 helps illustrate one of the ways in which critical companionship can be used in everyday practice.

Box 6.1   The lunchtime walk: a brief story of critical companionship

The two of them (Cassie & Alex) often met in the staffroom at lunchtime. They had got to know one another over the previous few months and would discuss how their day was going. Alex was an experienced educator and facilitator, Cassie on the other hand was quite new to the educator role. Conversations would often steer towards the environment in which they worked and the perceived lack of support for educators. Other staff often joined in these conversations and added differing perspectives about the issue of who could support them in their desire for professional development when the focus of their job was to 'professionally develop' others. These lunchtime conversations tended to be recycled and usually failed to go beyond a cathartic expression of discontent.

One day Cassie and Alex decided to go for a walk instead of joining the lunchtime crowd. On the walk Cassie shared some of her concerns with Alex about the lack of opportunities for her own professional development, her level of motivation as well as her discontent about her job. Alex realised that their regular conversations were taking a new dimension and whilst she was able to listen to Cassie's concerns she also felt that together they may be able to move beyond the 'recycled' lunchtime conversations. She asked Cassie whether she wanted more than what was offered in the staffroom. Together they explored what a 'lunchtime walk' might mean for them if they were to go beyond catharsis and perceived inertia and move towards a more critical and reflective way of working and walking. Cassie agreed that this might help her look through the issues she was dealing with and they agreed on some principles of working/walking together and so their new journey begins.

Over the coming months the lunchtime walks usually occurred once or twice a week. During this time Alex was able to help Cassie explore her feelings of uneasiness about her position. This helped uncover that Cassie often felt ill-prepared for her position as an educator, especially when she was asked to do things that did not sit well with her values about practice and care delivery. She often felt unsupported by some of her colleagues and in particular her manager who often pushed her in directions she did not want to go. This left her feeling vulnerable and eroded her self-confidence and belief in her ability to 'do the job'. As the layers around Cassie's issue began to unfold, Alex encouraged her (through a number of interventions) to reframe negative experiences into opportunities to act. This of course was not easy to achieve but with consistent approaches and supportive interventions Cassie was able to critically reflect on her own actions and inactions and deconstruct how these were contributing to her feelings of helplessness and inertia.

Together they explored ways in which Cassie might overcome some of the barriers she herself had created. Alex worked with Cassie (sharing craft knowledge) to develop key strategies that would enable Cassie to act in situations where she felt vulnerable. Cassie learned to deconstruct and critically reflect on situations that confronted her. Over time she was able to challenge other staff when she felt they were asking her to do things outside her scope of practice or experience. In the past she would have done what was asked of her even though she might feel she did not have the skills, which left her questioning her value as an educator. After a few months of lunchtime walks Cassie built up the courage to discuss her concerns with her manager. During the conversation when the manager asked her a question, she took the time to take a deep breath (think) and then respond (act rather than react). This technique worked well for her. She was able to separate the emotion from the situation and discuss calmly processes and professional responsibilities. She no longer felt intimidated, she had found 'her voice' and was able to use it with great effect.

The lunchtime walks had been more than a chance to escape the staffroom. They provided Cassie and Alex the opportunity to develop a deep and meaningful relationship based on the critical companionship framework. Elements of the framework are highlighted throughout the journey as Cassie and Alex got to know one another (relationship domain), as Alex challenged Cassie to enable her critically reflect on her experience (rationality-intuitive domain), and as they worked together to deconstruct and reconstruct the issues to enable Cassie to act (facilitation domain). There were a lot of challenges for both of them on this journey but through these challenges came deep reflection, commitment to self-development, and the creation of new understandings about self, one another and working relationships.

Clinical supervision

Clinical supervision has been used in healthcare since the late 1980s (Mills et al., 2005). Its use as a reflective practice tool was promoted by the publication of a position paper on clinical supervision by the NMC in 1996 (Howatson-Jones, 2003). It can be configured in a number of ways, for example, one-on-one or in groups depending on the needs of individuals and the purpose for starting clinical supervision. The purpose will also inform the focus of the clinical supervision, for example, the focus might be on clinical practice, roles or professional development. The Clinical Supervisor may be someone you report to, such as your manager, or it may be facilitated by someone outside your clinical area. Sessions can be held as frequently as you choose, but research shows that meeting at least once per month in a location away from the immediate clinical area is more beneficial (Rafferty et al., 2003; Jones, 2001). Power relationships have been identified as important influences on the conduct of clinical supervision and these relationships need to be handled with great care and consideration (Jones, 1999). It is therefore of vital importance that the clinical supervision relationship is negotiated by all parties involved and due time and consideration are given to the development of that relationship. Care must be taken that sessions are not of a therapeutic nature but rather focus on developing skills and resolving complex clinical issues (Jones, 2001; Stevenson, 2005).

Patrick was a member of a clinical supervision group. Here he explores through a reflective conversation (with his critical companion) how clinical supervision helped him work through a 'crisis' he was having relating to his position (acting) as a Clinical Nurse Consultant. His conversation using a pseudonym is reproduced here with his consent.

Patrick's crisis

I felt safe that what I was saying was confidential and they weren't going to discuss it with anyone else because I felt like in a sort of precarious position ... I felt unsafe in my position, I didn't feel like I could disclose things about how I was feeling about work or how I was feeling about the service ... so there was a situation of comparative safety I guess ... with people who were outside the situation but in similar clinical roles, to me I guess, that might have been important that they were each in autonomous roles ... but mostly the fact that it was agreed that it was confidential and that seemed to be a ground rule that was stringently adhered to.

Why did I choose to dump it, yes, why did I choose to dump it with them, at the time that I did? ... I think I wanted colleagues to validate my feelings ... the reason I say validate my feelings was that I actually think that I had already made a decision that I didn't want to participate in the service anymore and I was looking for people to say 'its okay to change jobs' because I was in an acting CNC position which was likely to lead to a permanent position and so from my career point of view, being a CNC, some people see being a CNC as desirable and I think I saw it as desirable as well but I certainly didn't see it as desirable in the context that I was in, so I wanted them to say there are more important things than becoming a CNC just because you can.

I think it clarified for me about what the options in acting were so that having made the decision ... I could act sort of impetuously in a way and just go and do anything to get out of it, or consider what it is that I'd like to do and then work out strategies about how to get into that position or respond to advertised positions that I actually thought were consistent with the direction that I wanted to move in so that third option was what I took, I just think it was coincidence that it was so timely, or you know providence or whatever it was, you know what I mean? ... certainly the temptation was to behave reactively and sort of left to my devices, I might have done that ... the process helpful, yes the process was helpful, what made it helpful, it clarified for me, it kind of got rid of the emotions somehow, so that I was able to reason my way out of it rather than just drop the ball and run away ... in that sense it was safety issue as well because basing your decision exclusively on, or acting exclusively on your emotions isn't always in your best interest.

We can see from Patrick's narrative that clinical supervision gave him the time and space to critically reflect on his future actions. The safety (confidentiality) in the group was of vital importance to Patrick and enabled him to share his dilemma with others. Through Patrick's story we can see that he had already made some decisions about 'getting out' of his position, but was unsure how to act on this. Clinical supervision enabled him to extract the emotive element of the situation and validate his decision, in light of the fact that resigning from the position also meant him giving up his CNC status. This helped Patrick to explore solutions to the issue and he was able to identify three options, having rejected the fourth option, which was to stay in the position and try to improve the situation. The time and space within clinical supervision allowed Patrick to consider the options. He then acted on the third option, which was to apply for other positions that were of interest to him in rebuilding his career. He did this successfully and began work in another department where he is building his skills and knowledge with a new focus as he re-establishes his career. In his new position, he is a valued member of the team who actively contributes to critical challenge and support within the workplace.

Socratic dialogue

Socratic dialogue is a technique that may be used to facilitate exploration of a fundamental question of interest to a group of people. According to Fitzgerald and van Hooft (2000), it is a 'method of painstaking enquiry into the ideas, concepts and values that influence the real decisions we make in everyday life'. One or more participants in a group use real-life examples from their own practice so that the group can explore assumptions about everyday decisions, reflect on experiences and reach a collective judgement about their question (Fitzgerald & van Hooft, 2000). An example of how a group of nurses explored a question relevant to their ward is used here to highlight the principles of Socratic dialogue.

A Christmas tale

The nurses are members of a critical discussion group in a paediatric ward, which meets once a month. The group use a HC/HS framework to explore issues relating to their clinical practice and the environment in which they work. In a group session last year, one of the nurses raised the issue of 'decorating the ward prior to Christmas'. There had been a challenge put to the nurse that decorating the ward may not be an appropriate use of the units resources as it reduced the time they had available to provide nursing care for patients. The question considered by the group, therefore, was 'What is our purpose in decorating the ward for Christmas?' Hansten and Washburn (2000) describe strategies that may be used with a group undertaking Socratic dialogue to ensure that 'participants remain focused and engaged' (p. 186). These include seeking verification from individuals of what has been said by previous respondents or asking a participant to summarise what has been said in the group. The critical discussion group used a number of similar strategies to explore each participant's perspective and to challenge the assumptions that were emerging during the course of the discussion.

Each nurse in the group felt passionate about decorating the ward, many had done this over the years and felt it was a rewarding and satisfying activity. They wanted to explore in more depth the reasons (assumptions and perceptions) for this, to ensure that they could provide a considered argument for why they should be allowed to continue to spend time decorating the ward. Each participant listened attentively to contributions from the others and offered points of clarification where they felt it was necessary. The facilitator helped to keep the group focused on the intent of the discussion by asking critical questions relating to the question being explored. The group were able to identify that their passion for decorating the ward stemmed from the reaction of the children (whose faces would light up) to seeing the decorations, and provided the nurses with a sense of achievement and reward for the contribution they were making. They acknowledged that they considered patient care, safety and comfort of paramount importance in their role. With further questioning it became clear that during the decorating period, when they were called away to attend to direct patient care, parents would take over, becoming involved in the task of making decorations. This enabled parents to contribute to the work and helped foster a sense of teamwork between the parents and the nurses. They had a common purpose, to improve the environment for children who were unwell.

There was also acknowledgement that for many of them this activity was in addition to the everyday caring aspect of their nursing role. Nurses gave up their free time, when not on duty, to come to the ward to complete decorations. Their reasoning for this 'sacrifice' lay in their ability to make their ward a bright and wonderful place for children at a time of year that is focused on children and celebration.

Working in partnership with families and creating a child friendly environment are amongst the espoused aims of the ward. Undertaking the Socratic dialogue enabled the nurses to establish clear rationale for why they should continue to decorate the ward as a way of helping them to achieve these aims. Their desire to decorate the ward stemmed from a person-centred approach whereby they were contributing to outcomes for children, families and staff. They were creating an environment that would give pleasure to children, in doing so they were working together with families and providing support for one another at a time of the year when being in hospital is challenging for everyone.

Action learning

Action learning is a well-established strategy for reflective inquiry at an individual, collective and organisational level (Smith & O'Neil, 2003). It is based on the connection between reflection and action. It is a continuous process where set members work on real issues and take the time to reflect and learn from their own experiences (McGill & Brockbank, 2004). People learn from grappling with real-life issues and skills learned during this process can then be transferred into other areas (Revans, 1980; Raelin, 1997). It is also a process 'underpinned by a belief in individual potential: a way of learning from our actions, and from what happened to us, and around us, by taking the time to question, understand and reflect, to gain insights, and consider how to act in the future' (Weinstein, 1999, p. 3), and therefore provides the individual with the potential to learn more about themselves.

The learning potential of this approach is enhanced if participation is voluntary (Neubauer, 1995) and learning is explorative rather than prescriptive (Lee, 1999).

Action learning also has considerable emancipatory potential, especially if participants direct the issues rather than the facilitator or the organisation (Fenwick, 2003). The intervention strategies learned during action learning enable participants to increase their personal confidence resulting in them testing the boundaries of their practice (Rayner et al., 2003), overcoming the tendency to become passive when faced with workplace demands (Bourner & Frost, 1996) and to work towards achieving sustainable change (Inglis, 1994; Mumford, 1994).

Approaches to action learning vary according to the level of inquiry, reflection and organisational influence (Fenwick, 2003); however, they all have the characteristic of learning through experience (Smith & O'Neil, 2003). The type selected for implementation will depend upon the purpose of any given program (McGill & Beaty, 2001). The action learning in the example below is characterised by the development of critical reflection skills. It is based on perspective transformation as defined by Mezirow (1981). It incorporates elements of experiential learning based on Kolb's (1984) learning cycle (action, reflection, generalisation, and testing) and the learning process as defined by Pedlar et al. (1986), which encompasses experience, understanding, planning and action, and equates to the cycle of action research (McGill & Beaty, 2001). Learning emerges due to focus on the process of learning, whereby set members re-learn how to learn. In addition to this, it uses critical reflection to reflect on the assumptions and beliefs upon which practice is based. This type of critical action learning draws on the work of Argyris (1982), Schon (1983, 1987) and Senge (1990), and is related to the transformational effect of set members in achieving organisational change.

The following vignette helps explore what meaning action learning can hold for participants. The data highlighted within this vignette are a component of a PhD study that aimed to evaluate the impact and effectiveness of PD strategies implemented in a Special Care Nursery (Wilson et al., 2007). Julie was a member of an action learning set and here her story is told to highlight her experience.

What happens when you don't get to lunch on time?

Julie's issue

Julie came along to that first action learning set (ALS) to 'check it out'. She was unsure what 'presenting an issue' meant, and indeed she did not know what kind of things might be helpful to hear and explore within an ALS. Something had been troubling her since she came to work in the ward, but she was unsure if this was the kind of thing you might bring up in an ALS. As the first meeting grew closer she shared her tentative thoughts with another member of staff who encouraged her to present her thoughts on nursing handover.

Julie started off her 'presentation' by telling the group what happens to her when she 'doesn't get to lunch on time'. She explained that lunchtime was often delayed (which left her feeling light-headed and dizzy) and this upset her because handover seemed to go on forever. On the surface the issue might appear to be superficial and centred on Julie's desire to get to lunch. However, with questioning from the set members and as they got deeper into the issue it became clear that Julie's desire for a timely lunch was related to the fact that she did not value nursing handover. For Julie, handover was ritualistic and repetitive and provided her with little information on individual patients on which she could then make decisions and plan care. Her sense of frustration and uncertainty about the way in which the ward worked coupled with her lack of desire to 'rock the boat' meant that she articulated the issue as 'getting to lunch late'. The issue was motivated by a lack of relevance in the ritual-based handover, which could take around 40 minutes for even a small number of patients (usually between 8 and 12). Understanding this enabled Julie to develop some action points; the first of which was to check out how other staff felt about nursing handover. She talks about how that first meeting went:

> *Much to my surprise I felt supported and at the same time constructively challenged by the participants of the group. By the end of that meeting I had a set of action points that would start me on a journey of changing clinical practice.*

To Julie's astonishment most staff had similar frustrations and thoughts about the effectiveness of handover, yet none of them had raised the issue, far less discussed ways in which they could change things; it was an accepted 'way of working' in the ward. Over the coming months Julie continued to work on the issue with the help of the ALS and other staff in the ward. This led to an action research project aimed at improving the effectiveness of handover. Julie engaged in the process of the action research cycle, although in the early stages she did not know she was 'doing' research. Here she talks about her progress:

> *The group meetings and action points enabled me to progress the nursing handover debate. Action learning enabled me to reflect on current practice, to develop effective questioning techniques and to take action. I involved staff in the unit in reviewing handover practice, in the development of a handover tool and throughout the implementation and post implementation phase. The support and challenge that the group offered me was very important in overcoming the challenges and hurdles involved in the change process. Undertaking the action points that I set myself and having to report back to the group ensured that things progressed.*

Along the journey (through the process of action research and action learning) Julie developed research skills, learnt how to engage stakeholders, led a major change in practice, presented her work (with others) at conferences, and won a poster competition. Of vital importance for this journey was the parallel challenge and support that action learning offered Julie. Here she reflects on the significance of the experience:

> *Personally, joining the action learning group has been a huge learning experience, from not having the foggiest idea about where to begin, to reviewing the literature, data collection, developing a database, helping with the implementation of a nursing handover tool through to being involved in journal writing and presentations, it is . . . more than I ever thought possible.*

The combination of action learning and action research provided Julie and her colleagues with a powerful opportunity to learn about learning and about self as well as learning about processes and being systematic. All this was achieved through the challenge and support of the ALS as Julie explored the issue of why she 'doesn't get to lunch on time'.

Learning theory in practice development research and service development

PD research is a form of research that is characterised by its use of learning theories in the process of the research, and in so doing its intent is to not only create new knowledge but to view the research process as also a process of learning for those involved. This work has its origins in practitioner research and some forms of action research, and is characterised by three key issues.

Firstly, there is an emphasis on undertaking research that sets out to challenge assumptions of current practice (and in so doing disrupt present understandings of an issue). This requires an intimate engagement of practitioners themselves in the research process. Indeed, Somekh (2002, p. 90) describes how 'knowledge constructed without the active participation of practitioners can only be partial knowledge'. This is clearly evident in the work of Wilson et al. (2007) described above.

Secondly, the context-bound nature of practice is emphasised and embraced, rather than seeking to decontextualise an issue in order to investigate it, as highlighted by Somekh (2002).

Thirdly, the research aims to manage change and provide sustainability. Winter (2002, p. 27) describes action research as being committed to seeking to improve 'some practical aspect of a real situation as a means for developing our understanding of it'. It is, however, important to emphasise the continuity and sustainability of learning rather than necessarily or only continuing any changed actions. It is the continuing reflection and learning that will ensure optimal practice for the specific context. Similarly, Somekh (2002, p. 92) highlights reflective research as leading to 'the construction of knowledge with its enactment in practice'.

This emphasis on learning needs to be manifested at all stages of the research and change processes, and the following section serves only to provide a taste of how this may be achieved. It is a methodological field that has the scope for considerable further development and it is important to be open to ways in which this may be achieved. One example is the constructivist grounded theory approach described by Chenitz (2000), which creates the opportunity to develop theory (and learning) through sustained research engagement with participants. PD concerns the development of services as much as it does the development of individual practitioners, and the literature on organisational learning is very extensive. There are two methodological approaches that are particularly useful when working with organisations in PD research: soft systems methodology, which emphasises organisational development through an analysis of the social and political systems of an organisation and the constant comparison of developing theory with the 'real world' (full of the context dependency that characterises action research) (Checkland & Scholes, 1990); and appreciative enquiry, which identifies what works well in an organisation and seeks to extend those conditions that enable it to work well (Reed, 2007).

It is not only the overall design of a research study that needs attention to be given to learning, but can also be at the point of data collection as well. Two methods of data collection will be described here, each serving to illustrate different approaches to learning within research. The first is Collaborative Learning Groups, which have been developed and used in a number of studies by Clarke and colleagues (e.g. in dementia and continence care [Clarke & Gardener, 2002a, 2002b], integrated mental health team development [Gibb et al., 2002], nurse education [Clarke et al., 2003], risk management in dementia care [Clarke, 2006]). Collaborative Learning Groups share similar characteristics to the Reflective Practice Groups described by Cook (2004), which were modelled on Elliot's (1991, p. 52) approach to improving practice by 'developing the practitioner's capacity for discrimination and judgement in particular, complex, human situations (and to unify) inquiry, the improvement of performance and the development of persons in their professional role'.

Collaborative Learning Groups emphasise the learning of both the researchers (through data collection and analysis) and practitioners (through challenging assumptions around a particular issue in practice and together identifying development approaches). As such they are a hybrid between focus group interview and ALS. The model we have used has been to sample a group of practitioners (between 4 and 15) and hold a series of around five 2-hour sessions with the researcher facilitating exploration and problem-solving around a mutually agreed topic. Very often the discussion has been fuelled by discussing data collected at other points in the study; for example, in the dementia and risk study an excerpt from an interview with someone with dementia was enacted during one of the Collaborative Learning Groups and used to challenge assumptions of professional practice. Data have been recorded by tape recording the Collaborative Learning Groups, and as with focus groups it has been beneficial to use two recorders simultaneously to ensure as much conversation as possibly is captured.

A second approach to learning at the point of data collection has been in the context of one-to-one interviews with practitioners where attempts were made to facilitate analysis of a situation, rather than only a description of it. To achieve this, a conventional interview schedule of a list of questions was rejected and instead a limited number of key words were identified and presented to the person being interviewed who was invited to talk about the relevance, impact and interrelationship of the key word issues.

This approach was used in a study of the pervasiveness of PD within organisations (Clarke & Wilcockson, 2001, 2002) and in a study evaluating a Health Action Zone (Carr et al., 2006). In the former study, the key words were each written on a separate circular shaped card, which allowed the person being interviewed the opportunity to move them around independently from each other and so for each to be spatially located in relation to each other. In the latter study, key words were on a single sheet of paper, which was given to the person being interviewed. In this situation, the interviewer acts again as a facilitator, prompting and probing for further clarification and analysis. This approach appears to be particularly suitable for complex issues and to provide a framework for the person being interviewed to engage in a level of analysis that they may not have used previously (one person interviewed indicated that within an hour long interview she had been able to describe and articulate the complexity of the issues that had been 'buzzing around' in her head for the previous 2 years). This approach works well with a diverse sample because, as with any effective learning process, it allows the individual to choose their own starting point and articulate and build on what they already know within a reflective framework.

Conclusion

Learning theories and processes are essential to the development of practice and this chapter has sought to outline some of the key issues and approaches that may be used to promote learning. Many of these approaches build on ideas about reflective practice and the power of colleagues working together to problem solve. There is great scope to look beyond this and embrace learning theories within research methodology and methods, and in so doing create another level of PD activity that serves to develop care to meet patient need.

Acknowledgements

We would like to thank Margaret Kelly & Peter Lewis for sharing their personal learning journeys as part of this chapter.

References

Argyris, C. (1982) *Reasoning, Learning and Action: Individual and Organizational.* Jossey-Bass, San Francisco, CA.

Argyris, C. & Schon, D.A. (1996) *Organisational Learning II: Theory Method and Practice.* Addison-Wesley, Reading, MA.

Barnett, R. (1997) *Higher Education: A Critical Business.* SRHE and Open University Press, Buckingham.

Benner, P. (1984) *From Novice to Expert: Excellence and Power in Clinical Nursing Practice.* Addison-Wesley, Menlo Park, CA.

Boreham, N.C. (1994) The dangerous practice of thinking. *Medical Education.* **28**, 172–179.

Bourner, T. & Frost, P. (1996) Experiencing action learning. *Journal of Workplace Learning.* **6**, 11–18.

Brechin, A. (2000) Introducing critical practice. In: *Critical Practice in Health and Social Care* (eds A. Brechin, H. Brown & M.A. Eby). Sage, London.

Carr, S., Clarke, C.L., Molyneux, J. & Jones, D. (2006) Facilitating participation – a health action zone experience. *Primary Health Care Research and Development.* **7**, 147–156.

Checkland, P. & Scholes, J. (1990) *Soft Systems Methodology in Action.* Wiley, Chichester.

Chenitz, K. (2000) Grounded theory: Objectivist and constructivist methods. In: *Handbook of Qualitative Research* (eds N.K. Denzin & Y.S. Lincoln), 2nd edn, pp. 509–535. Sage, Thousand Oaks, CA.

Clarke, C.L. & Gardner, R.A. (2002a) Dilemmas, decisions – and continence care for people with dementia. In: *Dementia Topics for the Millennium and Beyond* (ed S. Benson). Hawker, London.

Clarke, C.L. & Gardne, R.A. (2002b) Therapeutic and ethical practice: A participatory action research project in old age mental health. *Practice Development in Healthcare.* **1**(1), 39–53.

Clarke, C.L., Gibb, C.E. & Ramprogus, V. (2003) Clinical learning environments: An evaluation of an innovative role to support pre-registration nursing placements. *Learning in Health and Social Care.* **2**(2), 105–115.

Clarke, C.L. & Members of the International Collaborative Research Network on Risk and Ageing Populations (2006) Risk and ageing populations: Practice development research through an international research network. *International Journal of Older People Nursing.* **1**(3), 169–176.

Clarke, C.L., Procter, S. & Watson, B. (1998) Making changes: A survey to identify mediators in the development of health care practice. *Clinical Effectiveness in Nursing.* **2**(1), 30–36.

Clarke, C.L. & Wilcockson, J. (2001) Professional and organisational learning: Analysing the relationship with the development of practice. *Journal of Advanced Nursing.* **34**(2), 264–272.

Cook, T. (2004) Reflecting and learning together: Action research as a vital element of developing understanding and practice. *Educational Action Research.* **12**(1), 77–97.

Cowley, S. (1995) Professional development and change in a learning organisation. *Journal of Advanced Nursing.* **21**(5), 965–974.

Davies, H.T.O., Nutley, S.M. & Mannion, R. (2000) Organisational culture and quality of health care. *Quality in Health Care.* **9**, 111–119.

Easen, P. & Wilcockson, J. (1996) Intuition and rational decision-making in professional thinking: A dales dichotomy? *Journal of Advanced Nursing.* **24**, 667–673.

Eby, M. (2000) Understanding professional development. In: *Critical Practice in Health and Social Care* (eds A. Brechin, H. Brown & M.A. Eby). Sage, London.

Elliot, J. (1991) *Action Research for Educational Change.* Oxford University Press, Buckingham.

Eraut, M. (1994) *Developing Professional Knowledge and Competence.* The Falmer Press, London.

Fenwick, T. (2003) Emancipatory potential of action learning: A critical analysis. *Journal of Organizational Change Management.* **16**, 619–632.

Fish, D. (1998) *Appreciating Practice and the Caring Professions – Refocussing Professional Development and Practitioner Research.* Butterworth-Heinemann, Oxford.

Fitzgerald, L. & van Hooft, S. (2000) A Socratic dialogue on the question 'What is Love in Nursing'? *Nursing Ethics.* **7**(6), 481–491.

Gibb, C.E., Morrow, M., Clarke, C.L., Cook, G., Gertig, P. & Ramprogus, V. (2002) Transdisciplinary working: Evaluating the development of health and social care provision in mental health. *Journal of Mental Health.* **11**(3), 339–350.

Green, J.M., Renfrew, M.J. & Curtis, P.A. (2000) Continuity of carer: What matters to women? A review of the evidence. *Midwifery.* **16**, 186–196.

Greenhalgh, T. (1999) Narrative based medicine in an evidence based world. *British Medical Journal.* **318**, 323–325.

Hammond, M. & Collins, R. (1991) *Self-Directed Learning: Critical Practice.* Routledge Falmer, London.

Hansten, R. & Washburn, M. (2000) Intuition in professional practice: Executive and staff perceptions. *Journal of Nursing Administration.* **30**(4), 185–189.

Howatson-Jones, I.L. (28 May 2003) Difficulties in clinical supervision and lifelong learning. *Nursing Standard.* **17**(37), 37–41.

Inglis, S. (1994) *Making the Most of Action learning.* Kogan Page, London.

Johns, C. (1996) Visualising and realising care in practice through guided reflection. *Journal of Advanced Nursing.* **24**(6), 1135–1143.

Johns, C. & Freshwater, D. (eds) (1998) *Transforming Nursing Through Reflective Practice.* Blackwell Science, Oxford.

Johns, C. & McCormack, B. (1998) Unfolding the conditions where the transformative potential of guided reflection (clinical supervision) might flourish or flounder. In: *Transforming Nursing Through Reflective Practice* (eds C. Johns & D. Freshwater), pp. 62–77. Blackwell Science, Oxford.

Jones, A. (1999) Clinical supervision for professional practice. *Nursing Standard.* **14**(9), 42–44.

Jones, A. (2001) Possible influences on clinical supervision. *Nursing Standard.* **16**(1), 38–42.

Kolb, D. (1984) *Experiential Learning: Experience as the Source of Learning and Development.* Prentice-Hall, Englewood Cliffs, NJ.

Kolb, D.A. (1995) The process of experiential learning. In: *Culture and Processes of Adult Learning* (eds M. Thorpe, R. Edwards & A. Hanson). Routledge and Open University, London.

Lee, N. (1999) Thinking reflectively: Solutions through action learning. *Nursing Times.* **49**, 54–55.

Manley, K. & McCormack, B. (2003) Practice development: Purpose, methodology, facilitation and evaluation. *Nursing in Critical Care.* **8**, 22–29.

McCormack, B. (1999) House conversions . . . nursing homes that offer students a learning and research environment are not just a dream. *Nursing Times; Nursing Homes.* **1**(3), 10–11.

McGill, I. & Beaty, L. (2001) *Action Learning: A guide for Professional, Management and Educational Development*, 2nd edn. Kogan Page, London.

McGill, I. & Brockbank, A. (2004) *The Action Learning Handbook: Powerful Techniques for Education, Professional Development & Training.* Routledge Falmer, London.

Meerabeau, L. (1992) Tacit nursing knowledge: An untapped resource or a methodological headache? *Journal of Advanced Nursing.* **17**(1), 108–112.

Meyer, J. & Batehup, L. (1997) Action research in health-care practice: Nature, present concerns and future possibilities. *Nursing Times Research.* **2**(3), 175–186.

Mezirow, J. (1981) A critical theory of adult learning and education. *Adult Education.* **32**, 2–24.

Mills, J.E. Francis, K.L. & Bonner, A. (2005) Mentoring, clinical supervision and preceptoring: Clarifying the conceptual definitions for Australian rural nurses. A review of the literature. *Rural and Remote Health.* **5**, 410. (http://rrh.deakin.edu.au)

Mumford, A. (1994) A review of action learning literature. *Management Bibliographies and Reviews.* **20**, 2–16.

Neubauer, J. (1995) The learning network. *Journal of Nursing Administration.* **2**, 23–32.

Pedlar, M., Burgoyne, J. & Boydell, T. (1986) *A Managers Guide to Self-development*, 2nd edn. McGraw-Hill, Maidenhead.

Polanyi, M. (1962) *Personal Knowledge: Towards a Post Critical Philosophy.* Routledge and Kegan Paul, London.

Quinn, F.M. (1998) Reflection and reflective practice. In: *Continuing Professional Development in Nursing* (ed F.M. Quinn). Stanley Thornes, Cheltenham.

Raelin, J. (1997) Action learning and action science: Are they different? *Organizational Dynamics.* **1**, 21–34.

Rafferty, M., Jenkins, E. & Parke, S. (2003) Developing a provisional standard for clinical supervision in nursing and health visiting: The methodological trail. *Qualitative Health Research.* **13**(10), 1432–1452.

Rayner, D., Chisholm, H. & Appleby, H. (2003) Developing leadership through action learning. *Nursing Standard.* **29**, 37–39.

Reed, J. (2007) *Appreciative Inquiry: Research for Change.* Sage, Thousand Oaks, CA.

Revans, R. (1980) *Action Learning: New Techniques for Management.* Blond & Briggs, London.

Roehler, L.R., Duffy, G.G., Hermann, B.A., Conley, M. & Johnson. J. (1988) Knowledge structures as evidence of the 'personal': Bridging the gap from thought to practice. *Journal of Curriculum Studies.* **20**(2), 159–165.

Rolfe, G. (1998) Advanced practice and the reflective nurse: Developing knowledge out of practice. In: *Advanced Nursing Practice* (eds G. Rolfe & P. Fulbrook). Butterworth-Heinemann, Oxford.

Schon, D.A. (1983) *The Reflective Practitioner.* Basic Books, New York.

Schon, D.A. (1987) *Educating the Reflective Practitioner.* Jossey-Bass, New York.

Schon, D.A. (1992) The crisis of professional knowledge and the pursuit of an epistemology of practice. *Journal of Interprofessional Care.* **6**(1), 49–63.

Senge, P. (1990) *The Fifth Discipline: The Art and Practice of the Learning Organization.* Doubleday Currency, New York.

Smith, P. & O'Neil, J. (2003) A review of action learning literature 1994–2000: Part 1 bibliography and comments. *Journal of Workplace Learning.* **2**, 63–69.

Somekh, B. (2002) Inhabiting each other's castles: Towards knowledge and mutual growth through collaboration. In: *Theory and Practice in Action Research: Some International Perspectives* (eds C. Day, J. Elliot, B. Somekh & R. Winter), pp. 79–104. Symposium Books, London.

Stevenson, C. (2005) Postmodernising clinical supervision in nursing. *Issues in Mental Health Nursing.* **26**, 519–529.

Stewart, M. (2001) Whose evidence counts? An exploration of health professionals' perceptions of evidence-based practice, focusing on the maternity services. *Midwifery.* **17**(4), 279–285.

Titchen, A. (2000) Professional craft knowledge in patient-centred nursing and the facilitation of its development. *University of Oxford DPhil Thesis.* Ashdale, Oxford.

Titchen, A. (2003) Critical companionship: Part 1. *Nursing Standard.* **18**(9), 33–40.

Titchen, A. (2004) Helping relationships for practice development: Critical companionship. In: *Practice Development for Nurses* (eds B. MaCormack, K. Manley & R. Garbett). Blackwell, Oxford.

Trinder, L. (2000) A critical appraisal of evidence-based practice. In: *Evidence-Based Practice: A Critical Appraisal* (eds L. Trinder & S. Reynolds). Blackwell Science, Oxford.

Weinstein, K. (1999) *Action Learning: A Practical Guide*, 2nd edn. Gower, Aldershot.

Wilson, V., Ho, A. & Walsh, R. (2007) Participatory action research and action learning: Changing clinical practice in nursing handover and communication. *Journal of Children's and Young People's Nursing*. **1**(2), 85–92.

Wilson-Barnett, J., Barriball, K.L., Reynolds, H., Jowett, S. & Ryrie, I. (2000) Recognising advancing nursing practice: Evidence from two observational studies. *International Journal of Nursing Studies*. **37**, 389–400.

Winter, R. (2002) Managers, spectators and citizens: Where does 'theor' come from in action research? In: *Theory and Practice in Action Research: Some International Perspectives* (eds C. Day, J. Elliot, B. Somekh & R. Winter), pp. 79–104. Symposium Books, London.

Winter, R. & Munn-Giddings, C. (2001) *A Handbook for Action Research in Health and Social Care*. Routledge and Open University Press, London.

7. An Exploration of Practice Development Evaluation: Unearthing Praxis

Val Wilson, Sally Hardy and Bob Brown

Introduction

This chapter captures how a cooperative inquiry undertaken as part of an International Practice Development Colloquium (IPDC) unearthed the notion of praxis evaluation. The specific aims of our group focused on the issue of evaluation and its relevance to practice development (PD). Our first steps involved a review of evaluation evident within the PD literature. We then focused on the significance of having an evaluation process that is core to all PD work. We have increased our understanding of evaluation in the context of PD through the development of a framework consistent with the intent of PD work. The ideas and critical questioning undertaken have led us to offer the notion of praxis evaluation as a critical creative framework suitable for the subtleties and triumphs of individual, team and organisational transformation within the healthcare context.

Praxis

The term 'praxis' is often referred to as a bringing together of theory and practice; however, interpretations of this sometimes place less important emphasis on 'practice' as the application of knowledge derived from 'theory'. Freire (1972, p. 28) defines praxis, as 'reflection and action on the world in order to transform it'. For Carr and Kemmis (1986) in praxis thought and action (or theory and practice) are dialectically related. They are 'mutually constitutive as in a process of interaction'. This chapter will consider the meaning of the term praxis in relation to PD and particularly PD evaluation. From a philosophical standpoint, we understand praxis as a continual interplay between thought and action. As Gadamer (1979, p. 275) has noted, praxis 'involves interpretation, understanding and application in one unified process'. Praxis in the context of PD evaluation requires a bringing together of prior knowledge, new understandings, action based on reflection and a commitment to engagement with others through a moral disposition to understand, search for truth, demonstrate respect for others, and nurture creativity, as a means of enabling human-flourishing.

Our intent in this chapter is to build on the work of our colleagues who have previously outlined the need for a clear evaluation strategy to underpin PD initiatives in order for it to be both systematic and rigorous (McCormack et al., 2004). McCormack et al. provide a number of critical questions that evaluators need to consider when developing an evaluation strategy. Their work identified a variety of approaches, methodologies and frameworks that can be used within PD. They suggested that whilst these are useful there was a need for clarity around the purpose of PD work in order to inform an evaluation strategy as well as to ascertain the most suitable approaches at the outset of the work. We believe that their work provides us with the foundation for considering further the role of evaluation within PD.

Praxis evaluation

We contend that 'praxis evaluation' reflects the six core components of effective evaluation of PD work: **p**urpose, **r**eflexivity, **a**pproaches, **c**ontext, **i**ntent and **s**takeholders. This first component focuses on understanding the purpose of PD work and how this then shapes the evaluation. Next, the importance of undertaking critical questioning and reflection about the evaluation process itself is an essential component and supports critical consideration regarding which approaches best 'fit' the evaluation. Further deliberation is given to the context in which the PD work is taking place and the potential impact of the context on the evaluation. This enables clarity regarding the intent of the evaluation itself and is clearly linked to the purpose of the PD work. Finally, there is a clear need to identify and work with the stakeholders for whom the PD work holds significance.

A visual depiction of praxis evaluation is best captured in a spinning gyroscope. As the evaluation begins, the emphasis is placed on bringing the individual components together and trying to maintain balance. Once momentum has begun, each element intersects revealing praxis evaluation within the core of the gyroscope. The sequence of each component becomes inconsequential as the evaluation begins to take shape. Think again of the gyroscope. It is made up of different parts that all come together and work in harmony to enable the gyroscope to function, keep moving and remain balanced. The movement that occurs reflects the evolving nature of evaluation and the energy generated by the continuing process. Whilst this in theory sounds simple, evaluation in practice takes skill to ensure that the gyroscope maintains momentum.

We now consider in more detail the elements that form the basis of a praxis evaluation.

Purpose relates to identifying clearly the purpose of the PD work (aims and objectives) and then developing an evaluation process that will help achieve clarity about and around that key purpose and common vision. Being clear about the purpose of the PD initiative will help in identifying which questions to ask to ensure that the approaches and methods used are effective in the evaluation. It also helps inform an audit trail of decision-making and data gathering. Being able to offer clear and transparent processes will enable participants to feel more included, as their expectations and fears can be allayed through clarification and understanding of a clear purpose of the project and their involvement within that process. Maintaining an audit trail makes explicit how data have been managed and interpreted. Having a clear purpose assists in identifying potential or anticipated outcomes.

Reflexivity within the context of understanding in more detail the component parts of praxis evaluation can be seen as relating to the notion of critical reflection and consideration of critical questions about the PD work, the evaluation process, participants' roles in that process, what drives and underpins the work, and how participants attend to that work. Being reflexive also helps to identify theoretical links with practice change. It enables insight, consideration of alternative perspectives, increased understanding and personal transformation.

Approaches concern not only the kind of approaches being undertaken in the evaluation process, but also how these approaches 'fit' within the context of the purpose and the questions asked. For example, what are the aims/objectives to be achieved in the evaluation, who should be involved, how do participants/stakeholders want to work together. The answers to these questions may lead the participants towards certain approaches. Within praxis evaluation we propose the chosen approach for the evaluation needs to fit with both the values and beliefs of the participants (cf intent) and the purpose (as described above).

Context is taking the context within which the evaluation is taking place into consideration, ensuring that it is part of the evaluation process. By providing an understanding of the context, this helps others understand the purpose of the evaluation, as it relates to them. Context-specific information is important when considering the evidence needed for that particular environment or context. Context is taking into consideration the local knowledge that already exists around the inquiry as well as timing factors and resource issues. When engaging in evaluation it is important to recognise that there will inevitably be consideration needed of the political context within which the work is taking place. Paying attention to the context will help make sense of some of the cultural anomalies that influence how people think, behave and respond to the evaluation itself.

Intent goes beyond merely taking a surface view of what is happening. The intent is to look deeper and to create a more thorough understanding, through the evaluation process. The intent is to be critical in the way the elements of the research process are questioned and to be critical in how an evaluation process is established. Intent is also about being critical in the way participants work, and in the way participants handle the data/findings. And finally, intent is to be and remain critical in reviewing the outcomes of the evaluation. The intention behind all actions related to the evaluation is considered important in the interpretation of evidence. The intention is therefore linked with purpose, reflexivity and approaches. Being clear about intent will enable clarity for all participants. PD evaluation and indeed all emancipatory PD work has the intention of enlightenment, empowerment and emancipation, further enhanced through a process of critical creativity whereby human-flourishing and transformation can occur for those involved in the evaluation process.

Stakeholders is identifying the people with a stake or interest in the evaluation, and is key to the success of any evaluation; working with the stakeholders in order to establish what needs to be evaluated (purpose), how it will be evaluated (approaches and intent) and by whom it may be evaluated. Stakeholders of course may form part of the data collection process for evaluation and may be involved in interpreting the results of the evaluation. This should be undertaken not as a token gesture but as an integral component of the evaluation. Including stakeholders can be a lengthy process, but through a deliberate intention to include a wide representation of stakeholders, the outcomes of the evaluation can be more widely adopted.

Now that we have briefly outlined the key components of praxis evaluation it is time for us to share with you the process and critical thinking that led us to uncover this evaluation framework and to convince you of its relevance for the future of PD.

Evaluation and practice development

Evaluation of PD in nursing has tended to focus on evaluating outcomes by using experimental designs or evaluating emancipatory approaches where an in-depth understanding of the effectiveness of processes in a particular context was developed. These differing approaches have served a useful purpose in developing our understandings of facilitation (Harvey et al., 2002; Manley & McCormack, 2003), cultural outcomes (Manley, 2000a, 2000b, 2004), enabling processes (Titchen & Binnie, 1995; Binnie & Titchen, 1999; Titchen & Binnie, 2001), quality indicators (Taylor et al., 2002), effectiveness of person-centred care (McCormack & Wright, 1999; McCormack, 2001, 2003; Wilson et al., 2005) and the links between these. However, it is at the level of these linkages that existing evaluation frameworks are most vulnerable. The processes used in PD are multifaceted and multilayered and there is little evidence from either PD or emancipatory action research to identify which processes lead to which outcomes.

It has been noted previously that PD aims to increase levels of effectiveness in patient-centred care through promoting and facilitating change (Garbett & McCormack, 2004). PD is a continuous, systematic, rigorous and often transformational process, which is in fact a methodology that can contribute to the modernisation of health and social care services through its focus on improving workplace cultures (McCormack et al., 2006). This chapter will examine how successfully PD evaluation has been as a means of testing the quality and impact of PD work, as well as its contribution to developing PD theory and knowledge about the effectiveness of PD processes and outcomes. What we aim to capture is the process by which evaluation of PD is undertaken in a way that reflects the core values and principles of PD (Manley & McCormack, 2004) as well as contributing to our understanding about the processes used and the resultant outcomes of PD work.

Remaining consistent with PD values

We recognised that in order to understand effective PD, its application, impact and effects on delivering evidence-based, person-centered healthcare, the first step was to understand and develop our knowledge and skills about evaluation itself. Paying attention to the process of evaluation was seen as one way in which to enable us to progress our aim of developing and considering the notion of how best to evaluate the effectiveness of PD. This is consistent with the definition of PD articulated in Chapter 1 of this book in which the importance of embedding both the processes and outcomes of PD works in corporate strategy.

Our ultimate purpose throughout this work has been to identify an evaluation framework that was consistent with the idea and interest in PD (e.g. person centredness, collaboration and transformation), for a meaningful evaluation process that would capture the processes of PD (e.g. values clarification, concerns, claims and issues), whilst also taking into consideration the key principles and intended outcomes of PD (e.g. human-flourishing, skilled facilitation, collaboration, person centeredness, working from a sound evidence base, transforming cultures and contexts of healthcare).

The IPDC has also 'unearthed' the notion of *critical creativity* (McCormack & Titchen, 2006), which centers around the basic concepts of *human-flourishing* and *praxis* (see also Chapter 4). Within critical creativity, the concept of praxis is extended to include action that is also creative. Praxis is achieved through utilising creative thinking, thinking about thinking (meta cognition) and through critique, *blended* with creative imagination and expression. Such an understanding of praxis is a means through which human-flourishing (as a means and as a deliberate intention of transformation) is brought about and further understood. So, within critical creativity it is intended that human-flourishing should be the outcome, not only for those for whom the development or research and evaluation are intended, but also for those who carry out the work and engage in the process. Thus, human-flourishing is seen as both a means and an end to all PD work. We therefore wanted to reconsider what current evaluation approaches had to offer, what the key concepts were, including such things as social change processes, and how we might capture the individual, more subtle changes that occur in healthcare practice. In other words, we wanted to delve under the surface of evaluation to uncover the potential for developing an evaluation framework that would be consistent with the principles, process and context of PD work.

Through our own theoretical work and participation in a values clarification activity, we established the following value statements associated with undertaking an evaluation in PD.

1. Evaluation in PD work can help to
   (a) build PD theory,
   (b) generate knowledge,
   (c) inform and refine ongoing developments within action-orientated study.
2. Evaluation is required to measure
   (a) Sustainability,
   (b) transferability of ideas, processes and strategies,
   (c) what works and what does not work.
3. Evaluation enables researchers to

  (a) develop political savvy and skills (which can be used to support ongoing
      PD work),
  (b) develop 'kudos' for PD and in so doing
  (c) increase opportunities for funding projects by articulating and demonstrat-
      ing the process of change/transformation.
 4. The absence of evaluation risks PD becoming reactive, ad hoc and unsubstan-
    tiated.

Reviewing the literature

The next stage was to review the published literature in order to provide a foundational understanding of how existing PD forms of inquiry are evaluated. Alongside
this, we also wanted to capture our own learning and the ways in which we were
incorporating the experience of practitioner research and theory development,
working towards the ultimate aim of establishing a clear path towards unearthing
the notion of praxis evaluation.

Examination of the PD and practitioner-orientated literature was seen as a means
of assessing the level of importance given to evaluation within PD. In order to do
this in a systematic way, a framework of questions was developed by the group,
based upon our current knowledge of evaluation and where the gaps in knowledge
had been identified, through our initial look at the evaluation landscape. These
questions (highlighted below) were intended to assist in the review process and
aimed to further clarify the significance of evaluation for PD work.

Critical questions identified by the group to frame the literature review were as
follows:

 1. Has the rationale for the chosen evaluation strategy been identified and dis-
    cussed in the paper?
 2. Have any links been made explicit to PD theory, if so what are they?
 3. How has the author reviewed and brought into context relevant evaluation and
    PD literature.
 4. Is there evidence of rigor within the evaluation process (e.g. was it collaborative,
    inclusive and embedded in the change process from the beginning)?
 5. Have the strengths and limitations of the evaluation process been identified?
 6. Does the paper make a contribution to knowledge about evaluating PD?

Search areas included CINAHL and MEDLINE electronic databases. The search
terms included the following key words: practice development, practice development evaluation, action research, participatory action research, practitioner
research, pluralistic evaluation, appreciative inquiry, evaluation research, fourth
generation evaluation, stakeholder analysis, realistic evaluation and cooperative
inquiry.

Inclusion criteria are set to include all nursing studies undertaken with a research
focus, written in English and published between 1996 and 2006. Several hundred

studies were identified in this initial process. A brief review of these articles, using the critical questions framework, helped to eliminate studies that failed to answer at least one of the six questions posed (see Table 7.1). This left 20 studies using a range of practitioner research and evaluation approaches.

The studies are now discussed in more detail as a way of helping to identify the strengths in evaluation approaches undertaken and highlighting areas for further consideration and debate. Each paper is referred to in the text by the number given to the paper identified in Table 7.1.

Review findings

It became apparent from reviewing the literature that both the methods/tools used in evaluating PD as well as those methodologies/approaches used to support the evaluation were varied, multifaceted, complex, confusing and at times contradictory or ill-informed. A broad range of methodological perspectives were identified as underpinning the PD work in addition to the use of a variety of methods/tools as outlined in Table 7.2.

This array of approaches did little in the way of providing clear rationale or links within PD theory and evaluation. In fact, it caused more confusion about what was happening within PD but augmented our own concerns for greater critical debate about the issues around PD-based evaluation. The variety of tools and approaches being used within these studies merely added to a sense of confusion, particularly when only limited evidence was provided to suggest how and why specific tools were chosen and in what way this choice had been supported and influenced by the theoretical stance taken by the evaluators or stakeholders within their particular PD evaluation. There was an overall lack of connection between approaches (methodology) and the tools (methods) used in the studies and a failure to articulate the link (if there was one) to either PD or evaluation theory. This did little to promote the cohesion of the evaluation process. That being said, a number of studies did, however, justify these links clearly (11, 12, 14, 15, 16).

In only 4 of the 20 papers was there an articulation of the espoused connections to critical social science (1, 2, 12) and emancipatory PD (5). However, it was difficult to see how this impacted on the study or the approach taken to evaluation. One study did clearly identify the theoretical links between evaluation (realistic), critical social science and PD theory (15). Links were also identified between PD and action-orientated research (12, 16, 17), adult learning theory (11), experiential learning (19), fourth generation evaluation (14) and collaborative inquiry (12, 14). However, again it was difficult to establish a high level of relevancy and currency in PD evaluation when little information was produced on which any critique could be based.

Other studies revealed evidence of the links between methodology and methods used in PD (5, 6, 11, 12, 14, 15, 16, 18). This helped to provide some guidance on what may be considered as rigor in praxis evaluation. This may of course be due to the limitation placed on some publications (e.g. word limit or purpose of publication/journal) or, perhaps more disconcerting, a potential lack of understanding about the importance and relevance evaluation holds for PD.

Mixed method approaches were seen by a number of researchers to add strength to the evaluation (6, 8, 14, 15). However, there was concern that at times the methods

Table 7.1 Unearthing the findings

	Author	Title	Method(s)	1	2	3	4	5	6
1	Chenoweth and Kilstoff (2002)	Organisational and structural reform in aged care organisations: empowerment towards a change process	Participatory action research	L	L	Y	L	L	L
2	Kilgour and Fleming (2000)	An action research inquiry into a health visitor parenting program for parents of preschool children with behavioural problems	Action research	L	L	L	L	L	N
3	Gerrish et al. (1999)	Promoting evidence-based practice: managing change in the assessment of pressure damage risk	Action research	L	N	L	L	N	N
4	Clendon (2003)	Nurse-managed clinics: issues in evaluation	Fourth generation evaluation	L	L	L	L	L	N
5	Lindsey and McGuinness (1998)	Significant elements of community involvement in participatory action research: evidence from a community project	Participatory action research	Y	L	Y	Y	N	Y
6	Clarke et al. (2003)	Seeing the person behind the patient: enhancing care of older people using a biographical approach	Practice development project	Y	N	Y	Y	L	Y
7	Paley et al. (2003)	Practice development in psychological interventions: mental health nurse involvement in the conversational model of psychotherapy	Practice development project	L	N	L	L	N	N
8	Taylor et al. (2002)	The impact of a practice development project on the quality of inpatient small group therapy	Practice development project	L	N	N	N	N	L
9	Gerrish (2001)	A pluralistic evaluation of nursing/practice development units	Pluralistic evaluation	L	N	N	L	N	L

(cont.)

133

Table 7.1 *(cont.)*

	Author	Title	Method(s)	1	2	3	4	5	6
10	Holman and Jackson (2001)	A team education approach: an evaluation of a collaborative education and practice development in a continuing care unit for older people	Education and practice development project	N	N	N	L	N	L
11	Ward and McCormack (2000)	Creating an adult learning culture through practice development	Practice development project	Y	Y	Y	Y	Y	Y
12	Reed et al. (2002)	Going home from hospital – an appreciative inquiry study	Appreciative inquiry	Y	Y	Y	Y	Y	Y
13	Drennan (2002)	An evaluation of the role of the clinical placement coordinator in student nurse support in the clinical area	Mixed methods evaluation	Y	N	L	L	L	Y
14	McCourt and Thomas (2001)	Evaluation of a problem-based curriculum in midwifery	Realistic evaluation	Y	Y	Y	Y	Y	Y
15	Wilson et al. (2005)	Understanding the workplace culture of a special care nursery	Emancipatory PD and realistic evaluation	Y	Y	Y	Y	Y	Y
16	Dewing and Traynor (2005)	Admiral nursing competency project: practice development and action research	Emancipatory action research and PD	Y	Y	Y	Y	Y	Y
17	Carr (2005)	Refocusing health visiting – sharpening the vision and facilitating the process	Action research	L	L	L	L	N	N
18	Koch et al. (2004)	Chronic illness self-management: locating the 'self'	Participatory action research	Y	N	L	Y	L	Y
19	Dick et al. (2004)	Changing professional practice in tuberculosis care: an educational intervention	Qualitative evaluation	Y	Y	N	Y	L	Y
20	Forrest et al. (2004)	Evaluating the impact of training in psychosocial interventions: a stakeholder approach to evaluation – part II	Stakeholder evaluation	L	N	N	L	L	L

Y, yes; L, limited; N, no.

Table 7.2 Approaches and tools used in PD-orientated evaluation studies

Methodology (approaches)	Methods/tools
o Randomised control trials	o Clinical and survey audit
o Phenomenological study	o Team climate inventory
o Fourth generation evaluation	o Pre- and post-test measures
o Illuminative evaluation	o Interviews and focus groups
o Pluralistic evaluation	o Observation
o Emancipatory action research	o Stakeholder analysis
o Participatory action research	o Critical reflection
o Action research	o Questionnaires
o Case study	o Validated scales

chosen did not justify the objectives of the study (20) and that the rigor of the evaluation may, at times, be questionable (3, 6). Of particular concern was the fact that some studies, using an action research methodology, provided little evidence of how this informed the methods, findings or action related to the evaluation component of the action cycles (1, 17), or how the action research cycle led to any changes in practice (11).

The collaborative and inclusive nature of action-orientated work was identified as a strength (12). However, undertaking action-orientated work did not automatically lead to collaboration with some studies indicating that a lack of collaboration had a negative impact on the evaluation itself (3, 8). One paper outlined how a summative approach to evaluation, as opposed to process-orientated evaluation, failed to provide any insights into why changes in practice were or were not achieved as a consequence of an intervention (10).

From this brief overview, we suggest that orientating and mapping the evaluation framework prior to commencing the evaluation process can help to identify appropriate tools and approaches that will be sensitive to the context and ontological perspectives of stakeholders included in the evaluation process. Thus, the outcomes of the evaluation can also be identified and mapped against this process to provide clear rationale for change and where that change occurred, how it was influenced and by whom or what.

Only a small number of studies in this review provided enough evidence and relevant information on which to answer all six of our critical questions with any degree of accuracy. Whilst the majority of papers reviewed offered little new knowledge about evaluation within PD, they did confirm what we suspected was happening in practice. Evaluation was seen as integral to any PD initiative (8) and should be considered at the beginning of any project or study area (6, 8, 10). A sound evaluation requires a clearly articulated methodological framework (5, 6, 9, 10, 13) and should consider mixed method approaches (6, 9). There was recognition for the depth of understanding and commitment required to evaluate both systematically and meaningfully (14). The importance of having a well-planned and robust evaluation process (7, 13, 16, 19) in which rigorous evaluative methods are applied (20) results in gaining more meaningful data, which in turn can influence sustainable change. The evaluation itself needs to focus on the shared aims of the study and develop evaluation questions, methods and processes to ascertain whether these have been achieved (13, 16).

There is a need to consider the culture in which each study took place and the importance shared values and beliefs play in changing culture (8, 15). There was acknowledgement of the challenges in trying to effectively measure changes in culture (11, 15). Alongside these challenges there was an identified need to include stakeholders, to be inclusive in the approach to evaluation and ensure participation in the evaluation, whilst taking into account the issues of power relationships that can occur within any group (12, 13, & 15, 16, 19).

It is perhaps pertinent to provide practice developers with the means to incorporate all aspects of PD theory, tools and approaches within one evaluation framework, but a question remains as to whether this is possible. As suggested above, this review of the literature did not convey new knowledge about the effectiveness of evaluation within PD. It did, however, confirm suspicions that many evaluation studies are carried out without due consideration of stakeholder perspectives and the appropriate processes to capture transformation and change as these occur during the evaluation itself, whilst also making a clearer pathway to monitor and measure change throughout the evaluation, as well as capture clear objectives and outcomes.

Limitations of the review

The review has a number of limitations. First, restricting the sample to articles between 1996 and 2006 in English undoubtedly led to the exclusion of some articles that may have had a contribution to the discussion on evaluation of PD. Similarly by focusing on nursing alone, we failed to learn from PD publications in the fields of allied health, medicine and social care or education. Second, we did not have the resources to include grey literature (unpublished thesis, dissertations, conference papers, etc.). Thus we were unable to complete a thorough or comprehensive review, but nevertheless we were able to achieve our aim of testing the published evidence base and stimulating discussion on the quality of evaluation within PD. Third, the review raises issues of how PD evaluations are written up for publication; this may be linked to such things as word limits and the sometimes imposed structure of reporting in nursing journals. Each of the issues raised in relation to the limitation of the review had a direct impact on what information was available to us within the papers reviewed to enable us to answer our posed questions.

Subsequent review of practice development evidence

Following our small literature review, an extensive review of evidence relating to PD has taken place on behalf of NHS Education for Scotland (NES) and NHS Quality Improvement Scotland (NHS QIS). The findings of this realist synthesis agree that the methodologies used in PD work are diverse in nature and are drawn from a broad range of perspectives (McCormack et al., 2006). Whilst there appears to be little consensus about the most effective methodology within PD there is also a lack of evidence in relation to what we are learning about (effective) processes and how these are being translated from one study to another. Indeed, there is very little to correlate how measures of specific PD work may influence outcomes; in particular, facilitation strategies are poorly articulated and evaluated. As with our review, there is limited attention paid to the forms of knowledge underpinning the developments undertaken. The evidence in the realist synthesis confirms our notion that outcome measurement needs to correspond with the values in PD such as 'participation and collaboration' and to ensure that the evaluation processes themselves (such as data collection and analysis) form an essential part of the development itself. The recommendations of the report outline the need for evaluation frameworks (for PD work) that support participation, collaboration and inclusivity. Further to this, it is suggested that

> *A strategic level evaluation framework should be developed that is consistent with the theory of complex interventions and their evaluation. This would enable the evaluation of the impact of PD frameworks and generate new knowledge about the effectiveness of PD processes and outcomes derived*
>
> *McCormack et al., 2006, p. 8*

This report not only validates the findings of the small review we have undertaken, but it also adds vital integrity to our findings and expands our notion of praxis evaluation.

Evaluation of PD

As identified above, without drawing from sound methods and processes of evaluation, PD would become merely an ad hoc activity, with no clear aim, purpose or intention. Therefore we were now at a stage where we needed to review our progress to date, collate our thoughts and understandings and to develop a means of reviewing the state of play around us.

Owen and Rogers (1999) describe the objective of an evaluation as negotiating an evaluation plan, collecting and analysing evidence to produce findings, and disseminating the findings to intended audiences, for use in describing or understanding a program, or making a judgment and or decisions related to the program. They have suggested that evaluators utilise a range of questions to evaluate, for differing purposes and different stakeholders. For example, evaluation around a PD programme of work (such as implementation of action learning in an organisation) might include the following questions:

- *What is happening in this work programme?*
  This question could be aimed at the facilitator, participants, structure and content of the programme.
- *What is it like to experience such a programme?*
  This question could be aimed at the individual participants, the group as a whole and the facilitator.
- *What is it like to deliver and experience such a programme?*

This question could be aimed at the facilitator or service provider/deliverer.
- *How is the programme performing on a continuous basis?*
  Aimed at the facilitator, participant, organisation.
- *How could the programme be improved?*
  Aimed at the facilitator, participants, organisation, as well as for the people receiving the service.

However, what appears to be lacking or missing in this simple framework is a means of evaluating the outcomes of engaging in the programme and capturing the subtleties of what it is like to be a part of the programme in terms of how individuals, teams and the organisation might be benefiting or transforming their practice as a result of engaging in the programme. McCormack et al. (2004) note that whilst there appears to be common agreement in contemporary evaluation literature that evaluation designs need to embrace a range of questions, there remains a tendency to focus on objective truths (objective evidence as the sole criterion of truth), which then dominate the evaluation methodology. Various evaluation theorists, for example Pawson and Tilley (1997) and before them Guba and Lincoln (1989), have argued that objective evaluations (i.e. those that concentrate only on outcome) fail to capture the range of perspectives that comprehensive evaluation encapsulate, nor indeed does it reflect the range of stakeholder values implicit in an evaluation design that is of particular importance for practice developers. Kemmis (2005) has raised the challenge further by arguing that practitioners are becoming less critical, as they are being driven towards outcome-orientated evaluation rather than seeing evaluation as a crucial part of an intention to collective action aimed at changing practices, understanding those practices in detail and recognising the impact of the context within which those practices are taking place.

Evaluation processes, drawn from PD principles and underpinned by PD methodology, we suggest should capture and include the transformational aspects of being engaged not only in the program, for example, but also in the evaluation of that program. In order to provide some guidelines for practitioners, who may at times, like us, struggle with understanding the complexities that evaluation brings to PD, we have created a praxis evaluation framework that highlights key decisions around evaluating PD projects. This has emerged through our collective work as part of the IPDC and further informed through our literature search and review of the realist synthesis of PD (NHS Report). We hope this framework will offer guidance, opportunities for critical questioning, as well as providing a means by which the enormous potential for growth within evaluation and PD can be explored further. We therefore propose a case for exploring further the notion of praxis evaluation.

Exploring praxis evaluation

We now want to take into account the potential of praxis evaluation as a framework for making sense of all the aspects arising from PD. What we propose is that praxis evaluation offers an approach to undertaking evaluation that takes into consideration not only the evaluation process, but also the experience of being engaged in that process, as well as attempting to capture outcomes that will improve and impact on how healthcare is experienced. Praxis evaluation, as a deliberate intention, considers how evaluation processes can inform and develop practice at all stages (before, during and after) of the evaluation. This can be achieved through identifying and exploring what works, what has not worked, and what needs further investigation. This appears on the surface to be no different from all other forms of evaluation. Where praxis evaluation differs is in the types of evidence gathered, the ways in which it is gathered, and what is considered significant. Engaging in critical creative exploration of practice change and capturing the nuances of change that occur (in people's conversations, attitudes and behaviours) can all add to the richness of the evaluation and help to make links between how practice has or can be improved. Alongside attention to these elements comes an increased awareness for the participants engaged in the evaluation, of their own challenges, changes and experiences that will further enable them to articulate and substantiate their practice decisions and actions.

Praxis evaluation we propose is a critical approach, drawing on the theoretical underpinnings of critical social science (Fay, 1987), with the added intention of exploring in depth the issues that are often forgotten, hidden or taken for granted (i.e. overlooked) within evaluations taking place in practice settings. The evaluation therefore takes into account not only the outcomes of the work itself but also unpicks the processes used within PD to enable a greater understanding of the impact the processes have in bringing about practice change. This incorporates consideration of utilising critical creative methods in the evaluation process itself. There is a potential that fragments can be captured and identified as significant to understanding more of what happens within PD and its influence on healthcare, as well as outcomes that may or may not be achieved. When pieced together these fragments can provide valuable information on how healthcare practice is influenced and influencing the context within which it functions. These issues are now explored as we look at praxis evaluation in more depth.

Praxis evaluation we believe can contribute towards human-flourishing, not only through the outcomes of person centredness and evidence-based practice, but also intentionally through its processes (e.g. person centredness, critical inquiry, reflection through consideration of the consequences of all aspects of the evaluation process, and stakeholder collaboration). A praxis evaluation framework is therefore driven by the values underpinning PD, and uses inclusive, collaborative and facilitative processes. Thus praxis evaluation is complex and multilayered, whereby each fragment of evidence builds one upon another to reflect a clearer and more meaningful understanding of what is happening in practice. This requires participants to engage in critical reflexivity (deep self-reflection) to examine and critique their values at all stages of the evaluation process.

Effective PD contributes to practice-based theory, therefore the outcomes of action-orientated research should enlighten practice and form the building blocks of practice-based knowledge. A strong evaluation component helps to promote sustainable and transferable evidenced-based knowledge for practice while informing future PDs. This is achieved by making explicit the processes of change and highlighting the evidence base upon which changes take place. In so doing, policy makers and service commissioners are guided by a collective and contextually driven evidence base that offers credible recommendations for service planning and delivery.

Praxis evaluation is facilitated via a collaborative evaluation process that includes relevant stakeholders, at all stages of the evaluation process, taking into consideration all forms of data/evidence (including the use of artefacts, creative expressions for example) relevant to practice enhancement and understanding how practice can be improved for all engaged in healthcare. In keeping with a collaborative approach, praxis evaluation also considers how to utilise knowledge and expertise to inform the evaluation process and findings. This means that the people involved in the work will come from a variety of settings and backgrounds, brought together with a common aim of uncovering the evidence, whilst also aiming to further their own knowledge of practice transformation. We propose that a praxis evaluation framework remains integral to all stages of PD work and offers a means to monitor transformation at individual, team and organisational levels, whilst also providing evidence on which to judge the success or otherwise of a PD project or initiative. The evidence of such an exploration can then be linked to ongoing critical discussions and debate between stakeholders as they make further recommendations about potential future PD work.

An example of praxis evaluation

In the following example, we use the implementation of an action learning group (ALG) for nurse educators in a healthcare organisation to help explore what praxis evaluation looks like in reality. The intent of the ALG is to provide peer support for the nurse educators as they develop their roles within a variety of teams across the organisation. Prior to implementation of the ALG the nurse educators had highlighted issues of concern around how they were working as a team, the support and challenges they received from one another as well as others in the organisation. The resources and support for the ALG was sanctioned by the manager of the Nurse Educator Group. Now we take time to consider each component of praxis evaluation in order to create a framework to evaluate the effectiveness of the PD strategy, in this case an ALG for nurse educators.

Purpose

The ALG was initially created to provide peer support for the nurse educators. Whilst this purpose was outlined when establishing and recruiting participants into the group, it was through further exploration of individual, group and organisational needs that the purpose was redefined. The purpose of the group then evolved to incorporate the development of knowledge and skills in using a high challenge/high support approach in working with one another and facilitating education in the clinical setting. In addition to this, it was hoped that through peer support the nurse educators would gain more satisfaction from the work they were doing individually and collectively. Understanding the changing nature of the purpose and documenting these changes enabled this to be taken into account within the evaluation approach.

Reflexivity

The facilitators of the ALG developed the evaluation questions in consultation with the key stakeholders, who included the manager, the participants (Nurse Educators) and the facilitators. As the purpose of the group developed, there was need for critical questioning and the development of further aspects to the evaluation. The notion of critical reflection and the use of high challenge/high support questions also helped the facilitators and participants explore the links between what they aimed to evaluate and how this related to the theory of PD. This resulted in a clearer understanding about the purpose of the ALG itself as well as the purpose of the evaluation.

Approach

Involving the participants, facilitators (and manager) in decisions around the purpose of the group and why it was being evaluated helped highlight what their values and beliefs were around the ALG and the outcomes they anticipated from this. This enabled the facilitators to understand this within the context of creating a meaningful evaluation for all stakeholders. The approach to evaluation, how and when data could be collected and analysed, was then established by the ALG (participants and facilitators) and was clearly linked to their understanding of PD theory. This was not fixed and critical questioning enabled the ALG to consider the effectiveness of the evaluation process as it was evolving.

Context

The ALG was set within a specific context (the education department of a large organisation). It was important to take into consideration this context and the impact it may hold in relation to the evaluation itself (what was happening within the department), how (and how many) educators were involved in the ALG, what changes were occurring for individuals and the team. This resulted in collection of data about the context (the people, the environment both learning and social and the 'way things are done around here') in order to provide a starting point for the work, to measure any changes that occurred as a result of the work for individuals and the team and to take into consideration such things as changing roles and resources.

Intent

The intent in this study was to go beyond what we could see happening within the ALG, i.e. participants were developing their skills and knowledge about such things as high challenge/high support. If we look back at the **purpose,** an aspect of this was *the nurse educators would gain more satisfaction from the work they were doing individually and collectively* and we link this to **reflexivity** and *the need to explore the links between what the group aimed to evaluate and how this related to the theory of*

PD (in other words, whether the ALG was an effective mechanism to enable the participants to develop through processes of enlightenment, empowerment and emancipation) and the **approaches** taken to evaluation (in this case individual and group journeys captured through creative means such as creative art, imagery, poetry and theatre), we can identify that a **critical intent** of this study was to evaluate if the participants themselves were flourishing and transforming (accepted wisdom of PD) as a result of participating in the ALG as well as evaluating the effectiveness of the ALG.

Stakeholders

The participants of this ALG were themselves the evaluators of the ALG in conjunction with the facilitators. They were involved in designing the evaluation through critical questioning, collecting and analysing the data at each stage of the evaluation, making sense of what was emerging and finally in using the evaluation to lobby for further resources to continue the ALG after the study period. The manager as a stakeholder was involved in a more peripheral sense regarding the evaluation but did participate in setting critical questions for the evaluation and responding to the outcomes of the evaluation itself.

So to return to our image of the gyroscope, all of the above core components are needed to help construct a PD-orientated evaluation. Once the evaluation gathers momentum, only then do all of these interlinked elements work together. We propose that the axis, on which the evaluation spins, has a core intent for human-flourishing. If we go back to our example of the ALG, the elements of the evaluation were intertwined and dependent upon one another. Had any one of the elements been missing or fragmented, we believe that the overall evaluation would not be as systematic and rigorous as it could be.

The following list highlights a summary of key aspects of what we propose constitutes an inclusive evaluation strategy, keeping the notion of praxis evaluation at the forefront of our thinking. If you use this as a guideline to help you discuss and develop your own evaluation strategy, you will have taken the first step towards your own explorative evaluation journey.

Consider:

- The evaluation at the start of any project.
- Engaging key organisational personnel to ensure the evaluation remains a priority for the organisation.
- What your philosophical approach to the issue under investigation is.
- If your chosen approach fits with those of other stakeholders.
- Engage all stakeholders in a strategic and systematic approach to the evaluation.
- What tools and approaches best fit with the agreed philosophical stance chosen for the project/evaluation.
- Choosing a range of approaches and mixed methods that can increase the likelihood of making a successful find.
- The time and impact the project will have on participants and the context.
- What approaches are most likely to add benefit to a rapidly changing context of healthcare.

- Using and capturing creative approaches to data collection.
- What constitutes evidence.
- How the evaluation process itself is raising issues for participants.
- In what way the evaluation process is raising issues about PD theory and which evaluation methodologies enable transferability of PD findings.

There are certain processes that we have identified throughout this chapter that we consider to be pertinent to achieving a praxis-orientated PD-based evaluation. We aim to further refine and test the notion of praxis evaluation through using it in different settings. One of our first aims is to test the merits of praxis evaluation within the work of the IPDC and the work we have undertaken as a collaborative inquiry over the last 4 years. This is exciting and daunting as well as vitally important if we are to indeed grow, learn and share our knowledge of the progress being made within PD. What we do not want is for the ideas and intent of praxis evaluation to become just another theoretical musing. We hope that it can be of value to those engaging in PD work and help them to consider the importance of evaluation within the work they undertake. The merit of praxis evaluation can only be realised if it becomes a living and informing entity within PD work. For this reason, we urge you to consider it on your next PD adventure. We believe that it will deliver more than mere outcomes for the work but will also lead to transformation for those who choose to engage in the spiral.

Praxis unearthed

This chapter outlined the key stages and evaluation processes of our developmental explorative journey, as we aimed to further our understanding of the role, processes and impact of evaluation on effective PD. We have outlined a praxis evaluation framework that offers a collaborative process for evaluation of practice change and workplace cultures in order to further explicate praxis, using critical creativity (and multiple discourses), with the ultimate purpose of informing PD theory. We have not unearthed a polished and honed exhibit; on the contrary we are more than happy to continue exploring the role of praxis evaluation in supporting the potential for transformation of healthcare practice, of individuals, teams and entire organisations. Our aim has been to awaken the readers' senses to a new mode of understanding and working with PD evaluation. We have called this process *praxis evaluation*, which is both a process- and outcome-orientated method of evaluating PD initiatives. Praxis evaluation takes into consideration not only the evaluation process, but also the experience of being engaged in that process, as well as attempting to capture outcomes that will improve and impact on how healthcare is experienced. Engaging in a critical creative exploration of practice change and capturing the nuances of change that occur (in people's conversations, attitudes and behaviours) can all add to the richness of an evaluation and help to make clearer the links between how practice has or can be improved for people who experience healthcare.

We are now taking praxis evaluation into different settings to test its application, for example through the IPDC 5-day schools that occur in Europe and Australasia as well as to test the impact of action learning in practice changes both in Australia and in Northern Ireland. We are preparing to engage in statewide projects in New South Wales, Australia, where the aim is to consider whether praxis evaluation can help clinicians understand new models of care.

We would also encourage you to test the framework and in so doing acknowledge the framework as intellectual property of the IPDC. We challenge each of you to consider *praxis evaluation* within your own PD work, and to add to the work undertaken within this first PD orientated evaluation exploration.

We welcome your thoughts, critique and comments.

References

Binnie, A. & Titchen, A. (1999) *Freedom to Practice: The Development of Patient-Centred Nursing*. Butterworth-Heinemann, Oxford.

Carr, S.M. (2005) Refocusing health visiting – sharpening the vision and facilitating the process. *Journal of Nursing Management*. **13**, 249–256.

Carr, W. & Kemmis, S. (1986) *Becoming Critical: Knowing through Action Research*. The Falmer Press, Barcombe.

Chenoweth, L. & Kilstoff, K. (2002) Organisational and structural reform in aged care organisations: Empowerment towards a change process. *Journal of Nursing Management*. **10**, 235–244.

Clarke, A., Hanson, E.J. & Ross, H. (2003) Seeing the person behind the patient: Enhancing care of older people using a biographical approach. *Journal of Clinical Nursing*. **12**, 697–706.

Clendon, J.M. (2003) Nurse-managed clinics; issues in evaluation. *Journal of Advanced Nursing*. **44**, 558–565.

Dewing, J. & Traynor, V. (2005) Admiral nursing competency project: Practice development and action research. *Journal of Clinical Nursing*. **14**, 695–703.

Dick, J., Lewin, S., Rose, R., Zwarenstein, M. & Van Der Walt, H. (2004) Changing professional practice in tuberculosis care: An evaluation intervention. *Journal of Advanced Nursing*. **48**, 434–442.

Drennan, J. (2002) An evaluation of the role of the clinical placement co-ordinator in student nurse support in the clinical area. *Journal of Advanced Nursing*. **40**, 475–483.

Fay, B. (1987) *Critical Social Science: Liberation and its limits*. Polity, Cambridge.

Forrest, S., Masters, H. & Milne, V. (2004) Evaluating the impact of training in psychosocial interventions: A stakeholder approach to evaluation – Part 11. *Journal of Psychiatric and Mental Health Nursing*. **11**, 202–212.

Freire, P. (1972) *Pedagogy of the Oppressed*. Herder & Herder, New York.

Gadamer, H.-G. (1979) *Truth and Method*. Sheed and Ward, London.

Garbett, R. & McCormack, B. (2004) A concept analysis of practice development. In: *Practice Development in Nursing* (eds B. McCormack, K. Manley & R. Garbett). Blackwell, Oxford.

Gerrish, K. (2001) A pluralistic evaluation of nursing/practice development units. *Journal of Clinical Nursing*. **10**, 109–118.

Gerrish, K., Clayton, J., Nolan, M., Parker, K. & Morgan, L. (1999) Promoting evidence-based practice: Managing change in the assessment of pressure damage risk. *Journal of Nursing Management.* **7**, 355–362.

Guba, E. & Lincoln, Y. (1989) *Fourth Generation Evaluation.* Sage, Newbury Park, CA.

Harvey, G., Loftus-Hills, A., Rycroft-Malone, J., Titchen, A., Kitson, A., McCormack, B. & Seers, K. (2002) Getting evidence into practice: The role and function of facilitation. *Journal of Advanced Nursing.* **37**, 577–588.

Holman, C. & Jackson, S. (2001) A team education approach: An evaluation of a collaborative education and practice development in a continuing care unit for older people. *Nurse Education Today.* **21**, 97–103.

Kemmis, S. (2005) Searching for saliences. *Pedagogy, Culture and Society.* **13**(3), 391–426.

Kilgour, C. & Fleming, V. (2000) An action research inquiry into a health visitor parenting programme for parents of pre school children with behavioural problems. *Journal of Advanced Nursing.* **32**, 682–688.

Koch, T., Jenkin, P. & Kralik, D. (2004) Chronic illness self management: Locating the self. *Journal of Advanced Nursing.* **48**, 484–492.

Lindsey, E. & McGuinness, L. (1998) Significant elements of community involvement in participatory action research: Evidence from a community project. *Journal of Advanced Nursing.* **28**, 1106–1114.

Manley, K. (2000a) Organisational culture and consultant nurse outcomes: Part 1. Organisational culture. *Nursing Standard.* **14**(36), 34–38.

Manley, K. (2000b) Organisational culture and consultant nurse outcomes: Part 2, nurse outcomes. *Nursing Standard.* **14**(37), 34–38.

Manley, K. (2004) Workplace culture: Is your workplace effective? How would you know? *Nursing in Critical Care.* **9**, 1–3.

Manley, K. & McCormack, B. (2003) Practice development: Purpose, methodology, facilitation and evaluation. *Nursing in Critical Care.* **8**, 22–29.

Manley, K. & McCormack, B. (2004) Practice development purpose, method, facilitation and evaluation. In: *Practice Development in Nursing* (eds B. McCormack, K. Manley & R. Garbett). Chapter 3. Blackwell Science, London.

McCormack, B. (2001) Clinical effectiveness and clinical teams: Effective practice with older people. *Nursing Older People.* **13**, 14–17.

McCormack, B. (2003) Researching nursing practice: Does person-centredness matter? *Nursing Philosophy.* **4**, 179–188.

McCormack, B., Dewar, B., Wright, J., Garbett, R., Harvey, G. & Ballantine, K. (2006) *A Realist Synthesis of Evidence Relating to Practice Development: Executive Summary.* NHS Quality Improvement, Scotland. (www.nes.scot.nhs.uk/)

McCormack, B., Manley, K. & Wilson, V. (2004) Evaluating practice developments. In: *Practice Development in Nursing* (eds B. McCormack, K. Manley & R. Garbett), pp. 83–117.Blackwell, Oxford.

McCormack, B. & Titchen, A. (2006) Critical creativity: Melding, exploding, blending. *Educational Action Research: An International Journal.* **14**(2), 239–266. (http://www.tandf.co.uk/journals)

McCormack, B. & Wright, J. (1999) Achieving dignified care for older people through practice development: A systematic approach. *Nursing Times Research.* **4**, 340–352.

McCourt, C. & Thomas, B.G. (2001) Evaluation of a problem based curriculum in midwifery. *Midwifery.* **17**, 323–331.

Owen, J. & Rogers, P. (1999) *Program Evaluation: Forms and Approaches*, 2nd edn. Allen & Unwin, Sydney.

Paley, G., Myers, S., Patrick, S., Reid, E. & Shapiro, D.A. (2003) Practice development in psychological interventions: Mental health nurse involvement in the conversational model of psychotherapy. *Journal of Psychiatric and Mental Health Nursing.* **10**, 494–498.

Pawson, R. & Tilley, N. (1997) *Realistic Evaluation.* Sage, London.

Reed, J., Pearson, P., Douglas, B., Swinburne, S. & Wilding, H. (2002) Going home from hospital – an appreciative inquiry study. *Health and Social Care in the Community.* **10**, 36–45.

Taylor, R., Coombes, L. & Bartlett, H. (2002) The impact of a practice development project on the quality of small group therapy. *Journal of Psychiatric and Mental Health Nursing.* **9**, 213–220.

Titchen, A. (1993) *Changing Nursing Practice through Action Research.* National Institute for Nursing, Oxford.

Titchen, A. & Binnie, A. (1995) The art of clinical supervision. *Journal of Clinical Nursing.* **4**, 327–334.

Titchen, A. & Binnie, A. (eds) (2001) *Practice Knowledge and Expertise in the Health Professions.* Butterworth-Heinemann, Oxford.

Ward, C. & McCormack, B. (2000) Creating an adult learning culture through practice development. *Nurse Education Today.* **20**, 259–266.

Wilson, V., McCormack, B. & Ives, G. (2005) Understanding the work place culture of a special care nursery. *Journal of Advanced Nursing.* **50**, 27–38.

8. *Enabling Practice Development: Delving into the Concept of Facilitation from a Practitioner Perspective*

Theresa Shaw, Jan Dewing, Roz Young, Margaret Devlin, Christine Boomer and Marja Legius

Introduction

In this chapter, we, the authors, would like you to accompany us on a journey of exploration into the complex concept of facilitation as it applies within systematic practice development (PD), which we refer to as enablement. We hope to inspire readers to explore their own experiences and understandings of facilitation. To help prepare readers for the journey through this chapter, we begin by briefing identifying our key intentions. We plan to emphasise the following:

- Person centredness as a key concept underpinning every aspect of facilitation practice.
- The theoretical frameworks about person centredness that clarify the role of facilitation in PD.
- Other specific enabling factors, attributes and consequences of enablement derived from practitioner data informing a two-phase process of concept analysis.

In addition, we hope this chapter will inspire readers to develop key insights into their own facilitation practice that they may then test out for themselves.

Facilitation is a complex and multifaceted role referred to in a wide range of literature from education (Rogers, 1983), health (Titchen, 2000) and counselling (Rogers, 1951). In the PD literature, the role is seen to be a key element in PD frameworks (Manley, 2004; Simmons, 2003) and to enabling PD to achieve its purpose and goals, such as the transformation of practitioners and practices (McCormack et al., 2006). Yet the existing literature reveals several gaps in our knowledge about facilitation in the context of PD. For example, it is not known if facilitation within PD is in any way different or should be different to that in other activities concerned with working with groups in particular contexts (such as quality improvement, evidence-based initiatives and learning from work). Given that the purpose of PD is becoming increasingly connected with notions of transformations and emancipation, it would be reasonable to assume that something different is called for. In addition, we argue that the literature including PD, apart from a few exceptions such as Manley (2000a, 2000b) who focused exclusively on Consultant Nurses, does not capture the experience of being a facilitator and the experiences of being facilitated within PD. Rycroft-Malone (2004) raises a series of questions about the role and process of facilitation together with the skills and attributes of a facilitator in the context of implementation of evidence into practice and the Promoting Action in Research Implementation In Health Services (PARIHS) framework. To a large extent these questions continue to remain unanswered.

The International Practice Development Colloquium (IPDC) for theory development in PD is a group of practice developers, practitioner–researchers and educators from healthcare who, through a cooperative inquiry methodology (Heron & Reason, 2001), are undertaking theoretical advancement of PD. Over the course of the last 2 years, as a sub-group of the colloquium we (the chapter authors) have undertaken a collaborative journey exploring the concept of facilitation within PD. This exploration grew from an earlier concept analysis within the whole colloquium group, which raised the possibility that 'enabling' or 'enablement' was a concept that could embrace and account for the complexity of PD facilitation. On this basis, the authors of this chapter decided to examine the literature to see what, if any, theoretical work had been undertaken in this area to date. As indicated above, we discovered that the literature on facilitation in PD work was limited. A total of five concept analyses of facilitation (Cross, 1996; Burrows, 1997; Kitson et al., 1998; Harvey et al., 2002; Simmons, 2003) were found, of which only one (Simmons, 2003) specifically focused on PD. This initial delving into the literature helped us (as a sub-group) to establish long-term aims that would contribute to the colloquium's work; specifically to

- clarify our current knowledge about the concept of facilitation,
- add to our existing understanding of the concept,
- explore and define the concept of enabling as an approach to facilitation in PD,
- provide a rigorous theoretical basis for a set of standards on enabling facilitation for use in systematic or emancipatory PD work.

Whilst committed to undertaking advancement of our knowledge on facilitation in the context of PD (which we term enabling) and hopefully devising a theoretical framework for enabling, the group wanted to embed their inquiry in and from healthcare practice. For this reason, we adopted an inductive method that drew on group members' personal experiences of facilitation and practitioners' ideas on the nature of enabling.

This chapter shares some of our work to date. Specifically, we present and discuss the data shared with us by different groups of practitioners regarding enabling and enablement, as this is building on a method used by others in concept analysis work in the field of PD (Garbett & McCormack, 2001).

Concept analysis approach

A concept analysis serves as the foundation for identification and evaluation of a concept, in this case the concept of facilitation (and enabling) within the context of PD. The initial phase in a concept analysis is to analyse the level of the concept's maturity. However, influenced by Hupcey and Penrod (2005) we recognise that disentangling concept analysis from techniques for concept advancement is critical to enhance the utility of concept-based research. This argument is based on the notion that concept analysis most aptly reveals the current state of the science in a precise form, while concept advancement techniques add to the existing body of knowledge through the synthesis of new knowledge. Subsequently, techniques for advancing a concept are a form of theory building (Hupcey & Penrod, 2005). Concept advancement in this instance pushes the concept of facilitation towards an increased level of scientific clarity and refinement. In common with numerous others attempting to analyse concepts related to nursing and other healthcare professions, the framework proposed by Walker and Avant (1995) was used. The concept of enabling was analysed through identifying the antecedents or conditions that precede the manifestation of enabling, the attributes or characteristics associated with the concept of enabling and the consequences or outcomes related to the concept (Walker & Avant, 1995).

Ridner (2004) indicates that multiple methods can be used to analyse a concept. In this conceptual advancement work, the approach outlined above by Walker and Avant was combined with two other processes. The first process involved consultation, over three phases, with a range of international practitioners engaged in PD work. The three phases that took place between 2006 and 2007 included the following:

1. Initial discussions with a number of UK practitioners involved in PD.
2. Collecting and collating contributions from delegates attending *The 6th International Practice Development Conference* in Edinburgh, Scotland in 2006.
3. Opportunistic collation of data from groups of nurses in England, Northern Ireland and The Republic of Ireland, all engaged in some form of PD after the Scotland 2006 conference.

During the collection of data during the three phases, we asked practitioners about facilitation in general and specifically inquired about enabling and what it meant to them. It might be argued that approaching nurses we worked with in this opportunistic way could have placed undue pressure on them to participate. Reflecting back on this we believe that the nurses participated willingly as we took care to explain our work with the colloquium and how the information would be used. Figure 8.1 demonstrates the contributions gathered at *The 6th International Practice Development Conference* in Edinburgh.

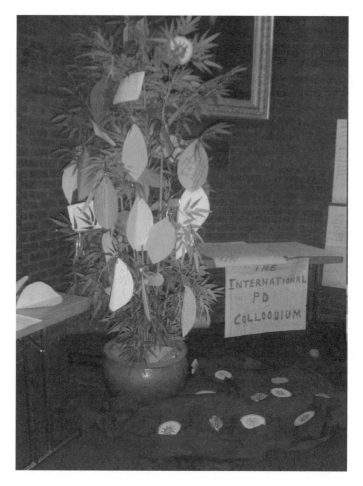

Figure 8.1 Collecting contributions from nurses at the international conference, October 2006.

The second process involved using the methodological framework of critical creativity (Chapter 4) to examine, combine and theme our experience and the data collected to date (see Figure 8.2).

Both processes have enabled broader insight into the emerging concept of enablement. This concurs with Simons and McCormack's (2007) views that engaging with the arts enables a holistic engagement with learning and the emergence of embodied ways of knowing.

Apart from work by Titchen (2004) relating to a specific framework of facilitation referred to as critical companionship, the group felt that literature reviewed thus far does not capture practitioner experience with skilled facilitation in PD and agreed that it would bring value to the analysis to include an inductive element.

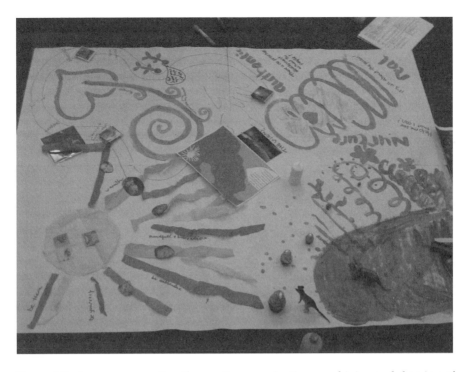

Figure 8.2 Image representing the creative examination, combining and theming of conceptual data.

This would also demonstrate commitment to valuing practitioner experience and practice-generated knowledge.

Synthesising the practitioner data on enabling

Conceptual themes emerged following a critical analysis of all of the practitioner data. The data were analysed by the group and then again independently by two group members (TS and JD). Through ongoing critical dialogue the themes emerging were further synthesised as presented in Table 8.1. At this stage, we have not attempted to demonstrate any horizontal relationships between concepts across the three columns in the table.

Although not included in the above table the concept of person centredness pervaded the data from practitioners and was interwoven with the antecedents, attributes and consequences of enabling as both a vertical and horizontal theme. Whilst we still need to examine and establish the exact relationship between person centredness and the factors, we have selected person centredness for specific consideration, as we believe that it is fundamental in regard to enabling self and others to achieve the *consequences*. Therefore, we will discuss the contribution of

151

Table 8.1 Antecedents, attributes and consequences of enabling

Antecedents	Attributes	Consequences
o Vision for practice development	o Self	o Independence in practice development
o Preparedness	– Knowing own beliefs and values	o Interdependence in practice development
– Willingness to get involved	– Authenticity	o Responsibility for learning, growth and development
o Safety for learning and practice	o Working with clear principles	– Self
– People	– Philosophy	– Team
– Place	– Frameworks/models	– Others
– Time	o Knowledge and skill-set	– Organisation
o Work-based learning and formal education opportunities	– Building person-centred relationships, one to one and groups	o Value validation and self-worth
o Knowledge and skills in facilitation	– Establishing vision and ownership	o Perspective/vision
o Permission to begin practice development	– PD methods and processes	o Action orientated
	– Working effectively in differing context and cultures	– Creating possibilities
		– Doing
		– Making changes
		– Sharing good practice
		– Formal systems and processes
	– Accessing and using different types of evidence and resources	– Formal systems and processes
		o Collaborative leading

person centredness to enabling before returning to discuss the findings from the practitioner data.

The contribution of person centredness to enabling

In Chapter 2, person centredness (or closely related principles) is considered the pivotal concept in relationships between and amongst people in healthcare systems. The authors recognise the assumption that person-centred relationships and PD have a common focus in transforming individuals, teams and workplaces. Manley and McCormack (2003) suggest that transformation is required in order to create effective, sustainable cultures that are person centred and evidence driven. Consequently, person centredness is a core element of PD that contributes to progressing macro healthcare agendas. To date, it is unclear to what degree person centredness and/or transformation has to occur to achieve effective team and workplace cultures. There is increasing recognition that further work is needed on the application of person-centred concepts (Ashburner, 2005; Dewing, 2004; Mc-Cormack, 2004; Nolan et al., 2004; O'Connor et al. [see also Chapter 10]) Dewing (2004) proposes that despite the concept of 'person' being one of the foundations for nursing theories and models, greater clarity is still required on what is meant by person centredness.

Applying what we understand so far in the context of enablement, person centredness is based on the process of promoting personhood (i.e. the attributes of being a person). Enhanced personhood is proposed as an outcome of enablement. At the core of clarifying person centredness in PD lies a philosophical and theoretical appreciation of the nature of personhood. Kitwood's ideas (1997) have strongly influenced our previous understanding of personhood and to some extent have been accepted without critical review. Dewing (2007), in regard to gerontological nursing, calls for a revisiting of the concept of personhood, claiming it is reliant on a mind–body dualism that values cognition as the primary attribute of persons. The consequences of this approach for PD would be the devaluing of creative and other forms of learning and knowledge generation such as intuition and tacit knowing that are becoming more widely used in PD and facilitation methods (Coates et al., 2004).

McCormack (2004), in a review of the literature on person centredness, also in gerontological nursing, suggests that Kitwood's ideas lead to an understanding of person centredness that focuses on four modes of 'being' and which collectively provide a loose framework for person-centred relationships:

1. Being in relation: *recognise that persons exist in relationships with other persons.*
2. Being in social world: *persons are social beings and the nature of that social connection is articulated through beliefs, values, narratives and social relationships.*
3. Being in place: *persons have a context through which their personhood is articulated.*
4. Being with self: *being recognised, respected and trusted as a person impacts on a person's sense of self.*

Applied to PD, where the centrality of person-centred relationships is implied, there are subsequent implications for enabling and facilitation that has at its core the principle of enabling others to make sense of their context. Persons make meaning by trying to understand their world, by making integrated sense of it and through making connections. In the context of emancipatory PD, this could be a description of a facilitator at work, although a facilitator needs to understand that complete meaning can never be fully achieved with continuous changes in the four modes of being. Therefore, PD with its focus on the development of sustainable cultures of effectiveness that are person-centred needs to take account of these four modes of being and accommodate them within the ultimate purpose, attributes and consequences of PD. It is proposed that enabling processes will bring increased integration in and between these four modes.

Mayeroff's (1971) ideas on caring have parallels with enabling facilitation conceived through the philosophical frame of 'personhood'. We arrived at Mayeroffs'

(1971) work from the work of Swanson (1991, 1993) who, through empirical development and refinement of theory generated from three related phenomenological studies, proposes enabling as one of five caring processes. The other four are knowing, being with, doing for and maintaining belief. Swanson (1991) suggests that enabling is

> *facilitating another person's passage through life's transitions and unfamiliar events in order to expand the other's capacity to grow, heal or practice self-care.*

Although a useful starting point, Swanson's (1991) approach to facilitation, in the context of PD, is incomplete in that it focuses on the person being facilitated and not on both people in the relationship (facilitator and the person being facilitated). Turning to Mayeroff (1971), this imbalance is addressed as

> *a helping relationship, essentially one of enabling others and consequently self, through transitions to achieve growth/development and ultimately self-actualisation.*

It is important to acknowledge two points. Firstly that Mayeroff (1971), although he does not directly specify, is influenced amongst others by the ideas of Carl Rogers (1951) and John Dewey (2004). Secondly, our work has not yet fully assessed the contribution and transferability of Mayeroff's (1971) ideas to ensure that it is inclusive of all (i.e. practitioners and patients/service users). In the meantime, Mayeroff's (1971) theoretical description of enabling as caring recognises and accommodates the four different modes of being, in that it focuses on helping relationships, the importance of self and transition (which requires addressing issues of context) in order for growth/development to occur.

At this point in our work, we have arrived at a place where we consider person centredness, in the context of PD in healthcare, as a particular type of relationship between people. Within this relationship, there is an enabling of others and of self through transition, to achieve growth/development and transformation that ultimately enhances integration between the four modes of being. We now return to the factors that practitioners identified as needed to be present to nurture enabling in PD.

Presentation and discussion of practitioner data

Antecedents: conditions that precede enabling

Antecedents refer to the conditions that precede the manifestation of a concept (Walker & Avant, 1995), in this case enabling as a specific approach to facilitation in PD. By delving into the practitioner data, we were able to draw out seven key factors, which we argue, are significant for enabling to take place:

1. *Vision for PD.* The practitioner data revealed that in order for enabling to take place there needed to be a shared vision for the future. It is not clear whether

the vision needs to be owned by the whole organisation or whether enabling is possible if individuals or a group of people hold the vision. However, from the literature, it is evident that there are links between having a shared vision and effective PD (Manley & McCormack, 2004). A study by McCormack and Garbett (2003) has also identified that having the ability to create a shared vision is one of the essential qualities of practice developers. Being visionary is also identified, along with enabling, as one of six transformational leadership processes (Manley, 2001, 2004), linked to working within an emancipatory PD framework (Shaw, 2005). Schein (1985) argues that the impact of transformational leadership is more wide-ranging than just the development of individuals or single practice changes. It can influence organisational culture thereby creating a context more receptive and conducive to development and change (Schein, 1985), a consequence later referred to by practitioners.

2. *Preparedness.* Across the practitioner data there was a sense that for enabling to be successful a level of preparedness was required. Preparedness seemed to relate to actions and processes that encouraged involvement. For example, practitioners referred to involving stakeholders, creating opportunities, challenging and supporting each other.

As outlined in Chapter 1, McCormack et al. (2006) argue that the principles that inform the three dominant methodologies of participatory models, action research orientated models and pedagogical models are participation, collaboration and inclusiveness. It was felt that the data suggested that, whilst facilitators do not necessarily attain all of the enabling factors at one time, there was a range and in-depth level of preparation required by what is considered to be an 'enabling facilitator'.

The data also highlighted a more personal and individual perspective related to preparedness as exemplified in the following quote:

[H]ow much enablement I can accept or can cope with depends on several factors; my openness, my defences, the facilitator's skill.

Here the personal commitment required to be enabled and therefore, it may be assumed, developed and transformed, is significant. Commitment can be linked to some of the earliest work regarding facilitation in the context of client-centred therapy (Rogers, 1951) and student-centred learning (Rogers, 1983). In preparing for such interventions, the facilitator needed to take account of a whole range of factors that may influence participation including readiness to participate or learn on the part of the individual (Roger, 1951, 1983). Additionally, the facilitator has a responsibility to ensure that they are equipped (skilled) and prepared to work with and meet the needs of those they are working with (Rogers, 1983).

3. *Safety for learning and practice.* In some ways interlinked with preparedness, the practitioner data referred to the need to create a safe environment for learning and practice. For example,

I have enabled by ... providing a safe place for the individual to discover their core self and issues.

PD work includes creating the opportunity for practitioners to reflect on and challenge their own practice as well as the practice of others. The potential to feel threatened or exposed is high and the facilitator has a key role in supporting others on what can be an intense and personal journey towards change. Again referring back to Rogers (1983), when using experiential learning strategies the notion of a safe environment is essential, with attention given to the individual, the place and time.

4. *Work-based learning and formal education opportunities.* 'Learning and workplace education opportunities' was a factor that arose from a discussion between two group members when analysing the completed practitioner data (TS and JD). This discussion was initially sparked by a practitioner's contribution that there needed to be an empowerment culture in place for enabling to be present. Whilst not referred to by others, one practitioner did state that enablement meant empowerment and autonomy by allowing staff to deliver and develop patient care within their own scope of practice. From the discussion, we concluded that having a culture of empowerment characterised by access to learning and education was ideal, but from the data it seemed that most practitioners did not work in workplace cultures or organisations where they experienced a culture of empowerment. Therefore, we inferred that as a minimum, practitioners need access to the formal academic style of education and work-based learning opportunities, in order to be aware of the range of learning possibilities.

McCormack et al. (2006), reporting on a realist synthesis of the PD literature, identify cultures that have a commitment to learning in practice and have an impact on the outcomes of PD; however, the exact relationship remains unclear. McCormack et al. (2006) argue that literature that is more recent places significance on the development of a learning culture to support and sustain PD work and suggest that external facilitators provide an educational function. Titchen and McGinley (2003), Wright and Titchen (2003) and also Webster and Dewing (2007 in press) illustrate in their accounts of PD work where an insider works with support from an external facilitator. Our data did not reveal any differences between internal or external facilitators with regard to learning and education. Some literature identifies that internal facilitators such as Consultant Nurses can achieve a similar outcome (Manley, 2000a, 2000b; Dewing et al., 2006). We feel that there are implications in terms of acquiring the skills necessary to undertake PD in the workplace, as identified by Manley and Webster (2006). Outsider roles generally do not have a direct connection with the actual development of practice but instead adopt a largely facilitative and educational role supporting internal practice developers or others actively engaged in PD projects. The authority that comes with the outsider role is generally through expertise and credibility within professional networks. Internal PD roles are generally combined with or are a sub-role of other role functions, e.g. service or department manager, clinical educator. In many instances, internal facilitators do not (yet) have the all-round expertise required to be an outsider or external facilitator as they may have only worked within their own workplace or organisation. An attribute of skilled enablers is that they know about context and culture and how to offer enabling in a range of cultures and contexts. The impact that comes with combining insider and outsider roles appears to contribute to the effectiveness of PD. As a word of caution, McCormack et al. (2006) report that the combination of insider and outsider roles brings challenges for integration, with a danger that the facilitative function can be seen as an additional rather than an integrated role function.

If opportunities for learning supportive of PD are not in place, it would seem crucial that facilitators plan and deliver this themselves or access support from others in order to ensure that enabling is available. Ward and McCormack (2000), Bellman et al. (2003), Walsgrove and Fulbrook (2005), Dickinson et al. (2005), Pilcher and King (2006) all provide examples of a collaborative approach to facilitation, integrating the expertise of practitioners, academics, researchers and practice developers. Working in this way can contribute to the development of facilitation skills within individuals as well as reduce isolation for practice developers, which is acknowledged as an issue. The literature also suggests learning that takes place in the workplace can be useful for the purposes of PD (Ward & McCormack, 2000; Dewing & Wright, 2003). Hardy et al. (2006), from findings of a concept analysis, propose that learning taking place in the workplace (work-based learning) stimulates debate and discussion between workplace colleagues and is aimed towards enhancing effective working practices that are based upon sound evidence and patient need.

Interestingly, learning from patients or service users was not specifically mentioned by practitioners although the most commonly referred to definition of PD states that PD should be influenced by service users' perspectives (Garbett & McCormack, 2002). In addition, recognising that PD aims to enhance the person's experience of care, Hamer (2002) argues that insight into the perspectives of service users, their perceptions, needs, wants and expectations is key to the success of PD. Despite the fact that some practice developers have successfully involved service users (Dewar, 2003; Keady et al., 2005; Dewing et al., 2007) there are still concerns about how some service users can be genuinely enabled to actively participate in PD (Dewing et al., 2006; Dewing & Pritchard, 2004; Webster & Dewing, 2007).

5. *Knowledge and skills in facilitation.* The practitioner data frequently refer to the importance of facilitators needing to have knowledge and skills about facilitation. In particular, the notion that facilitators are 'trained' or prepared to undertake facilitation in the workplace reoccurs. Manley and McCormack (2003) amongst others argue that the philosophical and methodological perspectives of a practice developer will influence how they work. For example, they suggest that there are clear distinctions between how facilitators working with a technical approach would approach and work through certain PD issues compared with facilitators working with emancipatory intent. In the latter instance, the facilitator would work in a more enabling way, creating the best conditions whereby practitioners felt empowered to critique and reflect on their work, thus freeing themselves from obstacles or

limitations in their current ways of working to develop their own practice. Interestingly, when practitioners were asked to provide examples of enablement, they could all be located within emancipatory rather than technical PD principles. Thus it seems that enabling has a strong association with both transformation and emancipatory intent in practice. Further, we propose enabling is a form of complex facilitation expertise that, although developed from a set of knowledge and skills based on facilitation, can only be fully acquired and synthesised by continuous commitment to, and engagement in, facilitation concerned with the transformation and emancipation of others.

The PD literature contains a mass of information suggesting that a wide range of knowledge and skills are necessary to become an effective facilitator. McCormack and Garbett (2003), for example, identify skills and qualities practice developers need to have to do their work. As one might imagine the range is broad and includes vision, motivation, empathy, reflexivity and the ability to communicate effectively. The RCN Facilitation Standards also give an insight into the attributes needed by facilitators (RCN, 2006). Further, Titchen (2000) proposes a skill-set for critical companionship. Critical companionship has been used in several PD initiatives (Harvey et al., 2002; Dewing & Wright, 2003; Titchen & McGinley, 2003; Wright & Titchen, 2003) but little development and testing of the framework has taken place since its initial development.

The practitioners' data in this concept analysis work reveal the primacy of the relationship between the facilitators and others being facilitated but also the difficulty of capturing this. We suggest that much of the literature fails to capture the essence or the spirit of facilitation in PD. However, this data extract from one practitioner perhaps conveys some of the essence of enabling:

> *From my experience with this PD project, it's a very personal relationship with a facilitator and with a PD vision directed at growth in several areas, but ultimately to promote person-centred care. It requires trust and taking a leap of faith with the facilitator's skills and [their] ability to know the practitioner and their needs and with PD ideas.*

The space in which the type of relationship described above evolves has both a here and now and, we would argue, a future and hopeful orientation to it. Contributions by Titchen (2000), Mayeroff (1971), Heron (1989) and Rogers (1983) come closer to capturing something of the essence or even magical quality of such enabling relationships. However, working in a person-centred and emancipatory way can also be challenging for all concerned. The PD literature appears slow to recognising some of the discomfort or distress that enabling can 'spark' for some practitioners and indeed for some facilitators. Henderson (2004), Dewing and Traynor (2005), Webster and Dewing (2007) all report discontent in participants emerging from emancipatory methods. The facilitators in these studies or projects gave evidence of demonstrating genuine concern when the issue was identified, listened to participants' views and negotiated new ways of working, whilst remain true to the principles of PD.

Attending to one's own learning as a facilitator is vital. This can be done in a number of ways based on what the learning and development needs are. However, in reality it often depends on the local availability of resources including expertise. Establishing a relationship with a higher education institution can provide an important means of accessing education opportunities; another option could be to access personal supervision using a model such as critical companionship (Titchen, 2004). Fundamental to learning in PD (i.e. emancipatory and transformative) is the commitment to critical reflection, receiving feedback from others and co-facilitating with others (Binnie & Titchen, 1999; Titchen, 2004). Our experiences suggest that learning through experiencing and the doing of emancipatory PD is vital and should not be missed or omitted.

6. *Permission to begin PD.* Practitioner data referred to having managerial support for PD and sometimes the need to have authority to go ahead with PD work was mentioned. The data were no more specific than this. Concurring with this, the PD literature refers to the supportive role management can play in PD work (Manley & Webster, 2006). All the evidence suggests that involvement of managers in PD is crucial for successful implementation of PD processes and the sustainability of effectiveness and person centredness. However, in reality there is mixed support from managers at different levels for PD work (Dewing & Traynor, 2005; Webster & Dewing, 2007). We suggest that this is due to a lack of understanding in a healthcare world that is on the one hand driven by short-term agendas that use a different discourse and on the other by practice or workplace cultures that continue to be suspicious of managers who demonstrate either an interest in practice or try to unduly influence practice. Managers who do not understand PD, do not appreciate its relevance in regard to the service modernisation agenda. There is an urgent need for further clarity on the role management needs to play in PD work. Practice developers who develop shared ownership with managers can be more successful in overcoming contextual barriers according to McCormack et al. (2006).

At some point someone in management needs to give permission for PD work to go ahead or even to continue, and this is essential for good governance. The giving of permission does not necessarily need to be of a formal hierarchical nature. Instead, the giving of permission can be a ritual with benefits that enables PD to take place. Having a senior nursing manager (or otherwise) say to a group of practitioners 'I/the organisation wants you to do this, I want you to see how you can do things differently' and explain why it matters and how it can contribute to the organisation's strategic agenda can be extremely catalytic and act as a means of harnessing energy. This way of permission giving can also do much to dispel myths or assumptions (about the level of commitment from the organisation) that can float around as part of the workplace culture and that can deter practitioners from investing energies in PD.

Attributes of enabling

A vast array of characteristics associated with the concept of enabling (Walker & Avant, 1995) were identified within the practitioner data. These ranged from statements about what practitioners believed facilitators 'do' to a long list of skills and techniques, i.e. helping, supporting, listening, guiding, patience, empathy, openness and so on. In part, this almost endless list felt like an impersonal reeling of techniques and, whilst much matched the kind of characteristics found within the literature, there was a lack of clarity and consistency. One practitioner conveyed the challenge of explaining the characteristics of enabling:

> [I]t is often said to be about helping, but this is too simple. It's a multi-faceted complex set of interventions.

With closer examination, it was possible to identify three broad attributes under which specific activities, skills and techniques could be located:

(i) *Self*. From our experience and knowledge of the literature, we had anticipated that the data would reveal strong evidence for self-awareness and use of self as we believed this may be an element that discriminated enabling from other types of facilitation. With this in mind, we were surprised, as highlighted previously, to discover that overall little reference was made to the use of self. Whilst there were some comments about helping others to use or explore self, only one statement referred to using self. Self-knowledge is an essential aspect of enabling others to focus on continual development (Manley, 2004) and move towards becoming enlightened and empowered (Fay, 1987), both words being used by participants when asked about what enabling meant to them. The intentional use of self is implicit in the critical companionship framework where the facilitator works with mind, heart, body and creative imagination (Titchen, 2004) to help and enable PD.

Two characteristics suggesting that 'self' might be important were 'knowing values and beliefs' and 'authenticity:

- Knowing own beliefs and values:

As individuals, our actions and reactions are influenced by personal values, beliefs and experiences. These in turn affect our way of being and behaviour. Helping others to articulate their values and beliefs is a key starting point for developing practice, and the extensive work of Manley (2004) makes a strong case for working with values and beliefs in order to understand and transform workplace culture.

- Authenticity:

The practitioner's responses regarding their experiences of enabling suggest that enabling is achieved through authentic ways of working. For example, one participant referred to enabling as 'about personal integrity, honesty and transparency'. Additionally, authenticity was said to be a two-way process of 'trust and mutual respect'.

In our experience, demonstration of realness and authenticity is central to enabling others to develop emotional intelligence in order to achieve personal development, learning and transformation (Brookfield, 1986). In PD, the horticultural model proposed by Binnie and Titchen (1999) emphasises the importance of working authentically with respect, love and care to achieve real growth and development in practice (Binnie & Titchen, 1999). Furthermore, in the context of getting research and evidence into practice (although more recently linked to PD) Kitson et al. (1998) indicate the value of authenticity and respect for effective facilitation.

(ii) *Working with clear principles*. Practitioner data suggested that enabling facilitators work purposely and with clear principles that would support, help and enable the development of individuals and their practice. For example, there were many references to realising the potential of another, helping others to feel empowered, assisting others to achieve goals. Yet, it was notable that no specific reference was made to a particular philosophy. By underpinning practice, and in this case enabling, with a theoretical or philosophical basis it is proposed that practitioners are supported to respond more effectively. Manley and McCormack (2003) suggest that practice developers consider the theoretical/philosophical work-view influencing their approach to practice PD as this will influence not only the processes used but also the style and impact of facilitation. However, the data we reviewed indicated that practitioners may still find this challenging.

(iii) *Knowledge and skill-set*. Under the broad attribute of a knowledge and skill-set, five key themes reflected the practitioner data:

- Building person-centred relationships, one to one and groups:

This included the helping and supporting so often mentioned within the data and found in the literature. The influence of a workplace culture or context that embraces person centredness as an overall way of working has already been discussed. Being person centred in the way we approach facilitation seems a natural progression from Rogers' (1983) view of the facilitation role being student centred. This is a notion built on by others including Heron (1989), who sees facilitation as focusing on individuals enabling them to examine and change behaviours and attitudes.

Within nursing and healthcare, being person centred is key to the delivery of holistic nursing care (Binnie & Titchen, 1999). In PD, the notion of valuing the person contributes to successful facilitation of PD (Garbett & McCormack, 2001; Titchen, 2004), is an espoused outcome of PD that has emancipatory intent (Manley & McCormack, 2003) and may influence opportunities created for human-flourishing (McCormack & Titchen, 2006).

- Establishing vision and ownership:

Following the earlier discussion regarding the role of vision in helping enabling to take place, there was a strong emphasis in the practitioner data that facilitators have an essential role in working with individuals and teams to create and establish a vision for what can be achieved. Implicit within this is the notion of engendering a sense of ownership. Asked about how they enabled others, practitioners referred to

> [w]orking with people from where they are at ... to where they want to go. ... Helping them to identify their vision.

Sander's (2004) reflections on her role as a PD facilitator provide insight as the importance of their being a sense of vision and ownership. Whilst the development of a new way of working seemed collaborative, the underpinning technical–rational focus on evidence as the driver resulted in practitioners rejecting the change once it became a reality in practice (Sanders, 2004). In contrast, Dewar (2003) having

161

acknowledged that imposing a plan on a ward team would not be effective, enabled staff using action learning to come up with a project idea and implementation plan.

- PD methods and processes:

Across the practitioner data there was reference to the use of a range of PD methods and processes; for example, processes for exploring values and beliefs, such as values clarification and concern, claims and issues; processes for enabling learning in and from practice, such as, action learning and clinical supervision; and processes for systematic evaluation. We would argue that more consistency in the methods and processes involved in PD is required, as highlighted by McCormack et al. (2006).

- Working effectively in differing context and cultures:

In the data, practitioners referred to being able to work in different cultures and contexts and responding to varying needs. The kinds of skills needed were not referred to and as with other attributes it was not clear how judgments and decisions were made about ways of working in different settings. The PARIHS framework highlights the influence both context and culture have exerted on research implementation (Rycroft-Malone, 2004). It is interesting to note some parallels with the characteristics of low and high context and culture, and those of enabling. For example, relationships with others, attitudes to learning, and values and beliefs. Such frameworks could provide a useful starting point for enablers to assess context and culture and focus their action planning.

- Accessing and using different types of evidence and resources:

The practitioner data suggested that enabling involves using a repertoire of resources to support PD. This seemed to range from helping individuals assess opportunities for development including study days, action learning opportunities or clinical supervision to using specific tools such as values clarification or 360° feedback (Garbett et al., 2007). Within the literature practice developers have described themselves as 'gatekeepers' for professional development opportunities as well as being able to secure external resources to support PD (McCormack & Garbett, 2003).

Consequences of enabling

As a result of synthesising the practitioner data, seven factors emerged as consequences or outcomes for the concept of enabling: independence – interdependence; responsibility for learning, growth and development; value, validation and self-worth; vision and perspective; action orientation; collaborative leading.

(i) *Independence: Interdependence in PD.* Practitioners talked about becoming more independent in their practice. We sensed that they perceived this as a positive consequence in that practitioners saw themselves as having increased agency and autonomy. There appears to be parallels between independence and empowerment in that practitioners experienced a sense of freedom from control, or influence from others or systems. However, in PD it is important to achieve a balance between independence and being influenced by others, in order to act collaboratively within agreed values and beliefs to achieve a shared vision. PD does not advocate the 'lone ranger' approach to leading and as a result of our critical dialogue we added 'interdependence' to this factor. From our experience, we recognise that some practitioners will achieve a sense of independence and that this can be part of personal and collective transformation, which go no further. This often relates to PD work ending or to other factors within the person or the workplace. However, some practitioners will continue to progress with their transformational journey towards a state of interdependence, probably becoming facilitators of others en route.

Interdependence is an element of respectful relationships with persons (Mayeroff, 1971), which in turn is an attribute of person centredness. The person enabling others in PD recognises that there is reciprocity in the relationship. The enabler knows the other persons' needs to be cared for or enabled to open up and progress towards their goals, and in turn this is reciprocated by seeing learning and growth in others. The balance of reciprocity might not be equal in many enabling relationships as it takes time to mature. For this reason, enablers will need the necessary skills as well as seek out and support each other. At its best, interdependence between enablers and the enabled provides a deep-seated sense of being in place and of continued renewal for both (Mayeroff, 1971).

(ii) *Responsibility for learning, growth and development.* Increased learning, growth and development come through strongly as an outcome of enabling in the practitioner data. This appears to suggest that practitioners see PD as a means to achieving learning for themselves, their teams and organisation. However, given the purpose of PD is more than learning for oneself, it is important that learning is used, seen to be used, by other stakeholders and put into action. Through planned and systematic activity, PD is evaluated to ensure that outcomes are achieved and further learning initiated. To this end, McCormack et al. (2006) recommend that learning strategies are embedded in PD activities in order that PD processes and outcomes are sustained beyond the life of a particular project. Within the data, practitioners referred to the use of reflective practice and action learning when enabling others. From our experience, we also propose that reflective learning strategies and group learning approaches such as 'action learning' appear to have more to offer the sustainability of PD. Linked to this, Chapter 14 of this book discusses how active learning can contribute to the sustainability of a workplace learning culture and thus to the purposes of PD. As argued by Heron (1989), the most appropriate learning methods combined with enabling are paramount to helping individuals and groups of practitioners grow and move from dependence to independence and subsequently, we suggest, to interdependence.

(iii) *Value, validation and self-worth*. The data reveal that practitioners value getting something for self out of being enabled. Central to this is the importance of feeling valued, validation and self-worth. This perhaps serves to demonstrate that practitioners do not always feel that their fundamental needs as a person are met in the workplace. It may also illustrate that initial encounters with PD need to attend to nurturing practitioners before transformations can be seen in workplace culture and patient experiences of care. Skilled facilitators learn to appreciate that enabling others adds to one's own sense of self-worth, as Mayeroff (1971) suggests (and thus illustrates interdependence in action).

(iv) *Vision and perspective*. The data show that practitioners perceive this factor as a consequence of enabling in the workplace. The importance of having clarity of values and beliefs and a shared vision for practice is a recurring theme in the data and in the PD literature. How this impacts on PD work is largely dependent on clarity of focus amongst facilitators, practitioners and managers. As previously mentioned, having a common vision across stakeholders is key to ensuring that there is an agreed focus and targeted outcomes. A vision is a mental picture that attracts others who can develop a similar mental image themselves. In PD, enabling others to acquire their vision and build its detail is skilled work. The notion of perspective can be considered in several ways; for example, seeing both micro- and macro-aspects of workplace culture and PD work. It can also be seen in regard to being able to enable others to see possibilities and their consequences from multiple positions or perspectives. Thus, acquiring the expertise to create and enable others to work with multiple possibilities is a consequence of effective enabling.

(v) *Action orientated*. The data reveal that creating possibilities, doing, making changes, sharing good practice and formal systems and processes are experienced as a consequence of enabling. Through our critical dialogue, we summarise this as being action oriented. Creating possibilities is necessary as part of vision creation and seeing perspectives. Likewise, Pritchard (2002) describes PD as helping practitioners within their real world context find creative and positive ways forward through the demanding, often confusing and draining, day-to-day trials and tribulations of practice. Dewing (in Chapter 6) suggests that a central feature of (active) learning in PD is that it is action or doing oriented where action in the workplace is aimed at contributing to transformation of the workplace and patient care. Doing goes hand in hand with learning and both act as catalysts to personal transformation, which can progress into emancipatory ways of working in practice. This equates with making changes. The sharing of good practice evolves over time when practitioners feel a sense of value in themselves and what they are achieving through PD. Practitioners recognise that PD has the consequence of introducing and enhancing formal systems and processes. Fundamental to this, as seen in some of the literature (such as McCormack & Manley, 2004; Dewing et al., 2006), is that PD provides practitioners with the means to assess evidence, evaluate and learn from it and decide on emerging action in negotiation with other stakeholders.

(vi) *Collaborative leading*. Throughout the practitioner data there is evidence that enabling involved collaboration and partnership; albeit processes for achieving this were not mentioned. According to Garbett and McCormack (2002) and Manley (2001, 2004) it is teams who are or have been enabled to work together that transform the culture and context of care. Therefore, to enable teams to work effectively, a facilitator must first establish what the culture they are working in is, gaining a consensus of what the cultural norms are. This is often done through using well-recognised PD tools such as 'values clarification' (Warfield & Manley, 1990) and 'claims, concerns and issues' (Guba & Lincoln, 1989). Manley (2001) asserts that there are often differences between espoused values and those seen in practice. The facilitator must therefore enable practitioners to engage in critical dialogue and reflect on how it really is in their workplace.

Summary and concluding remarks

We fully acknowledge that our values and beliefs (although not set out here) and experiences influenced this concept analysis. We also acknowledge that our work is still to be completed, tested and refined within the IPDC. Our consultation with practitioners has grounded this concept analysis in everyday practice. Our work to date suggests that enabling is a form of complex expertise in facilitation, which

- is centred around the concept of person centredness as an enabling factor, process and outcome in facilitation;
- is a particular type of relationship between persons where there is an enabling of others and consequently of self, through transitions to achieve growth/development and transformation that ultimately enhances integration between the four modes of being;
- is built on a set of knowledge and skills about facilitation;
- can only be fully acquired and synthesised by a continuous commitment to facilitation concerned with transformations and emancipation of others in the workplace.

Getting to grips with knowledge and skill about facilitation, including facilitation in the context of PD, is a requirement for enabling, as is the actual experience of facilitating with others when PD has a clear transformational and/or emancipatory intent. We still need to test this emerging practitioner-generated conceptual framework against a similar framework derived from the literature, account for any differences and gaps, then weave and blend the two together.

Acknowledgements

The authors wish to acknowledge and thank all those practitioners and practice developers who contributed to the data collection process that has informed this chapter.

References

Ashburner, C.H. (2005) Person-centred care: Using systemic and psychodynamically informed action research. Unpublished Doctorate in Health Thesis, St Bartholomew School of Nursing and Midwifery, City University.

Bellman, L., Bywood, C. & Dale, S. (2003) Advancing working and learning through critical action research: Creativity and constraints. *Nurse Education in Practice.* **3**(4), 186.

Binnie, A. & Titchen, A. (1999) *Freedom to Practice: The Development of Patient-Centred Nursing.* Butterworth-Heinemann, Oxford.

Brookfield, S.D. (1986) *Understanding and Facilitating Adult Learning: A Comprehensive Analysis of Principles of Effective Practices.* Open University Press, Milton Keynes.

Burrows, D. (1997) Facilitation: A concept analysis. *Journal of Advanced Nursing.* **25**(2), 396–404.

Coates, E., Dewing, J. & Titchen, A. (2004) *Opening Doors Resources for Awakening Creativity in Practice Development.* RCN, London.

Cross, K. (1996) An analysis of the concept facilitation. *Nurse Education Today.* **16**(5), 350–355.

Dewar, B. (2003) Enhancing partnerships with relatives in care settings for older people. In: *Foundation of Nursing Studies Dissemination Series No. 2* (eds T. Shaw & K. Sanders), Vol 2, pp. 1–4. London.

Dewey, J. (2004) *Democracy and Education.* Kessinger, Whitefish, MT.

Dewing, J. (2004) Concerns relating to the application of frameworks to promote person-centredness in nursing with older people. *Journal of Clinical Nursing.* **13**(s1), 39–44.

Dewing, J. (2008) Personhood and dementia: Revisiting Tom Kitwood's ideas. *International Journal of Older People's Nursing.* **3**(1), 3–13.

Dewing, J., Brooks, J. & Riddaway, L. (2006) Involving older people in practice development work: An evaluation of an intermediate care service and it's multi-disciplinary practice. *Practice Development in Health Care Journal.* **5**(3), 156–174.

Dewing, J., McCormack, B., Manning, M., McGuiness, M., McCormack, G. & Devlin, R. (2007) The development of person-centred practice in nursing across two continuing care settings for older people. *Final Programme Report.* Nursing Midwifery Planning and Development Unit, Dublin-Leinster Health Service Executive, Tullamore.

Dewing, J. & Pritchard, E. (2004) Including the older person with a dementia in practice development. In: *Practice Development in Nursing* (eds B. McCormack, K. Manley & R. Garbett). Blackwell, Oxford.

Dewing, J. & Traynor, V. (2005) Admiral nursing competency project: Practice development and action research. *Journal of Clinical Nursing.* **14**(6), 695–703.

Dewing, J. & Wright, J. (2003) A practice development project for nurses working with older people. *Practice Development in Health Care.* **2**(1), 13–28.

Dickinson, A., Welch, C. & Ager, L. (2005) improving the health of older people: Implementing patient- focused mealtime practice. *Foundation of Nursing Studies Dissemination Series*. **3**(10), 1–4.

Fay, B. (1987) *Critical Social Science: Liberation & Its limits*. Polity, Cambridge.

Garbett, R., Hardy, S., Manley, K., Titchen, A. & McCormack, B. (2007) Developing a qualitative approach to 360 degree feedback to aid understanding and development of clinical expertise. *Nursing Management*. **15**, 342–347.

Garbett, R. & McCormack, B. (2001) The experience of practice development: An exploratory telephone interview study. *Journal of Clinical Nursing*. **10**(1), 94–102.

Garbett, R. & McCormack, B. (2002) *A Concept Analysis of Practice Development: An Executive Summary*, pp. 1–6. RCN Institute, London.

Guba, E.G. & Lincoln, Y.S. (1989) *Fourth Generation Evaluation*. Sage, London.

Hamer, S. (2002) Innovation in practice. *Practice Development in Health Care*. **1**(2), 66.

Hardy, S. Garbarino, L. Titchen, A. & Manley, K. (2006) A framework for work-based learning. In: *Workplace resources for Practice Development*, pp. 8–56. RCN, London.

Harvey, G., Loftus-Hill, A., Rycroft-Malone, J., Titchen, A., Kitson, A., McCormack, B. & Seers, K. (2002) Getting evidence into practice: The role and function of facilitation. *Journal of Advanced Nursing*. **37**(6), 577–588.

Henderson, L. (2004) Critical application of Johari window in the development of clinical nurse specialists practice, utilising narrative inquiry. Unpublished MSc Thesis, University of Ulster, Belfast.

Heron, J. (1989) *The Facilitators' Handbook*. Kogan Page, London.

Heron, J. & Reason, P. (2001) The practice of cooperative inquiry: Research with rather than on people. In: *Handbook of Action Research: Participative Inquiry and Practice* (eds P. Reason & H. Bradbury), pp. 179–188. Sage, London.

Hupcey, J.E. & Penrod, J. (2005) Concept analysis: Examining the state of the science. *Research and Theory for Nursing Practice*. **19**(2), 197–208.

Keady, J., Williams, S. & Hughes-Roberts, J. (2005) Emancipatory practice development through life-story work: Changing care in a memory clinic in North Wales. *Practice Development in Health Care*. **4**(4), 203–212.

Kitson, A., Harvey, G. & McCormack, B. (1998) Enabling the implementation of evidence based practice: A conceptual framework. *Quality in Health Care*. **7**(3), 149–158.

Kitwood, T. (1997) *Dementia Reconsidered: The Person Comes First*. Open University Press, Buckingham.

Manley, K. (2000a) Organisational culture and consultant nurse outcomes: Part 1: Organisational culture. *Nursing Standard*. **14**(36), 34–38.

Manley, K. (2000b) Organisational culture and consultant nurse outcomes: Part 2: Organisational culture. *Nursing Standard*. **14**(37), 34–39.

Manley, K. (2001) Consultant nurse: Concept, processes outcomes. PhD Thesis, University of Manchester/RCN Institute, London.

Manley, K. (2004) Workplace culture: Is your workplace effective? How would you know? *Nursing in Critical Care*. **9**(1), 1–3.

Manley, K. & McCormack, B. (2003) Practice development: Purpose, methodology, facilitation and evaluation. *Nursing in Critical Care*. **8**(1), 22–29.

Manley, K. & McCormack, B. (2004) Practice development: Purpose, methodology, facilitation and evaluation. In: *Practice Development in Nursing* (eds B. McCormack, K. Manley & R. Garbett). Blackwell, Oxford.

167

Manley, K. & Webster, J. (2006) Can we keep quality care alive? *Nursing Standard*. **21**(3), 12–15.

Mayeroff, M. (1971) *On Caring*. Harper and Row, London.

McCormack, B. (2004) Person-centredness in gerontological nursing: An overview of the literature. *Journal of Clinical Nursing*. **13** (s1), 31–38.

McCormack, B., Dewar, B., Wright, J., Garbett, R., Harvey, G. & Ballantine, K. (2006) *A Realist Synthesis of Evidence Relating to Practice Development: Executive Summary*. National Education Scotland, Edinburgh.

McCormack, B. & Garbett, R. (2003) The characteristics, qualities and skills of practice developers. *Journal of Clinical Nursing*. **12**(3), 317–325.

McCormack, B. & Manley, K. (2004) Evaluating practice developments. In: *Practice Development in Nursing* (eds B. McCormack, K. Manley & R. Garbett). Blackwell, Oxford.

McCormack, B & Titchen, A. (2006) Critical creativity: Melding, exploding, blending. *Educational Action Research*. **14**(2), 239–266.

Nolan, M., Davis, S., Brown, J., Keady, J. & Nolan, J. (2004) Person-centred care and gerontological nursing. *Journal of Clinical Nursing*. 13 (s1), 45–53.

O'Connor, D., Phinney, A., Smith, A., Small, J., Purves, B., Perry, J., Drance, E., Donnelly, M., Chaudhury, H. & Beattie, L. (2007) Personhood in dementia care – Developing a research agenda for broadening the vision. *Dementia*. **6**(1), 121–142.

Pilcher, M. & King, L. (2006) Changing practice in continence assessment. *Foundation of Nursing Studies Dissemination Series*. **3**(7), 1–4.

Pritchard, E. (2002) RCN news: Gerontological nursing programme. Practice development trials and triumphs. *Nursing Older People*. **14**(5), 28.

Ridner, S.H. (2004) Psychological distress: Concept analysis. *Journal of Advanced Nursing*. **45**(5), 536–545.

Rogers, C. (1951) *Client Centred Therapy: Its Current Practice, Implications and Theory*. Houghton Mifflin, Boston.

Rogers, C. (1983) *Freedom to learn for the 80s*. Charles E. Merrill, Columbus, OH.

Royal College of Nursing (2006) *Accredited RCN Facilitation Standards*. RCN, London. Available from http://www.rcn.org.uk/downloads/practicedevelopment/accredited_rcn_facilitation_standards.pdf.

Rycroft-Malone, J. (2004) Research implementation: Evidence, context and facilitation – the PARIHS framework. In: *Practice Development in Nursing* (eds B. McCormack, K. Manley & R. Garbett). Blackwell, Oxford.

Sanders, K. (2004) Developing and implementing a family health assessment: From project worker to practice developer. In: *Practice Development in Nursing* (eds B. McCormack, K. Manley & R. Garbett). Blackwell, Oxford.

Shaw, T. (2005) Leadership for practice development. In: *Effective Healthcare Leadership* (eds M. Jasper & M. Jumaa). Blackwell, Oxford.

Schein, E.H. (1985) *Organisational Culture and Leadership*. Jossey Bass, San Francisco.

Simmons, M. (2003) 'Facilitation' of practice development: A concept analysis. *Practice Development in Health Care*. **3**(1), 36–52.

Simons, H. & McCormack B. (2007) Integrating arts-based inquiry in evaluation methodology: Opportunities and challenges. *Qualitative Inquiry*. **13**(2), 292–311.

Swanson, K.M. (1991) Empirical development of a middle range theory of caring. *Nursing Research*. **40**(3), 161–166.

Swanson, K.M. (1993) Nursing as informed caring for the well-being of others. *Journal of Nursing Scholarship*. **25**(4), 352–357.

Titchen, A. (2000) Professional craft knowledge in patient-centred nursing and facilitation of its development. DPhil Thesis, University of Oxford. Ashdale, Oxford.

Titchen, A. (2004) Helping relationships for practice development: Critical companionship. In: *Perspectives on Practice Development* (eds B. McCormack, K. Manley & R. Garbett), pp. 148–174. Blackwell, Oxford.

Titchen, A. & McGinley, M. (2003) Facilitating practitioner-research through critical companionship. *Nursing Times Research*. **8**(2), 2–18.

Walker, L.O. & Avant, K.C. (1995) *Strategies for Theory Construction in Nursing*, 3rd edn. Appleton and Lange, Norwalk, CT.

Walsgrove, H. & Fulbrook, P. (2005) Advancing the clinical perspective: A practice development project to develop the nurse practitioner role in an acute hospital trust. *Journal of Clinical Nursing*. **14**(4), 444–455.

Ward, C. & McCormack, B. (2000) Creating an adult learning culture through practice development. *Nurse Education Today*. **20**(4), 259.

Warfield, C. & Manley, K. (1990) Developing a new philosophy in the NDU. *Nursing Standard*. **4**(41), 27–30.

Webster, J. & Dewing, J. (2007) Growing a development strategy for community hospitals. *Practice Development in Health care*. **6**(2), 97–106.

Wright, J. & Titchen, A. (2003) Critical companionship part 2; using the framework. *Nursing Standard*. **18**(10), 33–38.

9. Being Culturally Sensitive in Development Work

Cheryle Moss and Jane Chittenden

Introduction

He Tangata, He Tangata, He Tangata ... Tis People, Tis People, Tis People

There is an important Maori saying that provides guidance for our daily practice: **tis people, tis people, tis people** reminds us of the centrality of people to any human endeavour. In this chapter, Jane and Cheryle draw on their experiences and reflections as they discuss the importance of being culturally sensitive in practice development (PD) work. However culturally sensitive practice progresses, valuing the centrality of people is a core value.

A group of staff in a small hospital in the North Island of New Zealand decided that PD would be helpful to them. Cheryle (an academic working in an university) and Jane (a Clinical Nurse Leader in the hospital) teamed up to support staff in developing their skills in PD. Since then a lot has passed between Jane and Cheryle as they shared, worked and gathered more experience in PD. In the beginning, they established a pattern of using reflective practice (Street, 1991; Johns & Freshwater, 1998; Taylor, 2000) and critical companionship (Titchen, 2001, 2003; Wright & Titchen, 2003) to explore PD and their clinical experiences (Manley, 1999; Manley & McCormack, 2003), to think about and consider the contextual landscapes of the work (Wenger, 1999; Wenger, et al., 2002), and to lift to consciousness their local theories (Smyth, 1986, 1987a; Tripp, 1987) of PD. Even though several years have passed and they work in different settings they still meet to discuss their work, practices and knowledge-in-action (Schön, 1983; Carr & Kemmis, 1983; Schulz, 2005). The ideas conveyed in this chapter were primarily derived from these systematic processes.

A place of beginning: Cultural sensitivity and development work

After a busy day working as PD facilitators Cheryle and Jane share their work over coffee. Jane begins:

As I work with people the more I realise that the effectiveness of what we do is highly connected to the ways in which we relate to and understand each other... we really cannot do development work without being in touch and touching the base of our culture.... Who we are and how we engage with others matters.... How can we take a journey together without acknowledging each other in the places we stand in the fullness of ourselves as history and as future?... How can we undertake the difficult work of attending to core issues without self-acknowledgement, respect in our place of connection, and commitment to our broader communities?

Responding to this, Cheryle muses:

Development work has as its heart person centredness, and cultural sensitivity is intrinsic to this.... In our practice communities what do we believe and what do we do in the expression of cultural sensitivity within person centredness?

And so, the two agree to watch and reflect on their practices and practice contexts and to share their insights with one another.

Positioning

Working as the people we are, doing what is at the heart of our work, in the context of our work and in relation to others, is something that we all experience in the workplace. Whether working as a practitioner at the bedside or using our skills as PD facilitator, we face the same opportunities and challenges in being 'person centred' (Binnie & Titchen, 1999; McCormack, 2004) and growing our 'cultures of effectiveness' (Manley, 2004). In a book extending theoretical and practical ideas about PD, it is important to address aspects of the inside work that takes place when we are seeking to grow, evolve and reform our working cultures.

In this chapter, we pose a series of questions and use our reflections to ponder the relationships and connections that are present between the practice of cultural sensitivity and the practice of PD. Whilst our reflective work is situated in New Zealand context and culture, we believe that the ideas expressed in this chapter hold applicability for international contexts and cultures.

Our processes

How does cultural sensitivity sit within PD and facilitation work?

We engaged in reflective conversations examining our own explanatory frameworks (Argyris & Schön, 1974; Schön, 1987) and theories of action (Smyth, 1986; Tripp, 1987; Smyth, 1987a, b; Street, 1991) and explored these ideas in relation to the literature and to our lived experiences in practice. In keeping with the tenets of theories-in-use, these have been extracted through critical reflection, conversation and exploration of what happens in practice with a view to articulating the important elements for facilitation of sustainable development (Argyris & Schön, 1974; Carr & Kemmis, 1983; Bernstein, 1985; Caputo, 1987; Bernstein, 1988; Street, 1992a, 1995; Manley, 2004).

Local theories are explicated by reflecting on action, and considering the underlying beliefs and reasoning and rationale that gave rise to the choices-in-action taken during the action (Smyth, 1987a; Street, 1992b). For example, if the practice beliefs are conscious when taking action, a practitioner in recounting this might say,

because I believe in 'a' and 'b', and I could see this situation needed something to make a difference. I could see that if I applied a bit of 'a' and a bit of 'b' then some of the underlying issues in the situation might be exposed and we might all gain some clarity around what was going on here. And so I did this and it did make a difference, although I could see if I did more of this...

This form of reflection exposes the local or practical theory that is in use during the action. This type of theory is helpful because it reveals how we make things work, and enables us to consider the principles of the explanatory framework underlying the actions and choices we make in particular contexts. This frees us up to apply these with discretion once again in other local situations requiring our actions.

A beginning point for our conversations in relation to cultural sensitivity was to consider a range of definitions.

Definition of cultural sensitivity

Many contemporary authors (Kim-Godwin et al., 2001; Purden, 2005; Wells, 2000; Burchum, 2002; Chrisman, 2007; Dreachslin, 2007; Leininger, 2007) note the importance of cultural competency in nursing. There are varying definitions and conceptualisations of cultural sensitivity; for instance, Kim-Godwin et al. (2001) describe cultural sensitivity as 'the affective aspect of care (respectful attitudes towards another's culture)' (p. 920), and Wells (2000) describes it as 'the integration of cultural knowledge and awareness into individual and institutional behaviour' (p. 191). Some authors place cultural sensitivity as a precursory element of cultural competence (Doyle et al., 1996), others as a step on a continuum in development of cultural competence (Rorie et al., 1996; Boyer, 2006), or alternatively as one of a number of aspects associated with culturally competent care (Gustafson, 2005; Jirwe et al., 2006). Some view cultural sensitivity as being the middle of a continuum between cultural awareness as a precursory step and cultural safety as a higher order process (e.g. Papps, 2005). Cultural satisfaction may be an outcome of culturally competent care, in that those on the receiving end of our actions and communications feel satisfied that they have been understood and that their cultural identity and meanings have been supported. Internationally, there are some interesting differences in discourses about what cultural competency is, how it is practised, and how we can continue to evolve our knowledge/knowing and cultures of practice (Jirwe et al., 2006).

In New Zealand, there has been strong investment in the development of cultural safety as a core cultural competency and practice (Ramsden, 1993, 2002; Wepa, 2003, 2005). Several iterations of the definition of cultural safety have highlighted different elements within this practice. A key feature of cultural safety is the intention that safe service is defined by those who receive the service, effective practice

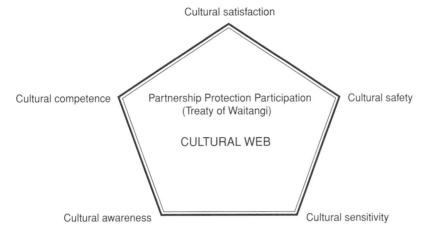

Figure 9.1   A depiction of our cultural web.

is determined by the family or the person receiving culturally safe interaction, and that the nurse or midwife undertaking service 'will have undertaken a process of reflection on his or her own cultural identity and will recognise the impact that his or her personal culture has on his or her own professional practice' (Nursing Council of New Zealand, 2002, p. 7).

The cultural competence and safety literature often cite cultural awareness and sensitivity as related behaviours. In this chapter, the differentiation between these aspects was less important than a broad exploration of what cultural competence/safety/sensitivity/awareness and satisfaction mean in relation to effective practice and PD work. The context of our interest is not to pursue academic differentiation between different elements or pathways towards cultural competence or cultural safety, rather to consider a broader framing for everyday practice. We opted to apply a general understanding from the cluster of terms and to reflect common-sense meanings of an everyday word 'sensitivity', which is applied and generated in the context of people within our work. To support this, we constructed our reflections as a web to encompass these cultural terms (see Figure 9.1).

Within the New Zealand context this also led us to consider the Treaty of Waitangi with the accompanying principles of 'partnership, protection, and participation' as central to our cultural understanding. The question we pose for readers is 'What specific community or indigenous cultures lie at the centre of your web?'

We engage with each aspect of the web as we practise and undertake development work. No one aspect is more important than another and various aspects form an intricate cultural web of interconnectedness. This is similar to the ideas of Lutzen (1997), who identifies the practical need for context-sensitive approaches to understanding ethical issues and the need for thoughtful consideration of practice in terms of context-specific meanings, interests and culture. Indeed, we consider that for culturally attuned practices to occur we use skills that draw on each aspect. Throughout the rest of this chapter we generally use the term cultural sensitivity to encompass all the meanings housed in the cultural web, although at times we may highlight particular aspects of the web such as cultural safety.

Cultural safety and cultural sensitivity

There are two interrelated forms of culture in considering the relevance and application of cultural sensitivity to development work. The first form of culture is drawn from the broader social context of communities, indigenous peoples, and culturally located group, and the second form of culture considered is workplace culture. As our critical discussion continued, we identified that

> *many of the meanings of cultural sensitivity work within health services are informed by, positioned, and reside firmly within the broader social culture of our communities.*

We recognise the cultural mandate that the Treaty of Waitangi holds within the social context of nursing practice and development work, highlighting the centrality of partnership, participation and protection in the expression and operationalisation of different values. These core values provide a critical means of working to achieve health and social equalities, and cultural reform.

In the context of an international audience, the general principles of partnership, participation and protection potentially hold influence as powerful values generally for working with cultural sensitivity in development work and are supported by McCormack et al. (2007a–2007d) in their systematic review of the evidence underpinning PD.

The New Zealand context and the Treaty of Waitangi

In Aotearoa, New Zealand, awareness of concepts of culture has been forged by the history of its people; the merging of Tangata whenua (indigenous) and those who colonised the country, most significantly being the British in the late 1700s and early 1800s (Orange, 1987; Kawharu, 1989; Yensen et al., 1989; Ritchie, 1995). The journey to New Zealand's present position of cultural identity and understanding is remarkable in that it has consisted of all the good and bad that history has to offer when two independently developed value systems meet. A key element in this has been a history of powerful colonisation by dominant British/European cultural values, and these values have generated long-term negative effects on the health and position of the Maori (Tangata whenua) within the New Zealand social landscape. While this landscape is of colonisation it also encompasses the processes of assimilation and integration. Contemporary cultural work within our country (within our political, social and health systems) is seeking to redress these power differentials within the expression of these two value systems. A significant cultural means for working with this (the honouring and expression of Maori and Pakeha value systems) as a goal in our everyday society in meaningful ways is drawn through the power of the Treaty of Waitangi constructs: partnership, protection and participation.

In 1988 Royal Commission on Social Policy (Ramsden, 2002) found that the principles of 'partnership, protection and participation' were inherent in the treaty and since then there has been concerted effort and overt commitment to bringing this into our formalised and non-formalised social practices as a nation. For instance, there is an overt commitment by government, and our social institutions through policy, law, education, health to find effective cultural practices that honour, affirm and grow our communities through Maori and Pakeha value systems. Within our daily cultures of living, similar valuing occurs.

As we think about this reality for us living and working in New Zealand, we wonder what traditions and national values influence others working in PD and to what extent there is a need to explore and make explicit the values, cultural locations and cultural mandates of broader society as we seek to grow our local cultures of effectiveness.

Cultural influences on context of nursing work within New Zealand

Following this line of argument, such cultural locations have implications for the work and practices of health professionals and affects the shape of their healthcare interests. Take, for example, the context of the treaty and its influence on nursing work within New Zealand. For nursing and health work partnership, protection and participation are core processes in the workplace; they inform the direction of health and workplace reform and they provide framing for human rights and practical means for working with consumers and colleagues alike. The cultural competency of health professionals invokes the active participation and living of the treaty towards better health and reducing health inequalities (Ministry of Health, 2000).

The bearing that 'Te Tiriti' and its identified principles have had on nursing and its professional work, and our cultural awareness, has been significant. Alongside this sits the ongoing poor health status of Maori and the need for those who work within health delivery systems to understand the webs of cultural meaning that contribute to health/poor health for Maori.

A key literature, construct and process for the systematisation of this within health arose in the late 1980s from nurses working with these issues (Ramsden, 1993, 2000, 2002). Known simply as 'cultural safety' this complex construct emerged from 'hui' (meetings) where nurses raised concerns regarding Maori health and the ways in which health service cultures arguably were systematically contributing to this plight through the domination of some health and cultural values over others. These hui critiqued the systemic culturally unsafe practices of health professionals and services, viewed these as culturally reproducing health inequalities, and identified that we needed 'culturally safe' practices, processes and practitioners (Wepa, 2005).

Since then cultural safety has become a core construct within nursing, and an evolving and influential idea within broader New Zealand society. In nursing, the construct of cultural safety has been theorised (Ramsden, 2002), studied and discussed (Wepa, 2005; McEldowney et al., 2006), incorporated into policy (Papps, 2005), incorporated into nursing education (Wepa, 2003; Richardson & Carryer, 2005), and exists as phenomena of clinical practice (Wepa, 2005; Simon, 2006).

Most importantly, cultural safety now sits as a core competency of nursing practice for initial registration and ongoing certification of professional practice. The history of 'cultural safety' learning in New Zealand nursing has been eventful and is reflective of the broader society's conflicting values and beliefs. In 1992 The Nursing Council of New Zealand approved guidelines that grounded the educational framework for learning of cultural safety, Te Tiriti of Waitangi and Maori health; as a part of this process it was expected that nurses will

- examine their own realities and the attitudes they bring to each new person they encounter in their practice;
- evaluate the impact that historical, political and social processes have on the health of all people; and
- demonstrate flexibility in their relationships with people who are different from themselves.

Ramsden, 1992

New Zealand based nurses do strive to exhibit a high level of cultural awareness. While definitions of cultural safety within New Zealand continue to evolve, there is in the nursing community a general agreement on the bases of the sought reforms, and understanding of the interlinkages between cultural sensitivity, cultural appropriateness, valuing cultural expressions and difference and the impact that these have on the ways in which we work, engage, and sustain health.

It is our belief that partnership, protection and participation are three core symbols that nurses, other health professionals and healthcare consumers respond to, relate to, expect as rights and as processes within everyday life and health services. These shape the degrees of interpretation of cultural safety and the ways in which we expect to interact with each other in health services generally, and in our interpersonal relationships specifically. In this sense partnership, protection and participation do have overt meaning within our overall interactions at local levels with each other in our everyday practice. It is also expressed as political and practical mechanisms to reform the ways in which we shape and define our health services, and comes with overall intent to reverse entrenched patterns of discrimination and health inequalities.

In relation to the subject of this chapter, these contextual influences translate into our practice as nurses, as development facilitators, and in the ways in which we express cultural sensitivity within person centredness in our interactions and are central to effective care. They inform our clinical processes and the cultural landscapes in which we work and live. We consider that the relational connection to land and the cultural traditions of broader society to who we are and the ways in which we deliver care, and achieve health, is an important place for reflexive engagement by health professionals. It holds some keys to our effectiveness in achieving appropriate culturally satisfying healthcare and to supporting people to optimise their health and well-being.

Culturally sensitive development work in New Zealand may be informed by constructs and practices of cultural safety, and situated in the values of the treaty (partnership, protection, participation); however, wider appreciation of these as everyday values in our work internationally will strengthen the effectiveness of healthcare services. Multiple authors (Binnie & Titchen, 1999; Dewing, 2004; McCormack, 2004; McCormack et al., 2004) have identified person centredness and facilitation as two central components of effective development work. We believe that for these components to be effective practitioners and practice developers need to achieve culturally attuned practices and use a cultural web of skills that includes understandings of cultural competence, safety, sensitivity, awareness and satisfaction.

Cultural sensitivity and the workplace

We spent some time thinking about the expression of culture in communities and in the workplace. We were struck by

> *the social power that we exert by virtue of the many cultural nuances that we carry and respond to in our daily practice.*

Some reflections on the power of cultural messages

Culture is expressed through what we value and believe and through our social and personal identity (Jirwe et al., 2006) as well as our interpersonal interactions, through our thoughts and language, our actions, customs and rituals. When we consider ourselves in the context of our workplace, it becomes clear that our culture is expressed through our social, workplace, professional and personal identities (Carr & Kemmis, 1983; Benhabib, 1992; Barlow, 1996). It is also clear that this exists in individuals, groups, and organisational contexts and that there is natural exchange between these cultural contexts (Street, 1989, 1992b). Consider a team working in a clinical unit on a day shift; the individual beliefs and values of the members of the team influence the ways in which they work with patients, each other, and others outside of the unit. Similarly, individuals shape and are shaped by the collective culture that exists between the members of the group and within the organisational context (Carr & Kemmis, 1983; Bernstein, 1988; Street, 1995).

Consider also the experiences we have of group and unit culture when we are working on each shift. It is as if the moods and expression of the workplace etch into our being as we get on with what has to be done. The cultural expectations influence the ways in which we work, how we manage our time, when and how we converse, and so on. The coalesced beliefs and practices are held symbolically and expressively and in our understanding of what is okay and what is not okay.

There is an interesting paradox that exists whereby the power of one can influence and shape the culture of others, while the power of others can influence and shape the culture of one. Returning to our example of the team on the day shift, the values, beliefs and self-expressed cultural meanings of how one nurse practises may influence the ways in which another nurse or indeed the team practise. Conversely the ways in which a group of nurses work may influence the individual's practices, beliefs and actions.

In an open and responsive cultural system this co-constructing process is in dynamic flux – the cultures within shift and move in response to need, contextual influences and conscious intent (Flax, 1990, 1999). A social challenge that we face is how to keep the emerging cultures open and diverse rather than progressing them towards closed, merged and unified states.

Some writers (Fay, 1977; Friere, 1985; Habermas, 1987) suggest that cultural health is best served when these co-constructing forces are in balance with each other, and that issues arise when a particular directional force becomes too strong, unified and exerts a dominating influence over the other forces. These powerful directional forces might be expressed in various cultural analyses as overarching, dominant, colonising or marginalising and result in diminution, disempowerment, disattribution of meaning and expression of values and beliefs held by others.

When such forces exist within culture, or when the dominant position within the culture is so overarching and powerful, we tend to see it as the 'norm'; it can subtly or not so subtly assert itself as 'the way things are done around here' (Bate, 1994). This entices those new to the culture to adopt these as their own cultural stances and cultural practices. The social repercussions of not conforming to these dominant views are often negative, effectively limiting the power of non-conformists. This form of dominance can be identified as enculturating individuals and groups and viewed as 'systemic' forces that sustain the dominant practices, meanings, and social constructions in the everyday life. These systemic forces may be helpful if they assist how we interact, communicate and evolve our knowledge, learning and practices, and our humanness as individuals and groups. However, if they alienate us from our true heart, ways of being in the world, and from the things that refresh us and help us to grow, then they carry a powerful negative impact. When working effectively, a systemic culture generates a sense of inclusion, belonging, fitting; however, when the culture is dominating, these same forces can be experienced as alienating, limiting, and diminishing.

Sometimes to those sitting comfortably within the systemic and dominant culture, there is a dulling of awareness that others may experience the same culture as alienating and diminutive. Those who experience the negative impact of the culture cannot understand why those sitting comfortably in the culture fail to see the power they are exercising over them and others. Thus cultural processes of 'being done to' and 'doing to' are not high in our shared consciousness.

It is in this territory that social agendas for change and for cultural reform find voice and focus. Work in furthering our understanding of how to achieve cultural sensitivity, awareness, competence, safety and satisfaction is borne through seeking to raise awareness about our practices so as to reduce our hegemony, and our diminishment of others. Reform in our cultural practices and ways of engaging with others involves a form of praxis, the active investment of ourselves towards our conscientisation of our hegemony and advancement in our cultural sensitivity as individuals and as groups (Habermas, 1978; Bernstein, 1988; Caputo, 1987).

Within nursing and healthcare this is important. Many aspects of our everyday work-life carry systemic cultural messages. These messages, on the one hand, can help us with our sense of purpose, sense of community and the ease with which we can express ourselves and act in the workplace; on the other hand, we can experience these messages as demanding, demeaning, and as robbing us of our freedoms and our sense of relevance.

In a general sense, patients and families often experience health service cultures, and the clinical attitudes of teams as dominating and alienating (e.g. Schim et al., 2006, 2007). For example, to survive the culture of being an in-patient and to achieve what is best for themselves, patients often have to 'learn the rules' and 'play the game'. It is as if any powerful expression of being a whole person with experience, attitude, self-knowing and self-styling must be configured through what it means to be a 'good patient' and to suit the health professionals and health services. The consequences associated with departing from this hold threatening risk to receiving the health services and care that is needed.

We know from our experience that we do not intentionally set out to rob patients of their individuality and autonomy, nor do we seek to impose behavioural sanctions on them as bargaining points for the delivery of care, yet that we do just this in our prevailing clinical cultures is painfully obvious. There is considerable evidence from literature to suggest that patients and staff who also have other forms of difference (e.g. race, age, disability) often experience these powerful agendas for conformity and hurdles to care in multiple forms. The challenge for cultural reform is how to achieve our work in practical ways while advancing the ease and sponsorship of our patients' ways of being in the world in their cultural wholeness. The literature on person centredness (McCormack, 2004) is helpful; the attention to processes and concepts that support patients in their 'being in relation', 'being in a social world', 'being in place' and 'being with self' while participating in the social world of healthcare services gives us some guidance as to what and how to achieve this state in the everyday life. These processes give definition to the construct of person centredness and gain additional potency when we acknowledge them as situated in relation to cultural safety/cultural sensitivity and to the practices of partnership, protection and participation. An important aspect of facilitation may be in finding ways to support others to advance cultural satisfaction and to achieve cultural reform through active investment in cultural work.

Cultural sensitivity and person centredness

As PD facilitators we discussed the need for us to meet and work with people as 'the people that they are' with 'the ways they express themselves in their practice'. This core requirement is supported by a recent conceptual analysis of theoretical frameworks concerning cultural competence (Jirrwe et al., 2006). We reflected upon the following notion: if cultural sensitivity is intrinsic to person centredness and involves the unfolding of selves and practices in relationship, there is a need to consider how it happens, what we do, and how we do it. We posed the following question for consideration:

How is cultural sensitivity present in our everyday practice?

Over several weeks we gathered reflections on our theories of action, as we explored practices observed in our clinical areas. We identified a number of practices we believe support cultural sensitivity within person centredness such as

○ establishing webs of meaning and connections,
○ noticing and understanding core symbols of cultural identity and self-expression,
○ generating and strengthening in-tune-ness and
○ connecting with the person in relation to the symbols of the practice world.

Jane begins her discussion with Cheryle in which she poses some key critical questions (in bold) her observations have raised for her:

> *Last week a new member of staff commenced work in our unit and I found myself wondering* **'how do we as a team come to know this person?'** *I could see the team working hard to meet and greet Jean and help her to feel comfortable, and I could see Jean working just as hard to settle in, find out about the staff and to find out about the ways in which we work. What struck me was that because Jean was the newcomer to the unit, she was doing a lot more finding out about us and our practices than what we were doing of her. I guess a critical question for me as a member of the group is* **'how do we as a team make ourselves more open to learning about the history and practices of someone joining the team?**
> *... while I do think the team will gather this from Jean over time, I suspect that this will not happen fully until she has proved herself to the group. So another question I have is* **'what are messages that we send about acceptability – what makes a newcomer to the staff group acceptable to us as a group?'** *I wonder how much messages and gradations of acceptability permeate our culture and processes as a clinical team.*
>
> *I realised that because I was watching for signs of person centredness and cultural sensitivity I was taking more notice of our everyday practice than normally would and I was seeing our actions as a group in a different light. I know that Jean comes to unit with lots of experience, and that she has completed advanced study in this area of practice and that she comes to our unit with a reputation for being forthright and highly motivated. A question for me is* **'how will we as a team come to know and draw on Jean's skills and knowledge, and how will we adapt our group processes to value her personal style of interaction and engagement?'**

Establishing webs of meaning and connections

These observations speak to us of the subtlety of workplace and team cultures, and of the unspoken rules that we have for engagement. What struck us about this scenario was the movement and 'meaning-making' that need to go on between the members of the group and Jean to establish strong and reasonable threads of connection. To be culturally healthy they need to be reasonably reflective of the positions, culture, self-meanings that they each subscribe to. Cultural difficulties will arise if those meanings become distorted, or if the traffic to meaning and understanding becomes strongly unidirectional. It is as if both parties need to be free to be themselves and feel an openness of acceptance for this. We reflected that to be free to be themselves they needed to avoid making assumptions 'about' each other in order to enable them to be open 'with' each other through listening, acceptance and discovery.

Reflecting on this as facilitative practice and as a process of cultural sensitivity within person centredness opens the importance of remembering that 'a person's culture is their personal property, invalidate it and you invalidate the person' (Ritchie, 1995, p. 104). While Ritchie was concerned with managing the process of communication as a bicultural process, he alerts us to the essential integration of self-identity and cultural meaning. The process of opening oneself to the encounter and to the experience of other within the fullness of our cultural identities is, we believe, a significant element in the process.

Similar distinction was made by Buber (1958), in his exploration of I–thou and I–it relationships, and by nurse humanistic theorists Paterson and Zderad (1976). It is as though we philosophically and practically commit to the other as an open encounter. In some ways this is like meditative clearing. The space of readiness is actively prepared. As the encounter occurs what we are seeking is for the natural webs of meaning and interconnection to surface between us, and once these begin to surface the art is one of strengthening the expression of the other while not holding back on the authenticity of self (Ricoeur, 1992).

Noticing and understanding core symbols of cultural identity and self-expression

The importance of establishing genuine webs of meaning and connections is not about converting newcomers like Jean to the extant culture, but rather it involves a genuine opening and investment in creating the space for new and possibly divergent understandings to be present and legitimate. This process can be supported by attention to the practice of 'noticing and understanding core symbols of cultural identity and self-expression' that are central to the person. For example with patients this may involve seeking to understand wider expressions of self than those that are related to the socially constructed roles of patient and ill person.

This is achieved not only by direct questioning but also in the everyday taking an interest in hearing what is present and being said, noticing how things are expressed and checking out and responding positively to the person's preferred ways of thinking and acting. Awareness of diversity, awareness of ourselves, and awareness of others (Purnell & Paulanka, 2003; Richardson & Carryer, 2005; Wepa, 2005; Jirrwe et al., 2006) will help our practice and skills. In the realities of our everyday work it does not matter whether we start from the big picture of someone's history, cultural and personal map then considering them within the local context, or whether we work from the particular circumstances and expressions in the here and now, seeking then to understand what lies behind the person. The important point is that we are active in seeking to create opportunities for this to occur.

Challenges arise when the assumptions we make about others remain unchecked and unchallenged. Making assumptions prevents what McCormack (2004) described as 'being with self', that is, being comfortable in expressing one's own values. Insensitive communication with others may lead to trivialising or minimising the importance of another's values and beliefs and projecting our assumed understandings in inappropriate ways. The knowing we have of people does need to not hold them and restrict them in a place or at a particular level of maturity; people must be trusted to grow and change, and culturally entrenched or insensitive views of them should not restrict the possibility of this. It is therefore important as we seek to work in culturally sensitive ways that we generate sufficient energy to opening our awareness to the complexities and various perspectives that may be present in a situation, and sufficient openness to the sense of future possibilities that may evolve in people and be advanced through our person centredness and skills in facilitation.

Generating and strengthening in-tune-ness

To facilitate robust cultures there is the need to value engagement and to grow successful practices that generate and strengthen 'in-tune-ness' and establish common ground (Walsh et al., 2005). A powerful cultural pattern that we often encounter with teams is the habit of finding the place that divides and separates us rather than finding or generating the common area that brings us together. Take, for example, wards that fight and compete with each other, consider the ways in which their differences are often used to 'block' rather than facilitate development and evolution. Valuing complexity and diversity is important, but within this it is nearly always possible to find or to create common ground for working in and with partnerships. Once the common ground is identified, the art of facilitation is to build on this by strengthening the in-tune-ness that sits between people. The cost of failing to work in this way is high (Billett, 2004; Clarke, 2006; Chrisman, 2007). Failure to engage with this practice may leave us responding primarily to role-based images or to organisational discourses rather than in recognition of real people (Dreachslin, 2007).

Consider the ways in which people in the workplace may be 'othered' by roles or workplace positions, or by performing organisational duties (Street, 1992b; Carradice & Round, 2004; Wilson et al., 2005; Clarke, 2006). An example of this that we encounter is the common expression of health professionals that management 'does not care'. This sustains stereotypes, holds those in 'management' roles in ransom to the discourse, and sustains health professionals in a place of subjugation and of difference. The challenge is to understand the mechanisms in culture that reinforce the divides and to use our knowledge of cultural sensitivity, person centredness and facilitation to reform the practice of 'othering' and to advance points of genuine connection and in-tune-ness. Similar illustrations apply to our ways of responding to 'patient culture' (Labonte et al., 2005; Kleiman, 2006; Schim et al., 2006). It may be helpful to explore these relationships for presence of practices that support 'othering' and subjugation, and to consider how these could be reformed through practices that support cultural safety, cultural satisfaction and more productive partnerships.

Connecting with the person in relation to the symbols of the practice world

Supporting a person's connections and fit with the practice world is key to cultural sensitivity using a person-centred approach. Take, for example, working with Jean: it will be important that she is able to contribute her personality, knowledge and skills as a full-fledged member of the team. Facilitating this will require an investment in building Jean's connections and groundedness in the symbols of the practice world. For example, being able to work with the cultural and practice nuances, cultural ground rules and being able to contribute in and to the evolution of the practice culture will require attention to making explicit what is important and what is needed for the future. Failure to work at this is likely to result in less intertwining and investment in the future of the team or clinical developments (Billett & Somerville, 2004; Larsen et al., 2005). Person centredness needs to be realised in a way that gives primacy to the person. If we give greater value to external or group norms and respond to these at the cost of individual respectfulness and understanding, we can progress the tyranny of subjugating the person to dominant cultural standpoints (Liaschenko, 1999).

Cultural activism from the team is required as they hold the keys and functioning of opening the extant culture to new possibilities and to create responsiveness to Jean. As brokers of the dominant culture they need to protect Jean from being 'colonised' by them, to create opportunities for her participation and influence on their practice worlds, and to forge genuine and productive partnerships with her as they co-create a future. Anything less than this is likely to result in the reproduction of hegemonic and counter-hegemonic practices within the team. If the team are person centred and have good facilitation skills, this process of cultural brokerage is likely to occur quite comfortably and naturally. However, if the team have less skill in this area, then working with their level of cultural awareness and cultural sensitivity in relation to their workplace practices and culture may become an important development agenda.

Concluding discussion

We have shared our reflections, observations and local theories about supporting culturally sensitive practices in development work. We have argued by illustration the importance of considerations of the cultural locations and mandates of broader society as we engage in development work, and that these may have significant implications for the work and practices of health professionals. For instance, such mandates may require support and targeted evolution of healthcare practices in communities in ways that support dominant social cultures, or conversely the presence of significant social and cultural inequities may require health professionals to engage in specific actions that will sustain cultural reform. Skills in cultural sensitivity are needed to achieve such goals. We argued that cultural sensitivity can and should be embedded within person-centred practices and is a core competence associated with facilitation. The principles of partnership, participation and protection were identified as important cultural values in supporting cultural safety and culturally sensitive practices.

These ideas were developed in a wider discussion about the power of cultural messages and the importance of our active participation in the brokerage of cultural forces in our communities, in our workplaces and with people. We argued the centrality of our conscientisation of cultural hegemony and of our own participation in it as means by which we need to engage in active cultural reform and development. It is here that active development work around cultural sensitivity finds the heart of commitment and the spirit of justice.

These debates and ideas were extended to consideration of culture in the workplace. We argued that the principles of cultural sensitivity applied equally well to this context of culture. We shared our observations and theorising about cultural sensitivity in development work, where four sets of practices ('establishing webs of meaning and connections', 'noticing and understanding core symbols of cultural identity and self-expression', 'generating and strengthening in-tune-ness' and 'connecting with the person in relation to the symbols of the practice world') appear to support the facilitation of others in culture. These ideas were illustrated by drawing on situations in everyday practice.

This chapter makes it clear that contemporary writing around the construct of cultural sensitivity is strong and diverse, and that it is related to concepts such as cultural awareness, safety, competence and satisfaction. Culturally sensitive practice in development work may be best informed by considering these as an interrelated web of ideas/constructs that we can draw on to establish stronger practice and cultural reforms.

There is a need for more dialogue and investigation of this area of development work, with observational studies, theoretical work and explorations in relation to the cultural web being undertaken. Further work is needed into the relationship of person centredness and facilitation in the achievement of cultural sensitivity within healthcare practice, workplaces and in our communities.

PD work has at its heart working in context with people for more effective cultures and health outcomes. Cultural sensitivity along with its concomitant companions, cultural awareness, safety, competence and satisfaction are central ingredients in this mix. We encourage you to share your cultural stories, how you are achieving cultural reform, and what supports the attainment of cultural sensitivity in development work.

References

Argyris, C. & Schön, D. (1974) *Theory in Practice: Increasing Professional Effectiveness.* Jossey-Bass, San Francisco.

Barlow, C. (1996) *Tikana Whakaaro: Key Concepts in Maori Culture.* Oxford University Press, Auckland.

Bate, P. (1994) *Strategies for Cultural Change.* Butterworth-Heinemann, Oxford.

Benhabib, S. (1992) *Situating the Self: Gender, Community and Postmodernism in Contemporary Ethics.* Routledge, New York.

Bernstein, R.J. (1985) From hermeneutics to praxis. In: *Hermeneutics and Praxis* (ed R. Hollinger), pp. 272–296. University of Notre Dame Press, Notre Dame, IN.

Bernstein, R.J. (1988) *Beyond Objectivism and Realism: Science, Hermeneutics and Praxis.* University of Pennsylvania Press, Philadelphia.

Billett, S. (2004) Workplace participatory practices: Conceptualising workplaces as learning environments. *The Journal of Workplace Learning.* **16**(6), 312–324.

Billett, S. & Somerville, M. (2004) Transformations at work: Identity and learning. *Studies in Continuing Education.* **26**(2), 309–326.

Binnie, A. & Titchen, A. (1999) *Freedom to Practise: The Development of Patient-Centred Nursing.* Butterworth-Heinemann, Oxford.

Boyer, D. (2006) Cultural competence at the bedside. *The Pennsylvania Nurse.* December, 18–19.

Buber, M. (1958) *I and Thou* (Trans. Ronald Gregor Smith). Charles Scribner & Sons, New York.

Burchum, J.L.R. (2002) Cultural competence: An evolutionary perspective. *Nursing Forum.* **37**(4), 5–15.

Caputo, J.D. (ed) (1987) *Radical Hermeneutics: Deconstruction, Repetition and the Hermeneutic Project.* Indiana University Press, Bloomington.

Carr, W. & Kemmis, S. (1983) *Becoming Critical: Knowing Through Action Research.* Deakin University Press, Geelong.

Carradice, A. & Round, D. (2004) The reality of practice development for nurses working in an inpatient service for people with severe and enduring mental health problems. *Journal of Psychiatric and Mental Health Nursing.* **11**, 731–737.

Chrisman, N.J. (2007) Extending cultural competence through systems change: Academic, hospital and community partnerships. *Journal of Transcultural Nursing.* **18**(Suppl 1), 68S–76S.

Clarke, S.P. (2006) Organisational climate and culture factors. *Annual Review of Nursing Research.* **24**, 255–272.

Dewing, J. (2004) Concerns relating to the application of frameworks to promote person-centredness in nursing with older people. *International Journal of Older People Nursing.* **13**(3a), 39–44.

Doyle, E.I., Liu, Y. & Anacona, L. (1996) Cultural competence development in university health education classes. *Journal of Health Education.* **27**(4), 206–212.

Dreachslin, J.L. (2007) Diversity management and cultural competence: Research, practice and the business case. *Journal of Healthcare Management.* **52**(2), 79–86.

Fay, B. (1977) *Social Theory and Political Practice.* Allen & Unwin, London.

Flax, J. (1990) *Thinking Fragments: Psychoanalysis, Feminism and Postmodernism in the Contemporary West.* University of California, Berkeley, CA.

Flax, J. (1999) *The American Dream in Black and White: The Clarence Thomas Hearings.* Cornell University Press, New York.

Freire, P. (1985) *The Politics of Education: Culture, Power and Liberation.* Bergin & Garvey, South Hadley, MT.

Gustafson, D.L. (2005) Transcultural nursing theory from a critical cultural perspective. *Advances in Nursing Science.* **28**(1), 2–16.

Jirwe, M., Gerrish, K. & Emami, A. (2006) The theoretical framework of cultural competence. *The Journal of Multicultural Nursing and Health.* **12**(3), 6–16.

Johns, C. & Freshwater, D. (eds) (1998) *Transforming Nursing Through Reflective Practice.* Blackwell Science, Oxford.

Habermas, J. (1978) *Knowledge and Human Interests* (Trans. J.J. Shapiro), 2nd edn. Beacon, Boston.

Habermas, J. (1987) *The Theory of Communicative Action* (Trans. T. McCarthy), 2nd edn, Vols I & II. Beacon, Boston.

Kawharu, I.H. (1989) *Waitangi: Maori and Pakeha Perspectives of the Treaty of Waitangi.* Oxford University Press, Oxford.

Kim-Godwin, Y.S., Clarke, P.N. & Barton, L. (2001) A model for the delivery of culturally competent community care. *Journal of Advanced Nursing.* **35**(6), 918–925.

Kleiman, S. (2006) Discovering cultural aspects of nurse-patient relationships. *Journal of Cultural Diversity.* **13**(2), 83–86.

Labonte, R., Polanyi, M., Muhajarine, N., McIntosh, T. & Williams, A. (2005) Beyond the divides: Towards critical population health research. *Critical Public Health.* **15**(1), 5–17.

Larsen, J.A., Maundrill, R., Morgan, J. & Mouland, L. (2005) Practice development facilitation: An integrated and strategic approach. *Practice Development in Health Care.* **4**(3), 142–149.

Leininger, M. (2007) Theoretical questions and concerns: Response from the theory of culture care diversity and universality perspective. *Nursing Science Quarterly.* **20**(1), 9–15.

Liaschenko, J. (1999) Can justice co-exist with the supremacy of personal values in nursing practice? *Western Journal of Nursing Research.* **21**(1), 35–50.

Lutzen, K. (1997) Nursing ethics into the next millennium: A context sensitive approach for nursing ethics. *Nursing Ethics.* **4**(3), 218–226.

Manley, K. (1999) Developing a culture for empowerment. *Nursing in Critical Care.* **4**(2), 57–58.

Manley, K. (2004) Transformational culture: A culture of effectiveness. In: *Practice Development in Nursing* (eds B. McCormack, K. Manley & R. Garbett), pp. 51–82. Blackwell, Oxford.

Manley, K. & McCormack, B. (2003) Practice development: Purpose, methodology, facilitation & evaluation. *Nursing in Critical Care.* **8**(1), 22–29.

McCormack, B. (2004) Person-centredness in gerontological nursing: An overview of the literature. *International Journal of Older People Nursing.* **13**(3a), 31–38.

McCormack, B., Manley, K. & Garbett, R. (2004) *Practice Development in Nursing.* Blackwell, Oxford.

McCormack, B., Wright, J., Dewar, B., Harvey, G., & Ballantine, K. (2007a) A realist synthesis of evidence relating to practice development: Methodology and methods. *Practice Development in Health Care.* **6**(1), 5–24.

McCormack, B., Wright, J., Dewar, B., Harvey, G., & Ballantine, K. (2007b) A realist synthesis of evidence relating to practice development: Findings from the literature analysis. *Practice Development in Health Care.* **6**(1), 25–55.

McCormack, B., Wright, J., Dewar, B., Harvey, G., & Ballantine, K. (2007c) A realist synthesis of evidence relating to practice development: Findings from telephone interviews and synthesis of the data. *Practice Development in Health Care.* **6**(1), 56–75.

McCormack, B., Wright, J., Dewar, B., Harvey, G., & Ballantine, K. (2007d) A realist synthesis of evidence relating to practice development: Recommendations. *Practice Development in Health Care.* **6**(1), 76–80.

McEldowney, R., Richardson, F., Turia, D., Laracy, K., Scott, W. & McDonald, S. (2006) *Opening Our Eyes – Shifting Our Thinking: The Process of Teaching and Learning About Reflection in Cultural Safety Education and Practice: An Evaluation Study.* Victoria University of Wellington & Whitireia Community Polytechnic, Wellington.

Ministry of Health (2000) *The New Zealand Health Strategy.* Ministry of Health, Wellington.

Nursing Council of New Zealand (2002) *Guidelines for Cultural Safety, The Treaty of Waitangi, and Maori Health in Nursing and Midwifery Education and Practice*. Nursing Council of New Zealand, Wellington.

Orange, C. (1987) *The Treaty of Waitangi*. Allen & Unwin, Wellington.

Papps, E. (2005) Cultural safety: Daring to be different. In: *Cultural Safety in Aotearoa New Zealand* (ed D. Wepa), pp. 20–28. Pearson, Auckland.

Paterson, J.G. & Zderad, L.T. (1976) *Humanistic Nursing*. Wiley, New York.

Purden, M. (May 2005) Cultural considerations in interprofessional education and practice. *Journal of Interprofessional Care*. **19**(Suppl 1), 224–234.

Purnell, L.D. & Paulanka, B.J. (2003) *Transcultural Health Care: A Culturally Competent Approach*. F.A. Davis, Philadelphia.

Ramsden, I. (1992) *Kawa Whakaruruhau: Guidelines for Nursing and Midwifery Education*. Nursing Council of New Zealand, Wellington.

Ramsden, I. (1993) Cultural safety in nursing education in Aotearoa (New Zealand). *Nursing Praxis in New Zealand*. **8**(3), 4–10.

Ramsden, I. (2000) Cultural safety/Kawa whakaruruhau ten years on: A personal overview. *Nursing Praxis in New Zealand*. **15**(1), 4–12.

Ramsden, I. (2002) Cultural safety and nursing education in Aotearoa and Te Waipounamu. Unpublished PhD Thesis, Victoria University of Wellington, Wellington.

Richardson, F. & Carryer, J. (2005) Teaching cultural safety in a New Zealand nursing education program. *Journal of Nursing Education*. **44**(5), 201–208.

Ricoeur, P. (1992) *Oneself as Another* (Trans. K. Blamey). University of Chicago Press, Chicago.

Ritchie, J. (1995) *Becoming Bicultural*. Huia, Wellington.

Rorie, J.L., Payne, L.L. & Banger, M.K. (1996) Primary health care for women: Cultural competence in primary care services. *Journal of Nurse-Midwifery*. **41**, 92–100.

Royal Commission on Social Policy (1988) *The Treaty of Waitangi and Social Policy*. Royal Commission on Social Policy, Wellington.

Schim, S.M., Doorenbos, A., Benkert, R. & Miller, J. (2007) Culturally congruent care: Putting the puzzle together. *Journal of Transcultural Nursing*. **18**(2), 103–110.

Schim, S.M., Doorenbos, A.Z. & Borse, N.N. (2006) Cultural competence among hospice nurses. *Journal of Hospice and Palliative Nursing*. **8**(5), 302–309.

Schön, D.A. (1983) *The Reflective Practitioner: How Professionals Think in Action*. Basic Books, San Francisco.

Schön, D.A. (1987) *Educating the Reflective Practitioner*. Jossey-Bass, London.

Schulz, K. (2005) Learning in complex organisations as practicing and reflecting: A model development and application from a theory of practice perspective. *Journal of Workplace Learning*. **17**(8), 493–507.

Simon, V. (2006) Characterising Maori nursing practice. In: *Advances in Indigenous Health Care: Building Capacity Through Cultural Safety in Australia, New Zealand and North America* (eds E. Willis, V. Smye & M. Rameka), Vol 5, pp. 203–213. eContent, Sydney.

Smyth, W.J. (1986) *Reflection-in-Action*. Deakin University Press, Geelong.

Smyth, W.J. (1987a) *Teachers' Theories of Action (ETL 825)*. Deakin University Press, Geelong.

Smyth, W.J. (1987b) *A Rationale for Teachers' Critical Pedagogy: A Handbook*. Deakin University Press, Geelong.

Street, A. (1989) Thinking, acting, reflecting: A critical ethnography of clinical nursing practice. Unpublished PhD Thesis, Deakin University, Geelong, Victoria.

Street, A. (1991) *From Image to Action: Reflection in Nursing Practice*. Deakin University Press, Geelong.

Street, A. (1992a) *Inside Nursing: A Critical Ethnography of Clinical Nursing Practice*. State University of New York, Albany.

Street, A. (1992b) *Cultural Practices in Nursing*. Deakin University Press, Geelong.

Street, A. (1995) *Nursing Replay: Researching Nursing Culture Together*. Churchill-Livingstone, Melbourne.

Taylor, B.J. (2000) *Reflective Practice: A Guide for Nurses and Midwives*. Allen & Unwin, St Leonards.

Titchen, A. (2001) Critical companionship: A conceptual framework for developing expertise. In: *Practice Knowledge and Expertise in the Health Professions* (eds J. Higgs & A. Titchen), pp. 80–90. Butterworth-Heinemann, Oxford.

Titchen, A. (2003) Critical companionship: Part 1 (A framework for facilitating learning from experience). *Nursing Standard*. **18**(9), 33–40.

Tripp, D.H. (1987) *Theorising Practice: The Teachers' Professional Journal*. Deakin University Press, Geelong.

Walsh, K., Lawless, J., Moss, C. & Allbon, C. (2005) The development of an engagement tool for practice development. *Practice Development in Health Care*. **4**(3), 124–130.

Wells, M.I. (2000) Beyond cultural competence: A model for individual and institutional cultural development. *Journal of Community Health Nursing*. **17**(4), 189–199.

Wenger, E. (1999) *Communities of Practice: Learning, Meaning, and Identity*. Cambridge University Press, Cambridge.

Wenger, E., McDermott, R. & Snyder, W.M. (2002) *Cultivating Communities of Practice*. Harvard Business School Press, Boston.

Wepa, D. (2003) An exploration of the experiences of cultural safety educators in New Zealand: An action research approach. *Journal of Transcultural Nursing*. **14**(4), 339–348.

Wepa, D. (2005) *Cultural Safety in Aotearoa New Zealand*. Pearson, Auckland.

Wilson, V.J., McCormack, B.G. & Ives, G. (2005) Understanding the workplace culture of a special care nursery. *Journal of Advanced Nursing*. **50**(1), 27–38.

Wright, J. & Titchen, A. (2003) Critical companionship, Part 2: Using the framework. *Nursing Standard*. **18**(10), 33–38.

Yensen, H., Hague, K., McCreanor, T., Kelsey, J., Nairn, M. & Williams, D. (1989) *Honouring the Treaty: An Introduction for Pakeha to the Treaty of Waitangi*. Penguin, Auckland.

10. *Person-Centred Outcomes and Cultural Change*

Brendan McCormack, Tanya McCance, Paul Slater, Joanna McCormick, Charlotte McArdle and Jan Dewing

Introduction

The concept of 'person centredness' has become established in approaches to the delivery of healthcare and particularly within nursing. In the United Kingdom, person centredness is embedded in many policy initiatives (e.g. The National Service Framework for Older People [DoH 2001]). In a comprehensive review of the literature, McCormack (2004) identified 110 papers that related to aspects of person-centred practice, the majority of which originated from the United Kingdom. Whilst it appears that developments in person-centred nursing theory and practice are predominantly taking place in a UK context, comparisons can be drawn with other international nursing perspectives, such as the 'Quality Health Outcomes Model' (Mitchell et al., 1998; Radwin & Fawcett, 2002), the 'Synergy Model' (Curley, 1998) and a model of 'family-centred care' (Wilson, 2005a, 2005b).

Recent research into person centredness has attempted to clarify the meaning of the term (e.g. McCormack, 2004), explore the implications of the term in practice (Dewing, 2004) and determine the cultural and contextual challenges to implementing a person-centred approach (Binnie & Titchen, 1999). Evidence from Binnie and Titchen's research suggested that adopting this approach to nursing provides more holistic care. In addition, it may increase patient satisfaction with the level of care, reduce anxiety levels among nurses in the long term, and promote team working among staff. Binnie and Titchen (1999), however, did not test these assertions and were therefore unable to provide evidence of the suggested relationships.

Existing evidence is consistent with the view that being person centred requires the formation of therapeutic relationships between professionals, patients and others significant to them in their lives and that these relationships are built on mutual trust, understanding and a sharing of collective knowledge (Nolan et al., 2004; McCormack, 2001, 2004; Dewing, 2004; Binnie & Titchen, 1999). This evidence is also consistent with previous nursing literature on therapeutic caring where the concept of 'person' is central (for example, Leininger's theory of culture care [1988] Watson's theory of human caring [1985], Boykin and Schoenhofer's theory of nursing as caring [1993], and Roach's conceptualisation of caring relationships [1987]). McCance et al. (1999) further demonstrated the relationship between person centredness and caring by illustrating the centrality of concepts that are common to both, such as relationships, values, caring processes and the environment of care (context). This synergistic relationship between caring and person centredness was reinforced by Dewing (2004), who concluded that the use of humanistic caring frameworks in nursing practice enables person centredness to be realised.

Few studies, however, have attempted to evaluate the relationship between a person-centred approach to nursing and the resulting outcomes for patients and nurses. Whilst a number of conceptual frameworks for person-centred practice exist (e.g. Binnie & Titchen, 1999; McCormack, 2001, 2003, 2004) none of these have been used to evaluate the caring outcomes that may arise as a result of developing person-centred nursing. The project reported in this chapter aimed to promote effective person-centred nursing (PCN) within a framework for caring, thus building on previous work undertaken by McCormack (2001, 2003) and McCance (2003).

Methodology

The overall aim of the project was to evaluate the effectiveness of PCN when introduced into a range of clinical areas within an acute hospital setting. More specifically, three research questions were identified:

1. Does PCN make a difference to
   (a) patients' perceptions of caring?
   (b) nurses' perceptions of caring?
2. Does PCN make a difference to
   (a) patient outcomes of (i) satisfaction with care and (ii) involvement in care?
   (b) nurses' outcomes of (i) job satisfaction, (ii) morale, (iii) sickness and absenteeism, (iv) stress and (v) retention?
3. What are the experiences of the journey towards PCN?

A quasi-experimental design was adopted, with a qualitative element interwoven throughout in order to address the research questions. The research design comprised three major components:

- **A theoretical framework**, derived from previous conceptual frameworks developed by McCormack (2001, 2003) McCance et al. (2001) and McCance (2003).
- **A practice development (PD) intervention** based on a model developed by Garbett and McCormack (2002).
- **Measurement tools/evaluative approaches** used to evaluate differences over time on a range of dependent variables as a result of the PD intervention, and to map the experiences of participants during the course of their journey.

Sampling

A total of 10 wards and departments (8 participating sites and 2 control wards) were selected for participation in the study based on a broad set of inclusion criteria including effective leadership, nurse management support, evidence of some development work that focused on person centredness, and voluntary participation. Whilst the project team were keen to include a range of areas covering a variety of specialties within the hospital, all wards and departments were given an equal opportunity to become involved in the project. Wards and departments declaring an interest in participating were asked to demonstrate how they met the inclusion criteria. The participating areas included intensive care unit, sexual health clinic, older people rehabilitation ward, paediatric infectious diseases ward, medical admissions unit, general surgery ward, cardiology ward, and an operating room. The control groups were selected for inclusion based on a paired–matched technique as best as possible with clinical settings in the intervention group. The control groups comprised two (surgical and paediatric) clinical settings not involved in the project and allowed for the comparison of findings at the pre- and post-intervention stage.

Data collection methods

Several outcome measures were identified as dependent variables, which could be influenced by the PD intervention. These included job satisfaction, stress, staff retention, patients' satisfaction with care, patients' involvement in care, and nurses' and patients' perception of caring. The person-centred nursing index (PCNI) was generated from an amalgamation of key findings from an extensive literature review, focus groups and a pilot study. Its psychometric properties were tested and strong evidence of its validity and reliability was established (Slater, 2006; Watson et al., 2001). The PCNI was administered twice over a short space of time, prior to the intervention phase, in order to obtain an accurate baseline measure. Once the intervention stage had commenced, questionnaires were re-administered at four specific points over the 2-year intervention period.

Qualitative data were intertwined with the quantitative data to provide a comprehensive picture of the full impact of the intervention. The qualitative data were collected across all clinical settings in tandem with each of the questionnaire distribution time points. At each of the data collection points, nurses engaged in the collection of 2 hours of naturally occurring conversations between themselves, their peers and patients. This was done using electronic voice recorders and resulted in more than 200 hours of naturally occurring conversations being collected for analysis. Nurses were instructed in how to seek consent, and use of the electronic voice recorders. The data was transcribed and prepared for analysis using the software package Nvivo 2. Manual analysis was also used alongside the software package.

In addition to the questionnaire and naturally occurring conversation data, facilitators maintained field notes throughout the intervention period, documenting issues of note to inform development decisions, key milestones, particular successes/challenges and concerns regarding processes. These data were discussed at project team meetings and learning sets and used to inform decisions in subsequent stages of project planning.

Table 10.1 Response rates

Time point	Intervention group	Control group
Time 1	122 (76%)	35 (83%)
Time 2	121 (75%)	N/A
Time 3	67 (42%)	N/A
Time 4	90 (56%)	N/A
Time 5	86 (54%)	19 (45%)

The response rate

Table 10.1 illustrates the response rate of the participating and control sites. The control groups had a consistently lower response rate than the participating sites and only at data collection point 3 did the participating sites' response rate drop below 50%. This represents a consistently high response rate over the period of the study. Low response rates with the qualitative data at some time points meant that comparisons within some of the intervention groups at the same time points or across time points became non-viable.

Data analysis procedures

All quantitative findings were calculated using the software package SPSS 11.5. This was in two distinct areas: intervention versus control group and intervention group time analysis. The control groups were assessed at the pre- and post-intervention time points to compare with changes in the intervention groups as a result of the person-centred intervention. Comparisons of scores across the pre- and post-intervention stages show the direction and extent of change across the variables. Comparisons can be drawn between the intervention and control group. Two-tailed independent t-tests were used to assess the significance of the change in scoring for both the intervention and control group. Significant differences in scoring across the two time points were highlighted. Analysis of variance scores were used to compare the mean differences across the five time points of the intervention sample. This allowed for the comparison of construct mean scores sequentially. This analysis was at a group mean level rather than individually as not all respondents completed the PCNI at all five time points. Significant differences in scoring are highlighted where relevant.

The qualitative data produced a large number of lengthy texts. Because of this and that the broader based interests of person-centred practice were of more importance than the minutiae of conversation, it was decided to utilise a Discourse Analysis approach for data analysis (Wetherell et al., 2001). The PCN theoretical framework (see McCormack & McCance [2006] and an overview of the framework is provided in the next section) was utilised as a framework for analysis and reporting of data. After preparation, transcripts were read through several times. The episodes of conversation were then selected within each transcript. The episode was analysed for 'common-sense' meanings in relation to the four constructs of the PCN theoretical framework (Figure 10.1). This was followed by interpretation and

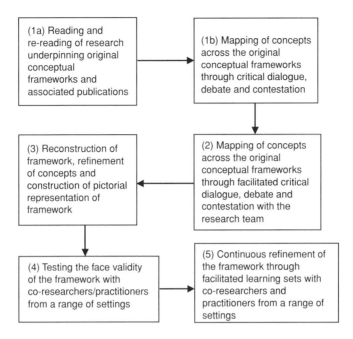

Figure 10.1   Processes used to develop the PCN framework.

meaning-making; specifically directed at making a decision about what type of conversation was going on as a whole, some idea of the context and how the parts of the conversation interconnected within PCN. Comparative analysis between different conversational episodes was undertaken, which led to 'collections' of both similar and different conversational content and processes for each nurse, between nurses in the same clinical area within the same and consecutive time lines and between nurses in different areas and over time. Descriptive reports for each time line of the project were prepared, which acted as the audit trail for the individual time points. A final summary report explored changes over the span of the project.

Theoretical framework for person-centred nursing[1]

The PCN theoretical framework (McCormack & McCance, 2006) originates from the combination of two existing conceptual frameworks derived from empirical studies that have their foundations in nursing practice (McCormack, 2003; McCance, 2003). McCance developed a conceptual framework to describe caring in nursing (as perceived by nurses and patients), whereas McCormack's conceptual framework focused on person-centred practice with older people derived from

---

[1] This section is derived from a previous publication (McCormack and McCance 2006).

a study of autonomy. The principles underpinning these two conceptual frameworks are consistent with human science principles such as those articulated by Watson (1985), including the centrality of human freedom, choice and responsibility, holism (non-reducible persons interconnected with others and nature), different forms of knowing (empirics, aesthetics, ethics and intuition), the importance of time and space, and relationships. Collectively, they represented a synthesis of the then available literature on caring and person centredness. The framework provides a unique perspective for nursing that conceptually links caring and person centredness.

The framework was developed through an iterative process and involved a series of systematic steps (Figure 10.1). Identifying the similarities and matched elements of each conceptual framework was an important first step and confirmed the strong relationship between caring and person-centred practice. For example, McCormack (2003) identified contextual factors that reflected many comparable elements captured by McCance (2003) under 'structures'. Similarly, the 'imperfect duties' described by McCormack (2003) incorporated elements of the process of caring described by McCance (2003). The second step involved the exploration of areas of difference using a critical dialogue with co-researchers ($n = 6$) and with lead practitioners from a range of clinical settings ($n = 16$) as a means of reaching agreement in relation to where these elements might fit within the new framework. The concepts underpinning both conceptual frameworks were then discussed. These conversations took the form of focused discussions using critical questioning techniques to unravel each concept. The original sources of literature and data were consulted in order to ensure shared clarity of meaning of key terms in each framework. These conversations were tape recorded and listened to after each discussion in order to identify key elements of each framework that needed to be retained or amended in the combined framework. Key concepts from both conceptual frameworks were listed and a first draft of the PCN theoretical framework was constructed.

A period of testing the framework was undertaken. Two focus groups were held – one with co-researchers ($n = 6$) and one with lead practitioners from a range of clinical settings ($n = 16$). The draft framework was presented and their views on clarity, coherence and comprehensibility sought. Prior to the focus groups, the individual frameworks (McCance, 2003; McCormack, 2003) were provided as background reading to enable discussion. The ease with which lead practitioners engaged with the framework and were able to contextualise elements within their clinical environments was clearly evident and was considered the most important indicator of its clarity, coherence and usability.

The PCN theoretical framework is presented in Figure 10.2 and comprises four constructs:

- *Prerequisites*, which focus on the attributes of the nurse.
- *The care environment*, which focuses on the context in which care is delivered.
- *Person-centred processes*, which focus on delivering care through a range of activities.
- *Expected outcomes*, which are the results of effective PCN.

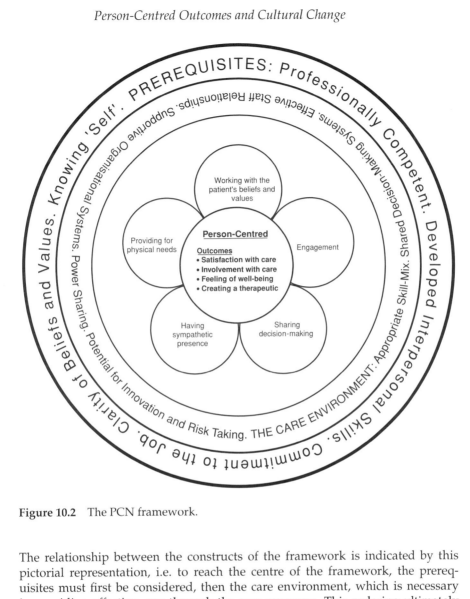

Figure 10.2 The PCN framework.

The relationship between the constructs of the framework is indicated by this pictorial representation, i.e. to reach the centre of the framework, the prerequisites must first be considered, then the care environment, which is necessary in providing effective care through the care processes. This ordering ultimately leads to the achievement of the outcomes – the central component of the framework. It is also acknowledged that there are relationships within and across constructs.

Prerequisites

The prerequisites focus on the attributes of the nurse and include being professionally competent, having developed interpersonal skills, being committed to the job, being able to demonstrate clarity of beliefs and values, and knowing self.

The care environment

The care environment focuses on the context in which care is delivered and includes the following: appropriate skill mix; systems that facilitate shared decision-making; effective staff relationships; organisational systems that are supportive; the sharing of power; and the potential for innovation and risk taking.

Person-centred processes

Person-centred processes focus on delivering care through a range of activities that operationalise PCN and include the following: working with patient's beliefs and values; engagement; having sympathetic presence; sharing decision-making; and providing for physical needs. This is the component of the framework that specifically focuses on the patient, describing PCN in the context of care delivery.

Person-centred outcomes

Outcomes are the results expected from effective PCN and include the following: satisfaction with care; involvement in care; feeling of well-being; and creating a therapeutic environment described as one in which decision-making is shared, staff relationships are collaborative, leadership is transformational, and innovative practices are supported.

The framework was used in several ways throughout the intervention phase. For example, it was used by facilitation teams to analyse underpinning barriers to change (arising, e.g., from differences in beliefs and values), focus on particular developments (e.g. the sharing of 'power' with patients) or evaluate developments as they progressed through the intervention (e.g. changes made to the care environment). The framework has been refined with co-researchers and project participants throughout the intervention period of the study and will continue to be tested through further PD work.

The intervention phase

The purpose of the intervention phase was to

1. enable participating sites to use the quantitative and qualitative data to identify where they were in relation to the PCN conceptual framework (McCormack & McCance, 2006);
2. support these sites in becoming more person centred.

The intervention phase consisted of a programme of individual PDs within the participating sites, guided by Garbett and McCormack's (2002) conceptual model of PD and the PCN conceptual framework (McCormack & McCance, 2006). Initial work by the facilitators with the clinical areas aimed to draw out individual areas for development. This work involved the following:

- Clarifying values and beliefs.
- Developing a collective vision in the clinical areas.

- Giving consideration to the culture and context of care in relation to the proposed interventions.
- Developing action plans with clear time scales, responsibilities and evaluation mechanisms.

Facilitation of the programmes of development incorporated the following methods:

- Working with teams
- One-to-one working
- Action learning
- Critical companionship
- Facilitators working in the clinical areas

At the start of the intervention phase a key question for facilitators was how to get all staff involved in the development work and keep them involved. The ward leaders were involved in action learning and regular meetings, but it was recognised that all the nursing teams needed to have ownership of the project to engage with it. Behaviours are heavily influenced by beliefs and values (Kotter & Heskett, 1992) and so identifying the beliefs and values of the participating teams assisted in giving direction to the project and creating a common purpose. All facilitators carried out values clarification exercises with staff in the participating sites in order to develop a vision statement.

A further piece of work was then completed to create a collective vision using the constructs from the PCN framework as a basis for discussion and the written statement developed from the values clarification exercise. The visioning exercise was completed using creative arts including collage, drawing, writing and painting to enable creativity. This statement then formed the basis for further work on creating a collective vision.

Examples of the intervention phase PDs within two clinical areas are illustrated below.

PCN developments in the intensive care unit (ICU)

At the time of the intervention phase, the ICU was a 15-bedded tertiary referral unit adjacent to a 5-bedded high dependency unit (HDU). One hundred and fifty whole time equivalent (WTE) nursing staff provided 24-hour, one-to-one care to patients (6.5 WTE nurses per bed). For managerial purposes, staff were divided into six teams led by a Clinical Nurse Manager. A self-rostering off duty was in place and 16 nurses were on duty each shift. One of these nurses coordinated the unit activity and allocated the other 15 nurses to care for any one of the 15 patients.

The senior nursing staff were interested in the project as a way of improving the job satisfaction of staff in such a large unit, recognising that an obstacle to development was the size of the unit/nursing establishment. With this in mind, one team of staff volunteered to be the sample for data collection purposes. Interventions, however, involved all the ICU staff.

A workshop was held with staff to explore the concept of PCN within ICU using a values clarification exercise. An underlying principle of person centredness is the therapeutic relationship; reflecting on this staff felt that they were more 'nurse centred' in terms of off duty and allocation of nurses to patients. In order to develop a therapeutic relationship, staff recognised the need to improve continuity of care to support the development of a therapeutic relationship with the patient/family This mirrors both the intentions, processes and the outcomes achieved in a study in critical care within the context of a primary nursing team (Manley et al., 1997). Along with discussion of the results of the baseline data, this work formed the initial intervention. The aims were to

- improve continuity of care, and
- develop closer (therapeutic) relationships with patients and their families.

Whilst the emphasis was on working towards these aims, it was envisaged that other benefits could be realised from the work, including improved communication and teamwork within the multi-professional team.

The plan for development focused on organisational/contextual changes to help achieve the aims. The unit was divided into five coloured 'zones' of three beds. The six teams of nursing staff were subdivided into the five 'colours' with their own off duty. These staff worked within each three-bedded 'zone' and provided continuity of care to patients/families. Timely feedback of data along with other contextual data such as new recruits, staff sickness, maternity leave and turnover, kept staff involved and allowed opportunity for discussion. Inevitably, changing the way organisation of care was managed highlighted a number of other issues that needed to be addressed. One-to-one working and the use of claims, concerns and issues exercises with groups of staff enabled these issues to be overcome and led to other strands of development flowing from the initial development, e.g. the changing role of the Clinical Nurse Manager and their deputy within the new 'zones'. Once values and beliefs were clarified within ICU, the focus of the intervention was very much within the care environment of the PCN conceptual framework (Figure 10.3). Supportive organisational systems were put in place to develop continuity of care, ensuring appropriate skill mix. Feedback from staff indicated more effective staff relationships as a result of the opportunity to work more closely with a smaller team of nurses – a finding also found in both Manley et al.'s (1996, 1997) studies of staff's perceptions and job satisfaction.

By time point 5, nurse–patient conversations showed an increase in the number of times families were talked about. Nurses talked about family members ringing up or when they would be next visiting and the nurses referred to family often in their conversations with patients regardless of their level of responsiveness. Data also showed nurses planning care and handing over care for their patients whilst they were away on breaks to ensure continuity.

PCN developments in genitourinary medicine clinic

The Department of Genitourinary Medicine (GUM) aims to provide a quality sexual health service for people throughout Northern Ireland. Services include

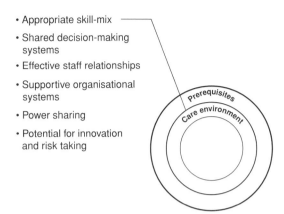

- Appropriate skill-mix
- Shared decision-making systems
- Effective staff relationships
- Supportive organisational systems
- Power sharing
- Potential for innovation and risk taking

Figure 10.3 Focus of PD in the ICU.

diagnosis, treatment contact tracing and counselling for patients affected by or concerned about sexually transmitted infections including HIV and AIDS. There are eight WTE nursing staff working with consultants at clinics, providing nurse-led clinics and carrying out disease-specific interventions.

Following the collection of baseline data a workshop using claims, concerns and issues was used to develop an action plan for the unit to take forward. The staff within the clinic were interested in developing therapeutic relationships with patients as often they work with the same patient group for many years. In order to develop more person-centred practice, staff felt that they needed more time to foster their nurse–patient relationships. During a busy clinic with many 'drop-in' patients this was not easy. Two main strands of work developed. The first strand involved dividing the nurses into two teams and within those teams each nurse took responsibility for providing a key worker role. This role involved reviewing the patient's clinical notes, ensuring that all tests had been reported and the results relayed to the patient. To do this, the nurses telephoned the patient introducing themselves if the patient did not already know them and explained the key worker role to them. This meant that any outstanding issues for the patient were addressed and they knew the name of the nurse responsible for their care at the clinic. The nurse–patient conversations in this setting tended to reflect attributes of the care environment in that it was a busy environment with short amounts of time for nurse–patient interaction. Analysis showed that nurses tended to remain with patients with few interruptions and took an overview of the tests and the process for reporting back results.

The second strand of work stemmed from the large number of daily telephone inquiries to the clinic from anxious patients. The steady stream of calls was taking the nurses out of the consulting room and leaving patients alone. A pilot project of the nurse triage system was introduced. A nurse was allocated this role for the duration of the day, a private room and telephone were provided and the receptionist provided clinical notes for the nurse while the caller was on the line.

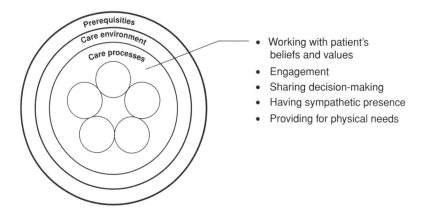

Figure 10.4 Focus of developments in the GUM clinic.

At further ward leader days (action learning) and through one-to-one working with the leader, this work was then linked back to the PCN model. Whilst several prerequisites and care environment attributes are required to enable these developments such as developed interpersonal skills and potential for risk taking and innovation, examining the care processes best highlighted what was achieved (Figure 10.4). Dedicated and planned time allowed the nurses to consider and work with the patient's values and beliefs. By doing so the nurses were able to engage with the patient and have sympathetic presence as a result of using their interpersonal skills to listen to and hear their voices.

Project outcomes

Twenty constructs were tested using independent t-tests to measure change between the pre-intervention and the post-intervention (henceforth known as time 1 and time 5 respectively). The intervention group reported differences on five constructs, all relating to nurse work stress and all decreasing during the intervention. This compares to four constructs in the control group, with mixed results (see Table 10.2).

Conversational analysis provided a different type of measure of change or movement towards person centredness in nursing practice. Overall, across all intervention sites, improvement in person centredness was seen over the course of the time points, but more so in some constructs than others and within certain areas of the constructs, such as developed interpersonal skills (prerequisites), engagement and sympathetic presence (processes). Whilst some areas such as working with patient's values and beliefs, sharing in decision-making and evaluation of satisfaction with care saw little change (processes and outcomes). Improvement towards person centredness was not always steady in all intervention sites. Conversations that were part of a hectic care environment or were challenging to the

200

Table 10.2 Pre- and post-intervention scores for the intervention and control groups, with statistically significant scores

Construct title	Intervention group (mean)			Control group (mean)		
	Pre	Post	Significance	Pre	Post	Significance
Workload	4.65 (1.06)	4.12 (1.17)	$t = 2.73$ $p = 0.01$	5.72 (0.94)	5.42 (0.92)	
Inadequate preparation	3.17 (1.10)	2.98 (1.10)		4.44 (1.16)	4.09 (1.58)	
Lack of staff support	3.32 (1.24)	3.04 (1.17)		4.5 (1.3)	3.82 (1.59)	
Conflict with other nurses	2.08 (0.86)	2.22 (0.96)		2.03 (0.93)	2.81 (1.72)	$t = 6.33$ $p = 0.037$
Uncertainty regarding treatment	2.55 (0.84)	2.3 (0.87)	$t = 0.14$ $p = 0.04$	2.73 (1.02)	3.3 (1.73)	
Work/home interface and social life	2.89 (0.97)	2.67 (1.00)		4.0 (1.18)	3.53 (1.76)	
Working environment	3.17 (1.2)	2.75 (1.0)	$t = 3.85$ $p = 0.01$	3.8 (1.13)	3.68 (1.54)	
Lack of communication and support	3.33 (1.09)	2.85 (0.99)	$t = 0.158$ $p = 0.002$	4.4 (1.23)	4.04 (1.67)	
Career development	2.68 (1.05)	2.38 (1.01)	$t = 0.487$ $p = 0.04$	3.64 (1.45)	3.75 (1.86)	
Satisfaction with pay and prospects	3.84 (1.43)	3.68 (1.48)		3.31 (1.34)	3.63 (1.58)	
Satisfaction with training	4.40 (1.42)	4.4 (1.62)		2.99 (1.5)	4.16 (1.92)	$t = 2.72$ $p = 0.017$
Personal satisfaction	5.25 (1.13)	4.97 (1.25)		4.53 (1.49)	4.46 (1.95)	
Professional satisfaction	5.04 (0.96)	5.22 (2.12)		3.90 (1.32)	4.62 (1.72)	
Control over practice	4.02 (1.00)	4.41 (1.09)		3.07 (0.93)	3.81 (0.99)	$t = 0.023$ $p = 0.009$
Empowerment	4.35 (0.88)	4.4 (1.22)		4.21 (1.17)	4.12 (1.70)	
Organisational support	4.42 (0.82)	4.6 (0.88)		3.80 (0.81)	4.43 (0.88)	$t = 0.245$ $p = 0.011$
Autonomy	4.39 (0.87)	4.54 (0.93)		3.87 (1.01)	4.22 (1.31)	
Doctor–nurse relationship	4.89 (1.1)	4.96 (1.07)		4.71 (1.24)	5.23 (0.89)	
Organisational commitment	4.45 (0.93)	4.56 (1.07)		3.98 (0.93)	4.22 (0.95)	
Intention to leave	3.56 (1.56)	3.7 (1.63)		4.63 (1.59)	3.88 (1.96)	

nurse for various reasons tended to revert to being less person centred and more nursing task centred.

Comparison between pre- and post-intervention phases

Twenty constructs measured the nurses working environment. These were on a seven-point Likert scale. The mean scores of each of the factors were compared at pre- and post-intervention for both the intervention and control group. Table 10.2 shows the mean scores; the statistically significant findings are highlighted for both intervention and control groups.

Generally, the intervention group nurses reported a more positive starting point than the control group on all of the 20 constructs. Stress levels were lower, job satisfaction higher and a more positive perception of the nurse working environment. This may be accounted for by the criteria of clinical setting selection (the presence of primary nursing, good leadership, etc.; see site selection criteria). At the end of the intervention phase these trends remained unchanged. Positive changes were reported in 15 of the 20 constructs with 2 remaining unchanged. Three factors changed negatively over the intervention period. Five of the fifteen positive changes had mean differences at a statistically significant level (see Table 10.2). The five statistically significant constructs were stress related with stress levels decreasing between the pre- and post-intervention measures.

Like the intervention group the control group reported positive change over time on 15 of the constructs. The remaining five constructs changed negatively. Four of the changes (positive and negative) were at a statistically significant level. The construct 'Conflict with other nurses' increased negatively, and the remaining three changed positively.

Intervention group scores

Analysis of variance scores were calculated to measure the statistical significance of changes over time. Transcriptions revealed a very low level, or in many instances, a complete absence of conversations where nurses talked about the care environment construct. This was probably a positive feature as most conversations were between nurses and patients; talk about the care environment was not an appropriate topic.

Nurse stress

Data from the intervention group collected across the five time points (baseline and intervention period) were analysed for change in scoring over time. This change may be attributed to the intervention. Figure 10.5 shows how the mean scores on each of the constructs relating to nurse stress changed over the intervention period. It is clear that each of the constructs reported small but consistent changes as the intervention progressed. Statistically significant changes were reported in the following factors: 'Workload'; 'Uncertainty regarding treatment'; 'Working environment'; and 'Lack of communication and social support'.

Measures of job satisfaction

Over the intervention period, there was relatively little change in the level of satisfaction on each of the constructs as measured by the 'Measure of job

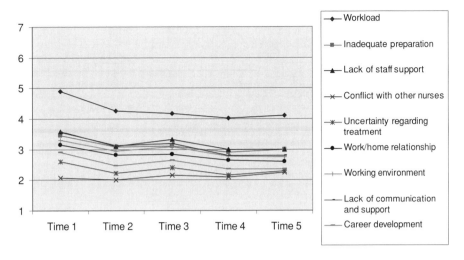

Figure 10.5 Nurse stress scale scores across five time points.

satisfaction' (Figure 10.6). The largest change in satisfaction was an increase in 'personal satisfaction' that changed significantly for the intervention group ($p = 0.032$). 'Professional satisfaction' and 'Satisfaction with training' also increased but not to a statistically significant level. 'Satisfaction with pay and prospects' did not change substantially over time. All changes were slow and constant over the data collection points.

Organisational-related traits

Statistically significant changes ($p > 0.05$) were reported for the organisational factors 'Autonomy' and 'Organisational support' (Figure 10.7). Both constructs' mean

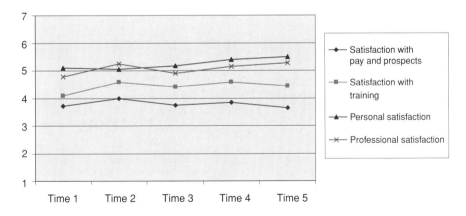

Figure 10.6 Measures of job satisfaction scores across five time points for intervention group.

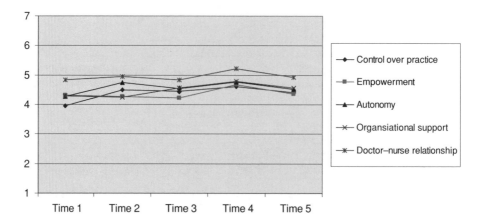

Figure 10.7 Organisational-related traits scores across five time points for intervention group.

scores increased across the data collection points, as did those of the other three constructs. This increase was from a neutral point regarding the constructs' presence on the ward/department to a more positive view of the constructs' presence.

Organisational outcome measures

There was a small increase in organisational commitment mirrored with a small decline in nurse intention to leave. The inverse relationship of these two variables is exemplified at time 3 where the steady movement in their respective directions is reversed before continuing on their trajectory (Figure 10.8). Over the five data collection points the gap between the two constructs increased (except at point 3). No change was statistically significant.

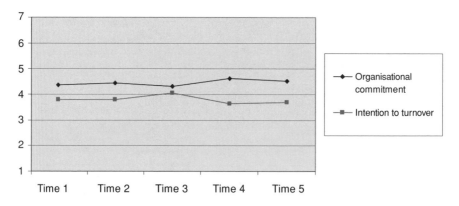

Figure 10.8 Organisational outcome scores across five time points for intervention group.

Table 10.3 Percentage scores of patients experience and satisfaction levels with being nursed

Clinical setting	Time 1		Time 2		Time 3		Time 4		Time 5	
	Exp	Sat	Exp	Sat	Exp	Sat	Exp	Sat	Exp	Sat
1	81	92	66.94	71.75	70.71	77.13	78.53	78.98	86.12	85.45
2	70.13	83.18	62.20	70.85	71.75	76.31	67.15	89.47	67.51	73.87
3	70	91	64.01	75.69	72.54	88.30	78.37	97.93	77.00	93.00
4	69.29	84.21	62.73	77.44	70.32	84.12	66.81	87.54	65.38	61.40
5	64.10	68.57	57.91	69.73	64.21	82.72	59.47	62.71	68.47	67.70
6	67.17	81.21	55.17	55.71	67.18	83.37	71.63	86.56	70.19	87.28
7	71.08	87.98	60.30	73.11	67.28	68.23	70.29	88.37	75.51	98.42
8	78.59	89.73	71.15	78.97	71.79	85.97	74.23	94.61	75.26	86.56
Overall	69.86	83.48	61.98	71.28	69.64	81.40	71.89	85.21	73.40	79.08
Control	70.66	78.75							72.94	86.73

Patients satisfaction with nursing

The patients' satisfaction with nursing scale comprises two scales: experiences of care received and satisfaction with that care. The tool has 26 items to assess the experiences of nursing and 19 items to assess satisfaction with nursing, both measured on a seven-point Likert scale. Scores on both experience and satisfaction ranged between 100% (perfect contentment) and 0% (perfect discontentment).

The scoring of the satisfaction scale is much the same as the experience scales (Table 10.3). Raw scores for the 19 items are converted into a percentage score. Interpretation of these scores is like that of the experience scales. However, the data need to be treated with caution as high scores are common on the wards, particularly so in the satisfaction with nursing scale. This was further compounded in clinical settings with low response rates that skewed the results.

Interestingly, conversation analysis at the baseline point showed that nurses rarely asked patients about satisfaction with care (an outcome construct). This was in two respects: satisfaction overall and satisfaction with particular aspects of care. This was a clear omission at the baseline across all settings. At time point 5, there was no real change seen with this construct. There were only a few examples of nurses asking patients to complete a questionnaire but the topic of satisfaction was not part of everyday conversation.

Experience of nursing

Experiences at all five time points were positively scored, the lowest at 62% (time 2) and the highest at 73% (time 5). A one-way analysis of variance was conducted to test for significant differences in patients' experience of being nursed and satisfaction with being nursed across the five time points. Both patient experience and

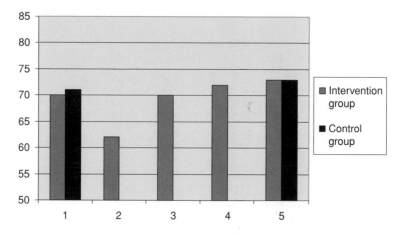

Figure 10.9 Percentage scores of patients' experience of nursing across time 1 to time 5.

satisfaction scores had statistically significant differences in scoring ($p = 0.001$) (see Figures 10.9 and 10.10).

There was a positive change in patients' experience of being nursed across all the clinical settings. All clinical settings reported an initial decline from time 1 to time 2 (see Table 10.3). Four clinical settings reported steady increases to time 5, and three reported mixed but generally positive findings. Only one clinical setting reported mixed but negative patient changes and this setting was not without its positive changes in scoring. Six of the eight clinical settings had increased scores from time 1 to time 5. The sample size limits the application of tests for statistical differences

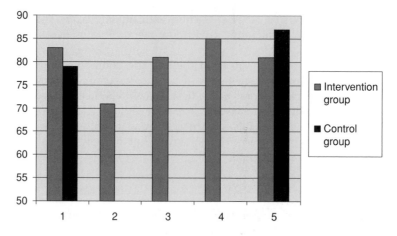

Figure 10.10 Percentage scores of patients' satisfaction of nursing across time 1 to time 5.

across clinical settings. However, applying an analysis of variance according to clinical setting across all 5 time points shows statistically significant changes in all but clinical setting 8 at a probability level of $p > 0.05$.

Satisfaction with nursing

Overall, patients were content with the level of care they received over the five time points. Satisfaction with being nursed decreased initially from time point 1 to time point 2 before increasing over time point 3 and 4 before finally settling at a score of 79% for time point 5. Statistically significant differences were recorded between time points 2 and 4 with time point 5.

The change in patients' satisfaction was less clear mainly due to a ceiling effect of high scores to begin with. Overall clinical setting scores increased across all latter time points from an initial decrease at time 2. At time point 1, one clinical setting had a score above 80%. This increased to five clinical settings at time 5, with two clinical settings scoring above 90%. Three clinical settings increased scores by time point 5 from their time 1 starting point. Six clinical settings increased satisfaction scores from time point 2 to 4 with three clinical settings increasing scores at time 5. An analysis of variance shows statistically significant differences in scoring in clinical setting 3, 4, 6 and 7 to a probability level of $p > 0.05$. The direction of the change can be seen in Table 10.3.

The qualitative data give a more in-depth, yet still a snap-shot, perspective of changes in person-centred constructs. As suggested earlier, findings from the conversation analysis show changes in some of the four constructs and the subconstructs indicating a move towards person centredness. The data findings seem to support the relationship between the constructs of the framework as outlined earlier in the chapter (Figure 10.2). It appears that the person-centred processes and outcomes at the centre of the framework saw the least and most inconsistent change.

Control group

The experience and satisfaction with nursing of the control group were assessed at time 1 and time 5. Mean scores for the two time points show a small change in experience of nursing in the control wards and a more pronounced change in satisfaction of nursing. Patients' experience of nursing rose from 71% at time 1 to 73% at time 5 and satisfaction rise from 79 to 87% over the same period. However, neither change was to a statistically significant level.

The experience of caring

Nurses and patients were asked to grade 35 statements relating to activities of nursing and to categorise them as caring or not caring. This instrument has proven statistical properties (Watson et al., 2001). Watson and colleagues classified the 35 statements into five areas: Technical; Supporting; Intimacy; Unnecessary; Inappropriate. The analysis of the data highlights only statements that were positively scored.

Nurses

Nurses had a clear idea of what constituted caring in nursing. Twelve 'core' statements were considered caring on all five data collection points. These statements related to technical and intimacy aspects of nursing duties, such as 'Listening to a patient or keeping relatives informed about a patient'. A further five items were scored by the nurses as caring on four of the five occasions, four statements on three occasions, two over two occasions and one statement once. Eleven statements were not considered as caring at any data collection point. Listening to a patient was scored as the most caring of all nursing tasks on all occasions. There was generally limited movement in the ranking of each of the 'core' statements over the five occasions, but as Table 10.4 shows tasks that had previously been considered as caring were being replaced by new statements towards the end of the data collection points, i.e. 'Getting to know a patient'.

Knowing what counts as caring and using those skills in everyday conversation are very different. At the baseline, conversations in many settings showed listening to patients' concerns and priorities were not as person centred as they could be. Midway in the time points, nurses tended to leave a space for patients to talk and thus gave the impression of listening more. However, nurses tended not to make use of the information contained within patients' talk in a direct way or simply moved the conversation on with no verbal acknowledgement of what was said. There may have been non-verbal acknowledgement, not picked up by the method. Towards the end of the project, data from some clinical settings indicated that listening and responding skills were improving.

Patients

Patients rated 2 of the 35 statements as caring on all five occasions. These were 'Involving a patient in care' and 'Providing privacy for a patient' (see Table 10.5). Unlike the nurses' responses, the variability in ranking and scoring was much more pronounced with patients. This is reflected in the distribution of items across each of the data collection points. This may be interpreted as reflective of the idiosyncratic nature of patients' views of what constitutes caring and that nurses, if wanting to act caringly, should attempt to learn what the patient considers as caring. This is supported by the presence of psychosocial functions such as 'Sitting with a patient' and 'Listening to a patient' among the statements identified by patients as being caring.

Summary of main findings

The data present a complex picture of movement towards PCN. Overall, however, in the quantitative data, the intervention had a positive impact on nursing to a statistically significant level. In particular, there was a statistically significant reduction in five of the nine stress-related constructs, suggesting that developing person-centred approaches to nursing helps nurses to manage their workloads more effectively and reduce associated stresses. This is further evidenced by the higher level of job satisfaction reported by participating nurses compared with those in the control group. The developments undertaken enabled nurses to experience a greater presence of positive organisational factors, such as autonomy, than at baseline and compared to the control group. Most significantly,

Table 10.4 Caring dimensions index: ranking and mean scores by nurses

	Statements	Construct	Ranking/time				
			1	2	3	4	5
1	Listening to a patient	Intimacy	1 (4.66)	1 (4.67)	1 (4.60)	1 (4.67)	1 (4.64)
2	Explaining a clinical procedure to a patient	Technical	5 (4.52)	4 (4.55)	2 (4.52)	5 (4.54)	4 (4.53)
3	Providing privacy for a patient	Intimacy	2 (4.57)	2 (4.64)	3 (4.51)	2 (4.58)	
4	Assisting a patient with an ADL	Technical		6 (4.52)	4 (4.45)	4 (4.56)	3 (4.58)
5	Being with a patient during a clinical procedure	Intimacy	8 (4.44)	5 (4.52)	5 (4.37)	10 (4.51)	6 (4.47)
6	Involving a patient in care	Intimacy	6 (4.51)	3 (4.57)	6 (4.37)	6 (4.54)	5 (4.49)
7	Measuring the vital signs of a patient	Technical	9 (4.43)	8 (4.47)	7 (4.35)	8 (4.53)	9 (4.45)
8	Consulting with a doctor	Technical	11 (4.41)	10 (4.41)	8 (4.34)	7 (4.53)	8 (4.46)
9	Getting to know the patient as a person	Intimacy			9 (4.34)	13 (4.30)	15 (4.30)
10	Reporting a patients condition to a senior nurse	Technical	14 (4.31)	9 (4.46)	10 (4.34)	12 (4.38)	10 (4.45)
11	Sitting with a patient	Intimacy	10 (4.41)		11 (4.32)		
12	Giving reassurances about a clinical procedure	Unnecessary	3 (4.54)		12 (4.32)	3 (4.57)	7 (4.47)
13	Being honest with a patient	Intimacy	12 (4.39)	7 (4.49)	13 (4.29)	9 (4.52)	12 (4.42)
14	Arranging for a patient to see a chaplain	Supporting	16 (4.25)		14 (4.18)	15 (4.28)	2 (4.63)
15	Instructing a patient about aspects of self-care	Technical	7 (4.47)	11 (4.39)	15 (4.17)	14 (4.30)	11 (4.42)
16	Observing the effects of medication on a patient	Technical	13 (4.37)	12 (4.27)	16 (4.15)	11 (4.41)	16 (4.29)
17	Making a nursing record about a patient	Technical	4 (4.52)	15 (4.14)	17 (4.12)	18 (4.16)	14 (4.33)
18	Being cheerful with a patient	Intimacy	17 (4.23)		18 (4.09)		13 (4.36)
19	Keeping relatives informed about a patient	Intimacy	15 (4.30)	13 (4.19)	19 (4.06)	16 (4.25)	17 (4.28)
20	Being neatly dressed when working with a patient	Technical		16 (4.11)	20 (4.05)	17 (4.18)	
21	Being technically competent with a clinical procedure	Technical		14 (4.18)	21 (4.03)	19 (4.13)	18 (4.18)
22	Putting the needs of a patient before your own	Technical	19 (3.71)		22 (3.89)	21 (3.62)	
23	Organising the work of others for a patient	Technical			23 (3.45)	20 (3.85)	
24	Attending to the spiritual needs of others	Supporting	18 (3.98)				

Table 10.5 Caring dimensions index: ranking and mean scores by patients

		Ranking/time				
Statement	Construct	1	2	3	4	5
1 Listening to a patient	Intimacy	4 (4.41)	4 (4.45)	1 (4.61)	7 (4.37)	
2 Explaining a clinical procedure to a patient	Technical	7 (4.40)	4 (4.45)		1 (4.51)	
3 Providing privacy for a patient	Intimacy	7 (4.40)	2 (4.55)	13 (3.93)	9 (4.36)	2 (4.51)
4 Assisting a patient with an ADL	Technical	19 (3.96)		10 (4.11)	19 (3.91)	6 (4.00)
5 Being with a patient during a clinical procedure	Intimacy	16 (4.13)	14 (4.13)	4 (4.35)	16 (4.07)	
6 Involving a patient in care	Intimacy	11 (4.33)	7 (4.36)	4 (4.44)	11 (4.31)	4 (4.35)
7 Measuring the vital signs of a patient	Technical	4 (4.41)		2 (4.44)	2 (4.49)	
8 Consulting with a doctor	Technical	2 (4.42)	6 (4.40)	6 (4.34)	4 (4.40)	
9 Getting to know the patient as a person	Intimacy	15 (4.14)	13 (4.16)	7 (4.32)	15 (4.11)	
10 Reporting a patient's condition to a senior nurse	Technical	12 (4.23)	11 (4.23)	12 (4.07)	12 (4.26)	
11 Sitting with a patient	Intimacy	16 (4.07)	16 (4.00)	3 (4.42)	17 (4.06)	
12 Giving reassurances about a clinical procedure	Unnecessary	1 (4.49)	1 (4.56)		3 (4.47)	3 (4.43)
13 Being honest with a patient	Intimacy	4 (4.41)	3 (4.47)		6 (4.39)	
14 Arranging for a patient to see a chaplain	Supporting		17 (3.68)		20 (3.86)	7 (4.00)
15 Instructing a patient about aspects of self-care	Technical	13 (4.21)	10 (4.27)		14 (4.20)	
16 Observing the effects of medication on a patient	Technical	10 (4.36)	8 (4.34)		9 (4.36)	5 (4.27)
17 Making a nursing record about a patient	Technical	16 (3.98)		11 (4.08)	18 (3.99)	6 (4.00)
18 Being cheerful with a patient	Intimacy	2 (4.42)		4 (4.35)	4 (4.40)	1 (4.60)
19 Keeping relatives informed about a patient	Intimacy	7 (4.40)	15 (4.12)		7 (4.37)	
20 Being neatly dressed when working with a patient	Technical		12 (4.22)			
21 Being technically competent with a clinical procedure	Technical	14 (4.18)	9 (4.31)	8 (4.25)	13 (4.23)	
22 Putting the needs of a patient before your own	Technical	18 (3.90)		9 (4.23)	21 (3.80)	
23 Organising the work of others for a patient	Technical	21 (3.79)		14 (3.89)	23 (3.16)	
24 Attending to the spiritual needs of others	Supporting		18 (3.09)			
25 Exploring the patient's lifestyle	Intimacy	22 (3.46)			22 (3.47)	
26 Keeping in contact with a patient	Unnecessary		19 (2.87)			
27 Praying for a patient	Unnecessary					8 (3.56)

participating staff indicated a lowered intention to leave with a statistically significant corresponding increase in organisational commitment. In terms of the patients' experience, the intervention had a significant impact on patients' experience and satisfaction with being nursed, with patients reporting that nurses addressed most, if not all, of the nursing duties considered by patients as caring. Incorporating qualitative data in this project has shown that movement towards person centredness can be evidenced across the four constructs of the PCN framework, through everyday nurse–patient conversations. It has also shown that the benefits of person centredness may be experienced more immediately and more significantly (as measured by the instruments used in this project) by nurses than by patients. It may suggest that more specific PD interventions are needed to ensure that everyday nurse–patient conversation is person centred regarding processes in order to address outcomes.

Lessons learnt and implications for practice development

The outcomes from this large-scale study have the potential to contribute to the existing knowledge base in a number of ways:

- It provides empirical evidence of the effectiveness of PCN across a range of indicators.
- It has led to the development and testing of tools that are tailored for use within PD projects such as the PCN framework and the PCNI.
- It demonstrates the impact of using a PD intervention to facilitate changes in practice cultures.
- It provides an insight into the challenges that are inherent in applying a quasi-experimental design in the real world of practice.
- It shows that everyday nurse–patient conversation is an area for PD interventions and evaluation.

In an attempt to draw out the implications of these outcomes to PD work, it is useful to reflect on the PD model presented by Garbett and McCormack (2002). The principle of PCN is at the core of this model, with the culture and context of the care environment and values and beliefs of practitioners enabling this style of practice. The development of the PCN theoretical framework has provoked increased clarity around 'person centredness', enabling practitioners to analyse and articulate their journey towards more effective person-centred care. Furthermore, the study demonstrates the strength of PD as an appropriate intervention through which practitioners can work with culture and context in order to deliver more effective PCN. The complementariness of the PCN framework with the underpinning principles of PD makes it a useful decision-making tool in PD work.

It is important to recognise that the outcomes described above were achieved in the context of a constantly changing care environment. Whilst this presented significant challenges for the project team, there were important lessons learnt along the way. In theory this was a 'simple' project framework, but in reality it proved to be complex and ambitious. This was due to a number of factors that in isolation were not insurmountable, but when combined created a significant challenge for the project team. The ambitious size of the project, both in terms of number of participating sites and the number of data collection points, was recognised as a challenge from the outset. This had implications for effective coordination and communication within the facilitation team, between the facilitation team and the project team, and with the participating clinical areas. Whilst clear roles and responsibilities were defined during the planning phase of the project, the constant turnover of staff from the participating sites and changes within the core project team led to some difficulties in coordinating the intervention phase and also data collection, particularly securing and collecting the recordings. This reflected the real world of practice focusing on the need for all participants to be creative in their response to changes in the practice setting. Leadership at all levels was therefore crucial to the success of this project, as was the sustained enthusiasm and commitment from the clinical teams. Whilst there was a visible team approach, there was always the risk of focusing on the eventual outcomes at the expense of the process. The need to demonstrate the espoused values of 'person centredness' in managing a complex project of this nature was recognised, emphasising the importance of, for example, developing ground rules, agreeing ways of working and identifying appropriate support mechanisms. Reflecting on the rich learning accrued by the project team throughout the process had led to the identification of some of the 'key ingredients' for a 'recipe' for facilitating similar projects.

Opportunities for the future development of PCN that can build on this research are being identified at local, national and international levels. The dissemination of this work locally and nationally has led to developments that aim to embed PCN into the strategic and policy direction for nursing and midwifery. The tools that have been developed such as the PCN framework and the PCNI are of international relevance and have sparked interest from colleagues in other countries providing important opportunities for further testing. The need, however, to draw out other key relationships that impact on the provision of effective PCN is paramount in order to continue to contribute to the knowledge base. This study provides a rich source of evidence on which to build future programmes of work in this area.

References

Binnie, A. & Titchen, A. (1999) *Freedom to Practice: The Development of Patient-Centred Nursing*. Butterworth-Heinemann, Oxford.

Boykin, A. & Schoenhofer, S. (1993) *Nursing as Caring: A Model for Transforming Practice*. National League for Nursing Press, New York.

Curley, M.A. (1998) Patient-nurse synergy: Optimizing patients' outcomes. *American Journal of Critical Care*. 7(1), 64–72.

Department of Health (2001) *National Service Framework for Older People*. Department of Health, London.

Dewing, J. (2004) Concerns relating to the application of frameworks to promote person-centredness in nursing with older people. *International Journal of Older People Nursing*. **13**(3a), 39–44.

Garbett, R. & McCormack, B. (2002) A concept analysis of practice development. *Nursing Times Research*. **7**(2), 87–100.

Kotter, J.P. & Heskett, J.L. (1992) *Corporate Culture and Performance*. The Free Press, New York.

Leininger, M. (1988) Leininger's theory of nursing: Cultural care diversity and universality. *Nursing Science Quarterly*. **1**(4), 152–160.

Manley, K., Cruse, S. & Keogh, S. (1996) Job satisfaction of intensive care nurses practising primary nursing: A comparison with those practising total patient care. *Nursing in Critical Care*. **1**(1), 31–41.

Manley, K., Hamill, J.-M. & Hanlon, M. (1997) Nursing staff's perceptions and experiences of primary nursing practice in intensive care 4 years on. *Journal of Clinical Nursing*. **6**, 277–287.

McCance, T.V. (2003) Caring in nursing practice: The development of a conceptual framework. *Research and Theory for Nursing Practice: An International Journal*. **17**(2), 101–116.

McCance, T.V., McKenna, H.P. & Boore, J.R.P. (1999) Caring : Theoretical perspectives of relevance to nursing. *Journal of Advanced Nursing*. **30**, 1388–1395.

McCance, T.V., McKenna, H.P. & Boore, J.R.P. (2001) Exploring caring using narrative methodology: An analysis of the approach. *Journal of Advanced Nursing*. **33**, 350–356.

McCormack, B. (2001) *Negotiating Partnerships with Older People – A Person-Centred Approach*. Ashgate, Basingstoke.

McCormack, B. (2003) A conceptual framework for person-centred practice with older people. *International Journal of Nursing Practice*. **9**, 202–209.

McCormack, B. (2004) Person-centredness in gerontological nursing: An overview of the literature. *International Journal of Older People Nursing*. **13**(3a), 31–38.

McCormack, B. & McCance, T. (2006) Development of a framework for person-centred nursing. *Journal of Advanced Nursing*. **56**(5), 1–8.

Mitchell, P.H., Ferketich, S. & Jennings, B.M. (1998) Quality health outcomes model. American Academy of Nursing Expert Panel on Quality Health Care. *Image: Journal of Nursing Scholarship*. **30**(1), 43–46.

Nolan, M., Davies, S., Brown, J., Keady, J. & Nolan, J. (2004) Beyond 'person-centred' care: A new vision for gerontological nursing. *International Journal of Older People Nursing*. **13**(3a), 45–53.

Radwin, L. & Fawcett, J. (2002) A conceptual model-based programme of nursing research: Retrospective and prospective applications. *Journal of Advanced Nursing*. **40**(3), 355–360.

Roach, S. (1987) *The Human Act of Caring*. Canadian Hospital Association, Ottawa.

Slater, P. (2006) Person centred nursing: The development and testing of a valid and reliable nursing outcomes instrument. Unpublished PhD Thesis, University of Ulster, Jordanstown.

Watson, J. (1985) *Nursing: Human Science and Human Care – A Theory of Nursing*. National League of Nursing Press, New York.

Watson, R., Deary, I.J. & Hoogbruin, A.L. (2001) A 35-item version of the Caring Dimensions Index (CDI – 35): Multivariate analysis and application to a longitudinal study involving student nurses. *International Journal of Nursing Studies.* **38**, 511–521.

Wetherell, M., Taylor, S. & Yates, S.J. (eds) (2001) *Discourse as Data: A Guide for Analysis.* Sage, London.

Wilson, V. (2005a) Developing a vision for teamwork. *Practice Development in Health Care.* **4**(1), 40–48.

Wilson, V. (2005b) Developing a culture of family-centred care: An emancipatory practice development approach. Unpublished PhD Thesis, Monash University, Victoria, Australia.

11. *Changing the Culture and Context of Practice: Evaluating the Journey Towards Family-Centred Care*

Val Wilson and Raelene Walsh

Introduction

This chapter will explore the changes (for patients, families, staff and the organisation) that have occurred in one special care nursery (SCN) as a result of the implementation and evaluation of an emancipatory practice development (EPD) programme of work. The study focuses on the experience of staff as they themselves clarify issues, develop ideas for change, and engage in practice development (PD) strategies as they work towards changing practice. The chapter begins by outlining the methods used and describing the implications of these methods for the study. The findings are then represented by comparing the pre- and post-implementation results together with relevant literature to highlight the case for achieving authentic family-centred care in the SCN and thereby achieving significant cultural change.

Methodology

The methodological structure of the study is based on realistic evaluation (RE) as developed by Pawson and Tilley (1997). The aim of RE is to evaluate the relationship between context (setting), mechanism (process characteristics) and outcome (arising from context–mechanism configurations) with questions framed around 'what (strategies) might work, for whom (may they work) and in what circumstances (will they work)?' This approach enabled the opportunity to focus on the pre- and post-implementation data with the view to identifying any improvements that may have occurred as a result of the implementation strategies and to highlight any changes in the culture of the SCN. An overview of the study is presented in Table 11.1.

215

Table 11.1 Overview of the study

Context	The study reported here is set in a SCN (in Australia) providing level 2 services for sick neonates and their families. The unit has around 30 nursing staff.
Aim	The study aimed to explore whether the implementation of EPD activities in the SCN influences the culture and context of care.
Methodology	Realistic evaluation informed by Critical Realism and Realism. Links made to emancipatory intent of practice development, which has its foundations in Critical Social Science.
Participants	Mainly nursing staff, although some activities also included medical, allied health and administrative staff. All nursing staff were female and the length of neonatal experience ranged from a few months to over 25 years.
Consent	The study site self-selected for inclusion into the study when a request for volunteers was circulated within the healthcare organisation. Participation in a variety of activities was voluntary and process consent was obtained at each stage of the study.
Emancipatory practice development activities	Choice of activities aimed at improving care in the unit such as participation in action learning, high challenge/high support mentoring and values clarification related to effective teamwork.
Key stakeholders	Nurses, other healthcare providers, patients, parents and policy makers.
Data collection and analysis	Multi-dimensional collection of data that reflected the attitudes and beliefs of a wide range of stakeholders. Analysis was informed by the principles of the study framework (methodology).
Overall research question	What works (in the practice development programme), for whom does it work (staff, patients, families) and in what circumstances does it work?

The practitioner–researcher

McCormack and Garbett (2003) suggest that 'credibility' of practitioner–researchers is a key factor in the success or otherwise of PD projects. The lead practitioner–researcher had both 'practice' and 'facilitation' credibility amongst staff and this enabled engagement with staff whilst simultaneously knowing the boundaries of such interactions in research practice.

Data collection and analysis

To systematically explore the aims of the study and capture the process and outcomes, several approaches to data collection were undertaken:

- Staff survey taken prior to implementation of (PD) strategies.
- Participant observation pre- and post-implementation of PD strategies.
- Field notes taken during the practitioner–researcher's clinical time on the unit.
- Interviews with staff pre- and post-implementation of PD strategies.

This multi-method approach provided the opportunity to use differing sources of evidence to assist with creating a more meaningful and deeper understanding of the changing context of the unit from a variety of perspectives. The multi-method approach enhances the validity and credibility of the findings (Patton, 1990). Change requires consideration of a way to monitor and evaluate its effectiveness (Bennett, 2003) and processes of evaluation need to consider how such changes have affected the individual, the patient (and family), the healthcare team and the organisation. Outcome-driven data collection is often a major part of this process and assists in reinforcing the longevity of the change in practice (Buonocore, 2004).

Cognitive mapping was used to manage and analyse data and is defined by Eden et al. (1983, p. 39) as a 'modelling technique which intends to portray ideas, beliefs, values and attitudes and their relationship to one another in a form which is amenable to study and analysis'. Thematic analysis was utilised in the process of map formation and refinement (Boyatzis, 1998). An independent researcher examined the labels and refinement of themes to enhance validity.

Exploring the context and culture of the SCN

Before commencing the implementation of EPD in the SCN an in-depth exploration and description of the SCN culture was required to provide a useful baseline against which changes in culture could be evaluated. Nursing staff were provided with this baseline data as a means of understanding the culture in which they worked. This also provided them with the opportunity to choose the PD activities (if any) they wished to be involved in. Figure 11.1 outlines the EPD activities selected by staff.

Four categories were developed from the pre-implementation data: teamwork; learning in practice; inevitability of change; and family-centred care. Values and beliefs connected the categories and were implicit in the unit's work. However, it was evident that values and beliefs were not clearly defined, often differed and were not universally adopted, resulting in recurring tension amongst staff. These findings have been published in detail elsewhere (Wilson et al., 2005); Table 11.2 contains an overview of the findings. Each category will be explored from pre- to post-implementation as a way of highlighting the changes that occurred in the SCN. Findings from the literature will be integrated into the discussion to illustrate the impact of the changes.

Teamwork

It was evident that teamwork, or lack thereof, created angst in the culture of the SCN in early 2002. This was evident by the constant tension that existed in the

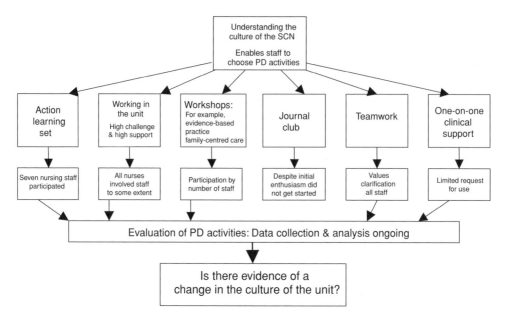

Figure 11.1 Overview of EPD activities in the study.

culture whereby staff felt judged, there was a need for new staff to 'fit in' with the existing culture, they were a team of 'individuals', and there appeared to be unrest and uneasiness amongst the staff. The members of the team held differing values and beliefs about how they worked together and this added to the complexity of the situation. Table 11.2 illustrates these tensions and gives examples of the contradictions between sets of values and beliefs. The resultant culture left some staff unhappy yet fearful of rocking the boat or challenging the status quo that existed amongst this group of people who struggled to form a cohesive and productive team. As one staff member highlighted: 'Teamwork, if you could get that going, breakdown barriers, it would be great, it could improve things'.

Staff were informed of the results as part of the process of PD. Findings were used to illustrate the tensions that existed between differing values and beliefs and the resultant effects this had on teamwork in the unit. Staff chose to focus on teamwork as part of the EPD programme. Part of this work was to develop shared values and beliefs about how they wished to work together and resulted in a shared philosophy statement being developed. The approach adopted has been discussed in detail elsewhere (Wilson, 2005). Developing their shared vision was only part of the process of achieving team effectiveness. The question remained: Were the team of the SCN able to realise their team values and beliefs in practice and to develop the kind of team they envisaged?

When undertaking the post-implementation interviews in 2004 the first question put to staff was 'What is it like for you to work in this unit?' The responses to this question were dramatically different to the interviews undertaken in 2002.

Table 11.2 The tensions evident between differing values and beliefs within the culture

Theme	Enabling pole		Opposing pole
Teamwork	**Cooperation** • Staff are there to help you. (1) **Judgemental awareness** • I don't want to get like that (judgemental) but it's endemic and I found myself almost doing it. (8) **Harmony** • We are like a family. (2)	↔ T E N S	**Individualism** • You do have to fit into their way of working. (8) **Judgemental blindness** • Judgements are made about families but I don't think it affects care. (7) **Disharmony** • There is an underlying feeling of unrest. (9)
Learning in practice	**Partnership** • I am now finding they (consultants) are listening to me and asking for my input. (7) **Questioning** • I am trying to challenge practice (3), challenging staff approaches to care in a non-threatening way. (4) **Team focused** • Sharing information and challenging one another; that's refreshing. (3)	I O N S ↔	**Subservience** • Nurses are not valued for their input, and have little involvement in the decision-making process. (3) **Rituals** • Keeping to the schedule (2), straight into tasks (3), always done this way (7), do my chores (4) **Self-focused** • Fear of new staff, disequilibrium, having to begin a teaching role. (7)
Inevitability of change	**Enablers** • I wanted change. I welcomed it. I'm getting on with it. (6) **New ideas** • The unit has come alive; it was stagnant. I love the change … we (older staff) just do the job, and they are asking questions, they want to know why we do it. (6)	↔ T E N S	**Barriers** • Some people are resistant, been here a long time, comfortable with where they are at. (7) **Old ways** • New versus old staff, the older staff want to hang onto everything they can, they are frightened of more change, vulnerable, they feel unsettled by new staff … they (medical staff) are hanging onto their old ways, they are concerned that things are going to change and they are not prepared for that. (8)
Family-centred care	**Empowerment of families** • I see myself as a co-partner in the babies' care, mum's need to feel it's their baby. (4) **Continuity** • Continuity of care increases parental confidence. (2) **Enabling environments** • Environments need to be less clinical and optimal for growth. (OJ)	I O N S ↔	**Ownership of babies** • Focus is on babies in my care … look after my babies. (4) **Discontinuity** • Some involve parents, others find it hard and just want to do it themselves. (7) **Busyness** • The image of busyness, parents don't want to disturb staff (8), staff remove cot covers, there are lights 24 h a day, noise levels are high (OJ)

Note: Numbers in brackets refer to the number given to each interview participant. OJ, observational journal.

All but one staff member had a very positive response using phrases such as 'I love it', 'great environment', 'very friendly', 'enjoy it', 'I really like it and the people', 'great to be working in a place like this' and 'nice to come to work'. The one staff member who was less positive indicated that this was due to her own sense of apathy towards work in general, rather than a reflection of the team or the environment that she indicated were positive. These responses indicated a dramatic turnaround in the teamwork culture of the unit with staff indicating that morale had improved and people in the unit appeared much happier. This resulted from the consensus achieved by the team about the ways in which they would work with one another (Avery, 2000). Staff felt a sense of belonging and indicated that there was 'a lot less tension' and a greater sense of collegiality, 'I feel like I am really part of a team'. The resultant reduction in tensions enabled staff to work together to improve relationships and to focus on creating an effective workplace culture (Cole & Perides, 1995; Shipley, 1995; Sullivan, 1998).

The work that staff undertook to review teamwork created significant learning in the unit, 'I think that when we did the teamwork thing, I think a lot came out of that', and a sense of accomplishment, 'getting the staff to work as a team has probably been one of the biggest achievements'. The creation of a teamwork philosophy based on shared values (Waughman, 1994) enabled staff to challenge one another about the ways in which they worked together rather than leaving issues to fester or go unresolved, which had previously resulted in tension and a simmering unrest in the unit. The unit developed a culture where staff were 'proud to work here and proud to be part of the team' and this helped to cement the sense of belonging and achievement. As a direct result of individual staff members now investing in the team's success (Pedersen & Easton, 1995; Katzenbach & Smith, 1999), the previous constraints placed on team function (by a small number of staff) were no longer evident (Chapman et al., 1995). The team moved from one where tensions within the team created an unhealthy work environment (Beattie, 1995) to a workplace where staff encouraged and supported one another. In creating such a positive team environment 'people who did not want change have now realised that the unit had to change ... it's positive because we are moving on we are updating, we are part of the team'. This has enabled staff to focus their energy on developing their practice rather than on keeping the peace or maintaining dysfunctional harmony within the team.

Effective teamwork is the key to the delivery of effective high quality care to patients (Minnen et al., 1993; Shortell et al., 1994; Young et al., 1998; Shortell et al., 2004; Wagner, 2004) and to increased patient satisfaction (Meterko et al., 2004). Teams who perceive themselves to be more effective become more involved in taking action to improve care (Shortell et al., 2004). Getting staff involved in how to improve team effectiveness is one way of achieving these improved outcomes for patients as well as staff (Temkin-Greener et al., 2004). Teamwork is a critical dimension of workplace culture (Shortell et al., 1995) and a culture that emphasises teamwork is associated with higher achievements in practice (Strasser et al., 2002). In order to change workplace culture, the SCN team had to change their everyday norms (Parker & Gadbois, 2000a) as they challenged long held and often cherished assumptions and resolved conflict within the team (Parker & Gadbois, 2000b). The team has achieved the three most valuable aspects of building an effective team: they established rules by which to work, they are clear about their roles and responsibilities, and they have created team goals (Larson & LeFasto, 1989; Glaser, 1994; Pearson & Spencer, 1995; Beebe & Masterson, 1997; Salas et al., 1999). Staff in the SCN embarked on the reshaping of their team in order to improve workplace culture. The results of this work suggest they have succeeded thus far and that whilst 'we can never achieve the ideal . . . we can achieve an approximation of the ideal' (Covey, 1998, p. 50). This is their measure of success.

Inevitability of change

With the development of a positive working culture, staff on the unit were able to review practice and move towards a culture that embraced rather than dreaded change. When this study first began, staff on the unit were in a constant state of anxiety about the changes that had occurred as well as the changes that were evolving. A synopsis of the tensions is contained in Table 11.2. Change generates anxiety and uneasiness and is often resisted to ensure that equilibrium within the culture is maintained (Peters, 2001; Porter-O'Grady, 2003; Nemeth, 2003; Buonocore, 2004). Whilst some staff members welcomed change, others were unsure about what this meant for them. There were feelings of resentment about the disruption to their previous peaceful existence, which Balfour and Clarke (2001) suggest can result in a type of bereavement.

Part of the EPD implementation was to work with staff on changing practice and this involved challenging and supporting them about changes that were occurring in the unit as well as changes that they themselves might wish to initiate. In order to enhance the sustainability of the change, it was important to use a structured approach (Buonocore, 2004) that was continuous and cyclical (Street, 1995), where practitioners owned the changes in practice (Balfour & Clarke, 2001). Before this could begin, some of the barriers to change had to be challenged. This was done by questioning assumptions about the effectiveness of existing practice and the process of clinical decision-making on the unit. The practitioner–researcher worked alongside staff using high challenge/high support techniques to ensure staff felt safe during the interaction and to develop a working 'with and for' rather than a 'working on' approach (Meyer & Batechup, 1997). Changing practice often adopts a technical approach (Carr & Kemmis, 1986); in EPD, however, changing practice is also about developing and empowering staff who are involved in the process thereby creating a transformative culture (Manley, 2001).

Generally, staff responded positively to these interactions and over time were able to build upon their skills in order to challenge and support themselves and one another. Staff demonstrated a readiness for change, which is an important factor in the overall success of changes in practice (Cockburn, 2004). Here one member of staff reflects on how this process has influenced practice: 'we didn't have a direction and a philosophy or anything like that we just came and did our work and that's it. Our education stagnated, our practices stagnated, nothing became updated or changed, there was no change'. Through the work that occurred on the unit, staff were able to move forward as they not only accepted the changing context of practice, but also embraced it as it became part of the everyday world of the SCN where 'everyone can express their feelings about what they would like to change', resulting in increased ownership and participation in the change process. When a cosmetic approach to change is adopted, it is doomed to fail; success is more likely when deep-rooted personal change drives practice innovation (Balfour & Clarke, 2001). This helped to reduce the barriers that had previously been constructed to prevent change from being effective as illustrated here:

> *I think once you start getting involved . . . everybody just then . . . it becomes like a rippling, everybody goes with the flow, and there is not that mindset that blocking, and I think it works and people are then all working towards the same and enjoying and not dreading it.*

This rippling effect meant that one small change could often lead to a myriad of changes. The more change that occurred the easier it became to implement such changes in practice. Over time, changes became part of the embedded values of the unit (Buonocore, 2004). Of course, not all barriers to change are easily overcome and there still remained a group of staff that were identified by others as happy to do basic care such as 'feeding, feeding, feeding' but did not want to engage in work that pushed them beyond their task orientated boundaries, to learn new skills or change their behaviour (Nemeth, 2003). Rogers (1995) describes staff who respond to change in this way as 'laggards' who want no part in the change process; however, this behaviour was now being challenged by other members of the team as they moved from the past to future orientated practice.

Changes were very much evident to staff as one nurse suggests:

> *If you look back over the last two and a half years you can see the changes that have happened . . . even though we are slow . . . we are progressing forward and we've made lots of positive changes so I see that as quite rewarding.*

This positive affirmation about the changes that were occurring served to increase confidence in the team's ability to take on significant cultural as well as practice changes as illustrated in this quote from a staff member who had very much been opposed to change in the past:

> *The changing environment, just learning by the change. I don't think I was as rigid, but I had been in that culture, and I think that it was important to not stay where I was at, and so just to accept . . . it is an enjoyable journey, you know you can fight it and it becomes stressful and dreaded or else you can just go with it and enjoy it.*

This resulted in personal as well as professional growth for staff in the SCN and a transition from a culture where change was a burden to a culture that not only supported change but also encouraged it. This, it is suggested, is the real key to lasting success (South, 2004). However, such growth needs to be sustained for a long term and it is increasingly recognised that the creation of a workplace environment that supports learning in practice is key to this sustainability (Wilson et al., 2006).

Learning

Consistently, the findings uncovered contradictions and tensions that were evident in everyday practice. These tensions created a distorted view of how learning was being managed within the SCN. The findings (Table 11.2) suggested that the team believed they were highly skilled, had ample opportunity to learn and were able to access information that would inform their practice. However, this existed alongside other opinions, which suggested that not all staff felt their learning requirements were being met. The learning culture underpinned by existing tensions ensured that little sustainable work was undertaken to change the workplace culture. Indeed, although there was significant evidence of people engaging in learning activities, there was very little evidence to suggest that this learning was impacting on the delivery of care. There appeared to be an overreliance on ritualistic practice with little evidence of nursing staff challenging their own practice or indeed members of the multi-disciplinary team.

The learning culture of the unit had been dominated by tensions that served to restrict the effectiveness of workplace learning. When these tensions were revealed, it enabled staff to look at their existing practice and to move forward as they engaged in EPD activities. In doing this, they were able to resolve the tensions and work towards a more effective learning culture. This was achieved by freeing the oppressive elements of the tension-laden culture, 'I'm feeling a bit more confident and I feel like people are looking up to me, asking me things . . . I think I was smothered a bit', as they worked towards being an effective team. They learned to be more self-assured, 'I ask questions, I never used to but now I just ask . . . I can ask and sort of challenge what they say instead of just agreeing all the time', as they became less subservient within the multi-disciplinary team whereas before they would 'have rolled out the red carpet' for medical staff. They now see themselves as working more collaboratively. Staff developed two essential characteristics that enable growth, change and ultimately transformation to occur, i.e. being open to personal learning as well as facilitating the learning of others (Dixon, 1999).

There was evidence of a positive learning environment with good teamwork (Levec & Jones, 1996; Denton, 1998) and a positive and supportive atmosphere (Senge, 1990; Quinn, 1995; Wilson-Barnett et al., 1995; Moss & Rowles, 1997; Denton, 1998), 'I feel most of the staff are supportive . . . if I need to do some further work . . . most staff are willing to help me', which enabled knowledge creation and transfer into practice (Denton, 1998) as well as sustained learning to occur (Senge, 1990). This was influenced by both internal factors such as the availability of facilitators who challenged practice (Ward & McCormack, 2000) and the individuals' desire to engage in learning (Squire & Cullen, 2001) as well as external factors such as the availability of formal courses (Huggins, 2004) to extend and challenge practice. The role of those in management positions was also key to enabling action to occur (Korhonen & Paavilainen, 2002) and ultimately influenced the success of the learning process (Eraut et al., 1998) and the outcome for the learning environment of the unit. A supportive learning culture emerged that was embedded within the environment, where learning about learning was seen as an important part of the context that enabled the development of the responsible self. Further details about the establishment of a learning culture can be found elsewhere (Wilson et al., 2006) In achieving this change in the learning culture, they were well equipped to deal with the changing context of care.

Family-centred care

The underpinning philosophy of care delivery in the SCN was said to be based on the principles of family-centred care. However, there was evidence (Table 11.2) of variations in care delivery, disempowering practice, and an image of busyness, all of which detracted from the efforts of family-centred practitioners and created a tension between them and staff who favoured a nurse-centred approach to care. Whilst nurses in the SCN espoused a philosophy of family-centred care, there was inconsistency in translating this into practice and this resulted in a disorganised approach to care delivery.

Since the implementation of EPD aims to improve the context and culture of care to ensure effectiveness in the delivery of patient-centred (or in this case family-centred) care, the tension-laden culture that existed in the SCN cried out for some much needed assistance. Staff worked together to improve teamwork, embrace change and develop a learning culture with the ultimate aim of improving family-centred care. This was by far the most challenging aspect of the work they undertook and it encompassed every aspect of care delivery and the way they worked together. Through a series of EPD activities (Figure 11.2) staff identified key areas that they wished to work on in order to achieve their aim.

All staff in the unit were involved to some degree in the high challenge/high support work that related to family-centred care. This formed the basis for challenging existing work practice, for engaging staff in practice change and supporting them as they undertook such changes. Participation in the workshops served to highlight the assumptions made about care delivery, the differences between the espoused and actual delivery of care, and the contradictions inherent in this practice as well as the evidence available that supports both family- and patient-centred care. This provided a good platform for reviewing current practice. Staff who participated in action learning also explored a variety of issues relating to the effectiveness of care delivery.

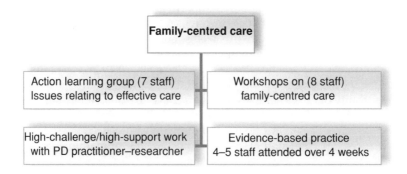

Figure 11.2 Improving family-centred care (EPD) activities undertaken.

Creating meaning: The impact on family-centred care

The findings of the study in relation to creating a family-centred culture are explored through two examples that relate to patients (the babies), parents and staff as well as the environment in which the context of care is based. These examples illustrate effective teamwork, ability to change and learning in and from clinical practice.

Baby what's your name?

On first entering the SCN, one of the things that struck me (practitioner–researcher) was the way staff discussed the babies in their care. These babies were always referred to either by their surname or as 'my baby'. To my ear this sounded disconnected and was neither patient nor family centred. When I asked about this practice, I was told that babies often had no Christian name while they were in the nursery; it was therefore easier for staff to refer to them by their surname. I could accept this rationale as appropriate when the baby had not been named, but questioned this practice with a baby who was now over 3 months old and asked staff to consider the implications of using surnames when the baby had been given a name by his/her family. What kind of message did staff send to families about the care of patients if every baby was known by only a surname or was referred to as 'my baby'? How did parents react to this type of language that served only to distance them from their baby and may have contributed to disempowering them further?

Challenging practice in this way enabled staff to think about what had become a routine ritualistic practice universally adopted by everyone within the SCN team. Raising awareness about the importance of language, the influence this may have on parents as well as where this practice may fit within a family-centred philosophy enabled staff to reflect on their own actions and inactions and how they may influence the way in which care is delivered. If they really wanted to adopt a family-centred care approach, then they would have to consider the significance of their own behaviour as a starting point. This resulted in staff wishing to change practice and to adopt an individualised approach to care, where babies were acknowledged for their uniqueness in the world and as a part of the family context. Changing this inherent behaviour was, however, not easy and several initiatives were used to assist staff in the transition such as the following:

- Informal discussion with EPD facilitator during meal breaks.
- Adopting a no-blame approach where staff were given gentle reminders about the importance of language such as 'oh you mean Joshua'.
- Positive affirmation.
- First names added to the handover sheet.
- Positive role modelling of desired behaviour.
- Challenge and support of each other.
- The name game that involved staff members addressing one another by their surnames and then discussing how this sounded; this was used to raise awareness of the impact of language.

Role modelling and reflection are considered effective strategies to teach family-sensitive care to nurses (Tomlinson et al., 2002). Involvement in these activities ensured that staff were able to change their behaviour as they adopted a more personalised approach to care as noted here: 'When I first came it was more like baby Smith, baby Jones . . . but now people are talking about Sam or Keisha . . . it is individual and very personal, that is why I think it is fantastic'.

Staff embraced this new way of working and made the effort to change, 'people are more aware of what they say', and remind one another about the way in which they speak, 'it's not your baby, it's the mother's baby', ensuring that the baby is placed within the context of the family. Fenwick et al. (2001) suggest that the way a nurse uses language is a strong measure of their capacity to provide facilitative care. The baby is recognised 'as being an individual' and as one nurse said that using the baby's given name is 'closer to the heart if you like . . . it's not sort of at a distance' thereby signifying to the family the connection between the nurse and the baby. This was especially important for longer term patients as it was not only knowing a name but connecting with the individuality of the baby as one nurse discusses here: 'like Chloe, as soon as she starts to squirm and stuff and you know she is not due for a feed, if you put the music on she will go straight back to sleep'. This illustrated not only this nurse's knowledge of Chloe, but also how this knowledge influenced the delivery of care. The nurse 'knowing' the child is important to parents and is a precondition of providing individualised care and establishing rapport with parents (Espezel & Canam, 2003).

The work in acknowledging babies' first names was not only about nursing staff changing behaviour, but it was also about nursing staff influencing other members of the healthcare team: 'I even say to the doctors . . . it is retraining them into thinking it as well . . . I think 90 to 99% of us have just about got it'. Clark (2001) noted that medical staff often referred to babies in the nursery as baby A, baby B, even when their names were clearly identified on their cots. He suggested that this created a barrier between the physician and the parents. This of course is not just about a name, it is about the delivery of care as this nurse here identifies: 'recognising it is the mother, it is her baby, that has come about I suppose by this Christian name business too. It is the mother's baby and you get her involved and help her look after the baby and make the decisions'. This then facilitates a more family-centred approach to care and the development of a family-centred environment.

Family-centred environment

Tension existed in the unit between the 'image of busyness' portrayed by some staff members and the desire for an 'enabling environment', which supports the growing child and the family (Table 11.2). The resulting chaos left parents unsure of their role within the unit and susceptible to the mixed messages conveyed by staff. Care delivery was inconsistent and babies were often subjected to a high level of environmental insult (such as light and noise) and not much in the way of appropriate developmental care. Robinson (2003) suggests that without consistent leadership and clear lines of accountability, developmental care is dependent on the beliefs of the individual, and under such circumstances the quality of care is inconsistent and is often unpredictable. The environment of the SCN unlike the womb is characterised by loud and unpredictable noise (Lotas, 1992). This is especially problematic for the premature neonate who lacks the mature function to deal with such trauma (Zahr & Balian, 1995). Noise is noxious and has been shown to have detrimental physiological effects on the premature infant (Catlett & Holditch-Davis, 1990), which can result in poor weight gain and reduced healing (Bremmer et al., 2003).

In recent years, healthcare staff have been striving to improve the environment for the premature and sick neonate in order to improve outcomes (Bowie et al., 2003). These issues were raised within action learning and subsequently became one of the major areas of change within the unit. Staff awareness of the issues was highlighted through undertaking literature searches, use of evidence to inform practice changes, challenge and support of one another, staff education and environmental advocates, all strategies that help facilitate the introduction of developmental care (Perkins et al., 2004). This has resulted in a more developmentally appropriate approach to care delivery that is influenced by a multitude of factors as outlined in Figure 11.3 below. These factors make up the basis of a developmental programme (Als, 1986) that incorporates family-centred care and promotes bonding (Byers, 2003).

Environmental stressors impact on the growth and development of the baby, disrupt sleep and wake patterns and negatively impact on family bonding (Field, 1990; Graven et al., 1992; Brandon et al., 1999). Once nursing staff were aware of the significant impact that the environment and they themselves had on the growing neonate as well as the family relationship, they were willing to review practice in order to make changes. This of course was not as easy as it sounds. Attitudes and

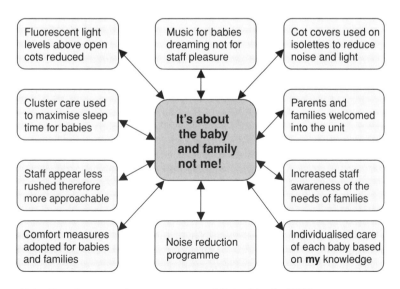

Figure 11.3 Developmental programme established in the SCN.

behaviours have been noted to be the greatest obstacles to reducing noise levels (Graven, 2000) whilst staff are more likely to respond to changes if they themselves are involved in the process of change (Bremmer et al., 2003). It has taken a concerted effort by a team of environmental advocates within the SCN to ensure adoption and sustainability of differing work practices. This team includes nursing staff who indicated an interest in environmental care as well as the unit manager, the nurse educators and myself. The work undertaken has had considerable influence on the SCN atmosphere and resultant impact for the baby, the family and staff:

> *it influences you...become more aware of things so you change the way you would normally do things... for instance about the noise in the isolette...bing bang everywhere...it is really a noxious environment...so when you have been educated...you keep the noise level down.*

Simple things like the introduction of cot covers serve to reduce the impact of noise inside incubators (Saunders, 1995; Walsh-Sukys et al., 2001) and is therefore beneficial for the premature infant (Elander & Hellstrom, 1995; Zahr & Balian, 1995: Robertson et al., 1999). Educating the team regarding how their behaviour impacts on noise has been shown to reduce noise levels (Bremmer et al., 2003). Staff have made a concerted effort to reduce noise levels in the unit as well as introducing 'a lot more music that is suitable for babies rather than suitable for the nursing staff...nice gentle music is good for everyone...it calms us all'. Light has also been shown to stress neonates (Shogan & Schumann, 1993) and disrupt the sleep–wake cycles (Brandon et al., 1999): 'it makes such a big difference turning the lights off because you instantly walk in the door and it's dark and quiet and you tend to be dark and quiet, you don't talk as loud, it makes a huge difference'.

Staff attitudes have also changed about care delivery where it is about 'remembering to cluster care together or look at what's best for the baby, not what's best for us'. This is an indicator of care that is transforming from nurse centred to patient centred. This transformation has not been easy as nurses have had to let go off their ritual-laden, tick-box approach to care and adopt one where care is informed by the behaviour and healthcare status of the individual baby:

> *I feel bad at handover because it looks like I have done nothing for the baby, like I haven't taken the temperature for 6 hours or changed its nappy for 6 hours, but I haven't touched the baby...it's been asleep the whole time and I think that is better than opening the doors every hour and fiddling with something because otherwise they don't have a sleep and they are awake all the time and they get stressed and they don't grow...I always keep my cot covers over their (incubator), keep it nice and dark, try not to bang the doors.*

Clustering care supports infant development by decreasing energy expenditure and increasing rest periods (Holditch-Davis et al., 1996; Als & Gilkerson, 1997; Als, 1998). It relies on the nurse providing care in response to the behavioural cues of the baby in order to deliver individual care in a timely and environmentally appropriate way (Als, 1997, 1998).

228

The two examples used to explore how meaning was created in the unit for patients, families and staff illustrate the depth of work that is required in translating an espoused philosophy of care into a reality of everyday practice. The work undertaken by staff did not occur in isolation and was accompanied by strategies aimed at improving care continuity and enabling families to become more involved in their child's care as well as the other initiatives discussed earlier in this chapter. On a recent visit to the SCN the newly appointed Director of Nursing (acting) remarked that the 'unit felt very friendly with a warm and welcoming environment ... I can see why the parents would feel at ease in the unit'. Whilst this is an indicator of the success of the work from an organisational stakeholder perspective, the stories of the families themselves give further credence to the notion of an authentic integration of family-centred care in the everyday practice of the SCN.

Stories from the SCN

By far the biggest measure of success for the PD work would be the evaluation of care undertaken by the families themselves. Here three short stories captured from thank-you cards and letters narrate the experience of care for families.

T was born in January 2005 weighing just 1000 g and was transferred to the SCN 3 months later for ongoing care her mother wrote:
To all staff at D SCN. Thank you for everything that you have done for T. You may say that you were just doing your job, but I have seen it as more than that. You gave me my baby back. It has been 15 weeks since T was born and it is only now that I am able to do normal mum things with her. This is what I have longed for, for quite a while now and you have helped make this happen for me. This I thank you for very much.

From the parents of a premature baby (Aug 2006):
A very heartfelt thank-you to all for the care and respect given in looking after our precious little gift.

The following is from a letter from parents who spent around 4 weeks in the SCN as their baby was treated for Neonatal abstinence syndrome (March 2006):
B and I would like to thank everyone at SCN for the outstanding, wonderful care and kindness that was continually shown towards us. From the very first moment that we arrived, we were greeted by staff that were truly professional and considerate in every way. Any questions or concerns that we may have had were dealt with in the friendliest, kindest manner. B and I cannot thank each and everyone at SCN who came into our lives enough. We truly respect all the wonderful help and advice that was given and shown to us ... We will never forget all the kindness, cuddles, bathing, playing and endless nappy changes, feeding and burping that everyone had performed while caring for P when we weren't there to do so.

These words are not only very touching, but they also illustrate that staff are making a difference; they are engaging families in care and helping them connect with their fragile neonate at a time when uncertainty is part of daily life. These stories convey that staff in the SCN are indeed achieving family-centred care in practice.

The influence of leadership

An integral component of the success of this work relied upon the influence and transformational leadership of the nurse unit manager who not only embraced the changes that were occurring but also challenged and supported staff to do likewise. In order to explore the role of leadership, Raelene (the nurse unit manager) shares her own PD journey (through a series of narratives).

Raelene's story: Narrative 1

Commencing in the Special Care Nursery unit was a great challenge for me. The unit had never had a permanent Nurse Unit Manager (NUM); in the past it had been managed by other units or short term managers. The staff who had been there for extended periods of time, were surviving as best they could under the circumstances. I could see from the beginning that a great deal of leadership and management skills would be required to achieve the aim of the unit in delivering high quality family centred care.

I had only been in the unit for about a month when I agreed for the unit to be involved in a practice development (PD) study. I didn't really know much about PD at that time but it sounded as if the study would be positive and could assist me with achieving some positive outcomes for the unit. Learning about the concepts of PD helped me to gain some valuable insight into the culture of the unit, the issues that existed and also the strengths that were evident. I could see that the changes would not occur overnight and that first I would have to learn about the unit, the staff, and also gain their trust and respect if I was to become the role model and leader that was required in this unit. As a manager I wanted to be approachable, to listen to staff, to be fair and consistent, to have high expectations for quality of care and to enable staff to develop.

I supported staff to look at the PD work as being positive, not as being threatening, but as a chance to look at where change was required and start making the changes. I was also able to act as a role model displaying the skills, actions and quality of care that was required.

From this narrative we can see that emphasis was placed on the future orientation of practice change in order to break down staff reliance on past practice as a means of informing present and future practice (Porter-O'Grady, 2003). Good leaders always challenge the status quo (Kotter, 1995) and good leadership skills are essential if nursing practice is to change (Watkins, 1997; Buonocore, 2004; South, 2004). Staff looked upon the manager as a role model, mentor, motivator, 'I look up to her, I do . . . I watch her the way she talks to the staff and the parents . . . she's listens to them', as well as expert nurse and patient and family advocate:

> *Her level of experience and the way that she deals with parents, the way she speaks to parents . . . I find really inspiring . . . she is always calm . . . she seems to get this all under control and calm . . . just her whole attitude, her whole attitude about babies coming first, but the family is so important to it.*

Raelene's story: Narrative 2

For me I see PD working hand in hand with management and leadership skills. Without demonstration of clear leadership and management skills, not only from myself but from the educators and other senior members of staff, the implementation of PD strategies would not be effective as integration would be more difficult and may never occur.

Staff locate their direction from leaders who demonstrate the enthusiasm, energy and commitment (Boyatzis et al., 2002) required to shift the perspective of staff (Porter-O'Grady, 2003). Leaders themselves need to embrace change within their own work practice if they expect to influence staff to accept significant change in the workplace (Bennis, 1990; Byram, 2000; Porter-O'Grady, 2003).

Raelene's story: Narrative 3

Learning about the concepts of high challenge and high support assisted me in being able to challenge nursing staff more but in a supportive way. Questions such as 'Is there a reason we don't have this policy?' 'Why do we do this test twice?' were often asked. It also enabled me to encourage them to challenge each other in a supportive way and this was discussed with each of them as part of their development plans. I encouraged them to develop their skills in this area to influence the changes.

High challenge and high support concepts also assisted me with the medical staff, some of them had become very ritualistic in their practice, and nursing staff had never before questioned this. Using this strategy helped me to role model ways in which nurses could challenge the ritualistic practice of medical staff. Medical and nursing staff now work as a team, and using protocols and policies developed from best practice we now have a high challenge/high support working relationship.

As the culture began to change more staff became involved in changing practice. Ideas about what we needed to do and innovative ideas were often discussed in team meetings. Once they had an idea it was then up to that team member to go out and research the idea, get a costing if it was going to cost money and then be the person to drive the change with support. For example a staff member asked 'Why don't we use sucrose for pain relief in neonates?' So I then asked 'Why don't you research and develop a protocol? From ideas such as this many changes have been made. We now have a policy/guideline for use of sucrose for pain relief. We have a nappy cream trial running, we are trialling a new neonatal admission form and care plan, we have handover database and guidelines for handover, just to name a few.

Throughout the work undertaken in the SCN the influence of the unit manager as the team leader was evident. She greatly influenced the EPD work that was being implemented and her support and encouragement of staff ensured their willingness to 'give it a go'. She also challenged and motivated staff to develop new skills and ideas about practice, encouraging them to perform beyond their own expectations (Bass & Avolio, 1994) and ensuring that they in turn drove practice change and helped create the solutions to problems they identified (Parker & Gadbois, 2000c). Her influence cannot be separated from the EPD work undertaken; indeed to try and do so would negate the very intent of the work. During the 2 years it took to conduct the project, the unit manager and I established a powerful and strong relationship based on the premise of EPD where our goal was always to improve the care of patients and their families. She took on board the philosophy of EPD and it then became integral to her own personal philosophy. In other words, the leader was able to transform herself and in doing so she became the inspiration for staff to transform themselves resulting in effective workplace change (Parker & Gadbois, 2000a). In this final reflection, Raelene shares her thoughts on PD and the changes that have occurred for her.

Raelene's story: Narrative 4

Being involved in PD assisted me to reflect on my own skills and abilities. When I commenced in the unit there was a great dependence on me to make all decisions. Being able to reflect on this assisted me to make changes and to start to challenge the staff to try and make decisions and become more independent. It assisted me in promoting the empowerment of the nursing staff. I started to ask them questions such as 'What do you think you should do?' and also supported their decisions or helped them to reflect on the decision and learn from it. I had to challenge myself to deal with issues as they occurred to assist with the continuing change of the unit. Often dealing with staff issues such as performance or resistance to change is difficult and time consuming. Knowing that these could be barriers to the change motivated me to keep going.

Learning about PD and becoming a practice developer has been a positive journey for me. The concepts of PD fitted with my own values and beliefs around change and promoting the empowerment of others to make changes as well as utilising staff knowledge and skills to identify change. The PD concepts assisted me to develop new skills and have some direction and planning about how to achieve our goal of delivering high quality family centred care. Through the work completed it also helped to challenge me personally and assisted me to reflect on how I could improve my own practice.

Working with the unit manager and fostering a partnership saw the bringing together of differing skills of facilitation (me) and leadership (nurse unit manager) in order to foster growth and to challenge and support one another (Titchen & Binnie, 1995). This enabled the unit manager to develop the necessary skills to become an effective EPD facilitator, to actively engage staff in the change process, and to implement strategies in practice to ensure that sustainable change was achieved long after the facilitator left the unit.

So what happens now?

Thor et al. (2004) suggest that facilitators help busy managers and teams by assuming reasonability for the many tasks involved in improving care and transferring insights across the organisation. They have clearly missed the point of effective facilitation with EPD work where the premise is to develop skills and expertise of those involved (Manley & McCormack, 2003) to ensure that staff can engage in meaningful work in everyday practice rather than always be dependent upon outside facilitation to drive and direct practice change. The learning that occurs whilst undertaking this type of work can then be used to inform other changes within this context as well as within the organisation.

The practitioner–researcher leaves the unit

Since the purpose of EPD is to introduce sustainable change in practice, it is fitting to take a look at what has happened since I left the unit. I spent some time with the unit manager reviewing the work that we undertook as well as looking at the changes that have been implemented since my departure. Table 11.3 highlights some of the changes that have occurred in relation to the major stakeholders, the patients, the families, the staff and the organisation.

Review of outcomes

These findings give credence to the notion that successful change is enhanced when driven by the those who implement care (Street, 1995) and that nurses are in the best position to ensure that changes are sustained (Balfour & Clarke, 2001). The combined strategies used in this and other studies (Haffer, 1986) have been shown to be successful in facilitating practice change and the range of opportunities for engaging practitioner-enhanced sustainability (Clarke et al., 1998). This has not only resulted in changes within the SCN but has also reached other parts of the organisation and impacted on practice changes elsewhere.

Whilst PD research is integrated into practice, the findings of this work require the capability to be transferred into other care environments (Clarke & Procter, 1999). Nursing staff have been involved with the dissemination of the work that has taken place in the SCN by presenting it at forums and conferences at a local, national and international level. One of the posters developed won first prize ($500) at 'International Nurses Day'. This money was then used to assist with the environmental changes in the unit. Participating in these activities has served to increase staff confidence, promote the reputation of the unit, as 'we've built up a name for the unit as well which is really positive. I have had feedback from different people . . . word gets around', as well as establish kudos for the PD activities undertaken. The work on values clarification has been repeated in three other units to date. Action learning has been utilised as a peer support strategy for nurse educators across the healthcare network. The process that resulted in changing nursing handover practice and developing a database for patient information has been translated into another adult-based unit. As a result of the significant work that has been undertaken on changing handover practice, the unit manager has now been asked to chair a committee that is reviewing the effectiveness of handover throughout the hospital.

Sustainability

PD is concerned with creating a culture that is not only sustainable but also one where developing practice is not dependent on any one individual (Garbett &

Table 11.3 Post-implementation changes

PD activity	Involvement by staff	Achievements	Impact factor
Working in the unit: High challenge/high support	All nursing staff involved with flow on effect to other staff within the SCN, e.g. medical staff	Babies are recognised as unique individuals Development of a supportive environment Introduction of care that is developmentally appropriate Increased awareness of how language and behaviour impacts on care Increase in problem-solving and critical thinking Family-Centred care drives nursing practice Nursing staff now proactive in changes in the unit Nurses participate in decision-making about care	Creation of an environment that supports the baby, the family and staff Emphasis on providing developmental care; families made to feel welcome and encouraged to participate in their babies care Nursing staff eager to suggest potential changes for improving practice Nurses less subservient and now act as advocates
Action learning set	Seven nurses participated	Various achievements based on the work of participants; details published in Wilson et al. (in press)	Multi-dimensional, impact on all aspects of teamwork, change, learning and FCC
Workshop: Evidenced based practice	A number of staff participated in the workshop	Developed skills is searching for evidence, reviewing research literature and using evidence in practice	Use of evidence to inform staff and to base practice changes such as 'reducing noise levels in the nursery'
Workshop: Family-centred care	A number of staff participated in the workshop	Staff clearer about the barriers to FCC as well as the difference between what we say we do and what we actually do in practice	FCC becomes the authentic philosophy that drives care
Teamwork: Values clarification	All staff in the unit involved	Developed a shared vision for teamwork; worked towards realising vision in practice; see Wilson (2005)	Improved teamwork, staff morale, sense of collegiality and multi-disciplinary communication
One on one clinical support	Limited use by a few nursing staff	Staff feel challenged and supported by the facilitator	Individual staff take on new challenges
Journal club	Not established	Nil	Nil

McCormack, 2004). It would therefore be a failure if the PD work ground to a halt once the practitioner–researcher left the unit as the emphasis is on developing practitioners who carry on the work long after the facilitator has left. This has resulted in staff continuing the change process: 'I think we have come a long way, it's positive . . . there is still lots we need to do and there will always be lots we need to do'. Since leaving the unit, many new initiatives have been implemented including such things as the 'hug a bub programme' where volunteers work alongside staff to reduce the distress of babies withdrawing for narcotic addiction. Working with the concepts of PD over an extended period of time has assisted with these concepts becoming embedded into the everyday culture and functioning of the unit. When asked a question recently about what PD activities the SCN still undertake, the manager's response was: 'it is now part of everyday practice and the concepts have been integrated into the culture of the unit. It's a part of how we work'.

Conclusion

This chapter has shared the journey of the changing context and culture of the SCN. Numerous EPD activities were undertaken by staff in order to facilitate the changes that occurred. There was the need for staff in the SCN to be cognizant of their own values and beliefs and the way they worked together in order to create the bridge between the espoused philosophy of family-centred care and translating this into practice. Through a PD process, staff were able to bring into the open the differences, tensions and conflict that existed for them with the team. Understanding and challenging their value system, establishing mutual respect and creating a shared meaning of teamwork were all important factors in the success of the team development. Cultivating a shared vision to underpin the cultural development of the SCN team was an essential step in the overall strategy of improving patient care. In order for teams to explore the effectiveness of the care they delivered, it was imperative that they first of all reflected on their effectiveness as a team. They were then able to adopt EPD strategies to review the existing state of play in the unit, freeing themselves from the oppressive elements of the tension-laden culture as they worked through a system of development opportunities that resulted in effective change. A supportive learning culture emerged that was embedded within the environment, where learning about learning was seen as an important part of the context that enabled the development of the responsible self. Each of these achievements, creating a supportive team, developing the responsible self and being responsive to change enabled the development of an authentic model of 'family-centred care' in the SCN. The significance of this work may go some way towards answering the question of how an espoused philosophy of care is realised in practice.

References

Als, H. (1986) A synactive model of neonatal behavioral organization: Framework for the assessment of neurobehavioral development in the premature infant and for support of parents in the intensive care environment. *Physical and Occupational Therapy in Pediatrics.* **6**, 3–55.

Als, H. (1997) Earliest intervention for preterm infants in the newborn intensive care unit. In: *The Effectiveness of Early Intervention* (ed M. Guvalvick), pp. 47–69. Brooks, Baltimore.

Als, H. (1998) Developmental care in the newborn intensive care unit. *Current Opinion in Pediatrics.* **10**, 138–142.

Als, H. & Gilkerson, L. (1997) The role of relationship-based developmentally supportive newborn intensive care in strengthening outcome of preterm infants. *Seminar in Perinatology.* **21**, 178–189.

Avery, C. (2000) How teamwork can be developed as an individual skill. *Journal for Quality and Participation.* **23**, 7–13.

Balfour, M. & Clarke, C. (2001) Searching for sustainable change. *Journal of Clinical Nursing.* **10**, 44–50.

Bass, B. & Avolio, B. (1994) *Improving Organizational Effectiveness Through Transformational Leadership.* Sage, Thousand Oaks, CA.

Beattie, A. (1995) War and peace among the health tribes. In: *Interprofessional Relations in Health Care* (eds K. Soothill, L. Mackay & C. Webb), pp. 11–30. Edward Arnold, London.

Beebe, S. & Masterson, J. (1997) *Communication in Small Groups: Principles and Practices,* 5th edn. Addison-Wesley Educational Publishers, New York.

Bennett, M. (2003) Implementing new clinical guidelines: The manager as an agent of change. *Nurse Manager.* **10**, 20–23.

Bennis, W. (1990) *Why Leaders Can't Lead.* Jossey-Bass, San Francisco.

Bowie, B., Hall, R., Faulkner, J. & Anderson, B. (2003) Single-room infant care: Future trends in special care nursery planning and design. *Neonatal Network.* **22**, 27–34.

Boyatzis, R. (1998) *Transforming Qualitative Information.* Sage, Thousand Oaks, CA.

Boyatzis, R., McKee, A. & Goleman, D. (2002) Reawakening your passion for work. *Harvard Business Review.* **80**, 87–94.

Brandon, D., Holditch-Davis, D. & Belyea, M. (1999) Nursing care and the development of sleeping and waking behaviors in preterm infants. *Research in Nursing and Health.* **22**, 217–229.

Bremmer, P., Byers, J. & Kiehl, E. (2003) Noise and the premature infant: Physiological effects and practice implications. *Journal of Obstetric, Gynecologic, and Neonatal Nursing.* **32**, 447–454.

Buonocore, D. (2004) Leadership in action. *AACN Clinical Issues.* **15**, 170–181.

Byers, J. (2003) Care and the evidence for their use in the NICU. *American Journal of Maternal Child Nursing.* **28**, 174–180.

Byram, D. (2000) Leadership: A skill, not a role. *AACN Clinical Issues.* **11**, 463–469.

Carr, W. & Kemmis, S. (1986) *Becoming Critical: Education, Knowledge and Action Research.* Falmer, London.

Catlett, A. & Holditch-Davis, D. (1990) Environmental stimulation of the acutely ill premature infant. Physiological effects and nursing implications. *Neonatal Network.* **8**, 19–25.

Chapman, T., Hugman, R. & Williams, A. (1995) Effectiveness of interprofessional relationships: A case illustration of joint working. In: *Interprofessional Relations in Health Care* (eds K. Soothill, L. Mackay & C. Webb), pp. 46–61. Edward Arnold, London.

Clarke, C. & Procter, S. (1999) Practice development: Ambiguity in research and practice. *Journal of Advanced Nursing.* **30**, 975–982.

Clarke, C., Procter, S. & Watson, B. (1998) Making changes: A survey to identify mediators in the development of health care practice. *Clinical Effectiveness in Nursing.* **2**, 30–36.

Clark, P. (2001) What residents are not learning: Observations in an NICU. *Academic Medicine.* **76**, 419–424.

Cockburn, J. (2004) Adoption of evidence into practice: Can change be sustainable? *Medical Journal of Australia.* **180**, 66–67.

Cole, R. & Perides, M. (1995) Managing values and organisational climate in a multiprofessional setting. In: *Interprofessional Relations in Health Care* (eds K. Soothill, L. Mackay & C. Webb), pp. 62–74. Edward Arnold, London.

Covey, S. (1998) The ideal community. In: *Community of the Future* (eds F. Hesselbein, M. Goldsmith, R. Beckland & R. Schubert), pp. 49–58. Jossey-Bass, New York.

Denton, J. (1998) *Organisational Learning and Effectiveness.* Routledge, London.

Dixon, D. (1999) Achieving results through transformational leadership. *Journal of Nursing Administration.* **12**, 17–21.

Eden, C., Jones, S. & Sims, D. (1983) *Messing About in Problems.* Pergamon, Oxford.

Elander, G. & Hellstrom, G. (1995) Reduction of noise levels in intensive care units for infants: Evaluation of an intervention program. *Heart and Lung, Journal of Acute and Critical Care.* **24**, 376–379.

Eraut, M., Alderton, J., Cole, G. & Senker, P. (1998) Learning from other people at work. In: *Supporting Lifelong Learning* (eds R. Harrison et al.). Routledge, London.

Espezel, H. & Canam, C. (2003) Parent-nurse interactions: Care of hospitalized children. *Journal of Advanced Nursing.* **44**, 34–41.

Fenwick, J., Barclay, L. & Schmied, V. (2001) 'Chatting': An important clinical tool in facilitating mothering in neonatal nurseries. *Journal of Advanced Nursing.* **33**, 583–593.

Field, T. (1990) Alleviating stress in newborn infants in the intensive care unit. *Clinics in Perinatology.* **17**, 1–9.

Garbett, R. & McCormack, B. (2004) A concept analysis of practice development. In: *Practice Development in Nursing* (eds B. McCormack, K. Manley & R. Garbett). Blackwell, Oxford.

Glaser, S. (1994) Teamwork and communication. *Management Communication Quarterly.* **7**, 282.

Graven, S. (2000) Sound and the developing infant in the NICU: Conclusions and recommendations for care. *Journal of Perinatology.* **20**, 88–93.

Graven, S., Bowen, F., Brooten, D. Eaton, A., Graven, M., Hack, M., Hall, L., Hansen, N., Hurt, H. & Kavalhuna, R. (1992) The high-risk infant environment. Part 1: The role of the neonatal intensive care unit in the outcome of high-risk infants. *Journal of Perinatology.* **12**, 164–172.

Haffer, A. (1986) Facilitating change. Choosing the appropriate strategy. *Journal of Nursing Administration.* **16**, 18–22.

Holditch-Davis, D., Torres, C., O'Hale, A. & Tucker, B. (1996) Standardized rest periods affect the incidence of apnea and rate of weight gain in convalescent preterm infants. *Neonatal Network.* **15**, 87.

Huggins, K. (2004) Lifelong learning – the key to competence in the intensive care unit? *Intensive and Critical Care Nursing.* **20**, 38–44.

Katzenbach, J. & Smith, D. (1999) *The Wisdom of Teams.* McKinsey, Boston.

Korhonen, V. & Paavilainen, E. (2002) Learning teams and networks. *Journal for Nurses in Staff Development*. **5**, 267–273.

Kotter, J. (1995) Leading change: Why transformation efforts fail. *Harvard Business Review*. **73**, 59–67.

Larson, C. & LeFasto, F. (1989) *Teamwork: What Must Go Right, What Can Go Wrong*. Sage, Newberry Park, CA.

Levec, M. & Jones, C. (1996) The nursing practice environment, staff retention, and quality of care. *Research in Nursing and Health*. **19**, 331–343.

Lotas, M. (1992) Effects of light and sound in the neonatal intensive care unit environment on the low-birthweight infant. *NAACOG's Clinical Issues in Perinatal and Women's Health Nursing*. **3**, 34–44.

Manley, K. (2001) Consultant nurse: Concepts, processes, outcome. Unpublished PhD Thesis, Manchester University/RCN Institute, London.

Manley, K. & McCormack, B. (2003) Practice development: Purpose, methodology, facilitation and evaluation. *Nursing in Critical Care*. **8**, 22–29.

McCormack, B. & Garbett, R. (2003) The characteristics, qualities and skills of practice developers. *Journal of Clinical Nursing*. **12**, 317–325.

Meterko, M., Mohr, D. & Young, G. (2004) Teamwork culture and patient satisfaction in hospitals. *Medical Care*. **42**, 492–498.

Meyer, J. & Batechup, L. (1997) Action research in health-care practice: Nature, present concerns and future possibilities. *Nursing Times Research*. **2**, 175–186.

Minnen, T., Berger, E., Ames, A., Dubree, M., Baker, W. & Spinella, J. (1993) Sustaining work redesign innovations through shared governance. *Journal of Nursing Administration*. **23**, 35–40.

Moss, R. & Rowles, C. (1997) Staff nurse job satisfaction and management style. *Nursing Management*. **28**, 32–34.

Nemeth, L. (2003) Implementing change for effective outcomes. *Outcomes Management*. **7**, 134–139.

Parker, M. & Gadbois, S. (2000a) Building community in the healthcare workplace: Part 3, Belonging and satisfaction at work. *Journal of Nursing Administration*. **30**, 466–473.

Parker, M. & Gadbois, S. (2000b) Building community in the healthcare workplace: Part 1, The loss of belonging and commitment at work. *Journal of Nursing Administration*. **30**, 386–390.

Parker, M. & Gadbois, S. (2000c) Building community in the healthcare workplace: Part 2, Envisioning the reality. *Journal of Nursing Administration*. **30**, 426–431.

Patton, M. (1990) *Qualitative Evaluation and Research Methods*, 2nd edn. Sage, Newberry Park, CA.

Pawson, R. & Tilley, N. (1997) *Realistic Evaluation*. Sage, London.

Pearson, P. & Spencer, J. (1995) Pointers to effective teamwork: Exploring primary care. *Journal of Interprofessional Care*. **9**, 131–138.

Pedersen, A. & Easton, L. (1995) Teamwork: Bringing order out of chaos. *Nursing Management*. **26**, 34–35.

Perkins, E., Ginn, L., Fanning, J. & Bartlett, D. (2004) Effect of nursing education on positioning of infants in the neonatal intensive care unit. *Pediatric Physical Therapy*. **16**, 2–12.

Peters, T. (2001) Leadership: Sad facts and silver linings. *Harvard Business Review*. **79**, 121–130.

Porter-O'Grady, T. (2003) A different age for leadership, Part 2. *Journal of Nursing Administration*. **33**, 173–178.

Quinn, F. (1995) *The Principles and Practice of Nurse Education*, 3rd edn. Chapman and Hall, London.

Robertson, A., Cooper-Peel, C. & Vos, P. (1999) Contribution of heating, ventilation, air conditioning airflow and conversation to the ambient sound in the neonatal intensive care unit. *Journal of Perinatology*. **19**, 362–366.

Robinson, L. (2003) An organisational guide for an effective developmental program in the NICU. *Journal of Obstetric Gynaecological and Neonatal Nursing*. **32**, 379–386.

Rogers, E. (1995) *Diffusion of Innovations*. The Free Press, New York.

Salas, E., Rozell, D., Mullen, B. & Driskell, J. (1999) The effect of team building on performance. *Small Group Research*. **30**, 309–330.

Saunders, A. (1995) Incubator noise: A method to decrease decibels. *Pediatric Nursing*. **21**, 265–268.

Senge, P. (1990) *The Fifth Discipline: The Art and Practice of the Learning Organization*. Doubleday Currency, New York.

Shipley, J. (1995) *Advancing Health in New Zealand*. Government Printer, Wellington.

Shogan, M. & Schumann, L. (1993) The effect of environmental lighting on the oxygen saturation of preterm infants in the NICU. *Neonatal Network*. **12**, 7–13.

Shortell, S., Marsteller, J., Lin, M., Pearson, M., Wu, S.-Y., Mendel, P., Cretin, S. & Rosen, M. (2004) The role of perceived team effectiveness in improving chronic illness care. *Medical Care*. **42**, 1040–1048.

Shortell, S., O'Brien, J., Carman, J., Foster, R., Hughes, E., Boerstler, H. & O'Connor, E. (1995) Assessing the impact of continuous quality improvement/total quality management: Concept versus implementation. *Health Service Research*. **30**, 377–401.

Shortell, S., Zimmerman, J., Rousseau, D., Gillies, R., Wagner, D., Draper, E., Knaus, W. & Duffy, J. (1994) The performance of intensive care units: Does good management make a difference? *Medical Care*. **32**, 508–528.

South, S. (2004) The 360 degrees nature of change implementation and the essential three Ds for successful and sustainable change. *Clinical Leadership and Management Review*. **18**, 107–111.

Squire, S. & Cullen, R. (2001) Clinical governance in action. *Professional Nurse*. **4**, 1014–1015.

Strasser, D., Smits, S., Falconer, J., Herrin, J. & Bowen, S. (2002) The influence of hospital culture on rehabilitation team functioning in VA hospitals. *Journal of Rehabilitation Research and Development*. **39**, 115–125.

Street, A. (1995) *Nursing Replay: Researching Nursing Culture Together*. Churchill Livingstone, Melbourne.

Sullivan, T.J. (1998) *Collaboration: A Health Care Imperative*. McGraw-Hill, New York.

Temkin-Greener, H., Gross, D., Kunitz, S. & Mukamel D. (2004) Measuring interdisciplinary team performance in a long-term care setting. *Medical Care*. **42**, 472–481.

Thor, J., Wittlov, K., Herrlin, B., Brommels, M., Svensson, O., Skar, J. & Ovretviet, J. (2004) Learning helpers: How they facilitated improvement and improved facilitation-lessons from a hospital-wide quality improvement initiative. *Quality Management in Health Care*. **13**, 60–74.

Titchen, A. & Binnie, A. (1995) The art of clinical supervision. *Journal of Clinical Nursing*. **4**, 327–334.

Tomlinson, P., Thomlinson, E., Peden-McAlipine, C. & Kirschabaum, M. (2002) Clinical innovation for promoting family care in pediatric intensive care: Demonstration, role modelling and reflective practice. *Journal of Advanced Nursing.* **38**, 161–170.

Wagner, E. (2004) Effective teamwork and quality of care. *Medical Care.* **42**, 1037–1039.

Walsh-Sukys, M., Reitenbach, M., Hudson-Barr, K. & Depompei, P. (2001) Reducing light and sound in the neonatal intensive care unit: An evaluation of patient safety, staff satisfaction and costs. *Journal of Perinatology.* **21**, 230–235.

Ward, C. & McCormack, B. (2000) Creating an adult learning culture through practice development. *Nurse Education Today.* **20**, 259–266.

Watkins, K. (1997) *Certificate of Management Course Handbook.* University of Newcastle, Newcastle upon Tyne.

Waughman, W. (1994) Professionalisation and socialisation in interprofessional collaboration. In: *Interprofessional Care and Collaborative Practice: Commission on Interprofessional Education and Practice* (eds R. Casto & M. Julia), pp. 23–31. Brooks/Cole, Pacific Grove, CA.

Wilson, V. (2005) Developing a vision for teamwork. *Practice Development in Health Care.* **4**, 40–48.

Wilson, V., McCormack, B. & Ives, G. (2005) Understanding the workplace culture of a special care nursery. *Journal of Advanced Nursing.* **50**, 27–38.

Wilson, V., McCormack, B. & Ives, G. (2006) Re-generating the 'Self' in learning: A practice development approach. *Learning in Health and Social Care.* **5**, 90–105.

Wilson, V., McCormack, B. & Ives, G. (2008) Developing healthcare practice through action learning: Individual and group journeys. *Action Learning: Research and Practice.* **5**(1), 21–39.

Wilson-Barnett, J., Butterworth, T., White, E., Twinn, S., Davies, S. & Riley, L. (1995) Clinical support and the project 2000 nursing student: Factors influencing this process. *Journal of Advanced Nursing.* **21**, 1152–1158.

Young, G., Charns, M., Desai, K., Khuri, S., Forbes, M., Henderson, W. & Daley, J. (1998) Patterns of coordination and clinical outcomes: A study of surgical services. *Health Services Research.* **33**, 1211–1236.

Zahr, L. & Balian, S. (1995) Responses of premature infants to routine nursing interventions and noise in the NICU. *Nursing Research.* **44**, 179–185.

12. *Becoming a Facilitator – The Journey*

Jacqueline Clarke, Helen O'Neal and Shirley Burke

Introduction

Our roles involve working with nurses, health professionals, other agencies and members of the public. To this end, it is necessary to be adaptable and flexible in the approaches we adopt as facilitators. Harvey et al. (2002) suggest that effective facilitation requires us to be adaptable in possessing and utilising the appropriate skills and attributes to meet the context and purpose and to recognise the requirements of individual situations.

In this chapter, we will share the individual journeys we experienced as we developed our facilitation expertise, through narratives of our reflective accounts, describing and highlighting the development of skills and knowledge as well as how these were used. We collectively explored our journeys, to identify common themes that we believe can enhance the development of facilitation skills or indeed may inhibit the process. In conclusion, we consolidate our feelings, learning and development making cognizant the supportive mechanisms that we became aware of as we undertook our facilitation journeys.

Facilitation is greatly dependent on the maturity of the learner, taking into consideration the culture and the environment in which the 'learning'/skill development is taking place. Throughout this chapter, some of these pertinent influences upon facilitation will be explored.

There are different modes of facilitation, for example those described by Heron (1989b) as hierarchical, cooperative and autonomous. Their use will be determined by the purpose of the facilitation and will also range along a continuum depending on this purpose (Grundy, 1982). In recognising what is significant we must be aware of what is of importance to us as the facilitators and what is salient to the co-learners (Titchen, 1999).

Before we present our narratives and exploration of the common themes, we share our biographies, so that you may gain a sense of who we are as 'persons'.

Biographies

Shirley Burke

Currently, I am working as the practice development (PD) leader at a large metropolitan paediatric health facility in Melbourne, Australia. This is a newly created role, which involves supporting the Director of Research and PD in implementing a hospital-wide PD strategic plan. The role involves working alongside a multidisciplinary team, including managers and practitioners to support them in facilitating and evaluating PD strategies. My journey will relate to my time as a nurse educator within another large healthcare facility and the co-facilitation of PD initiatives within that role and to my early work in the new role.

Helen O'Neal

I am a clinical support nurse within an intensive care unit of a large teaching hospital in the United Kingdom. My role is clinically based enabling new staff to develop their skills and competency as well as providing education and development for existing staff. I am supported and work closely in this role with a clinical nurse specialist in critical care, five PD nurses within general intensive care, and a team of four PD nurses from neuro-critical care. My key responsibilities are to manage the intensive care PD team and to participate in and disseminate trust-wide communication relating to PD. I am also responsible for supporting colleagues as they undertake activities including guideline development and coordinating study days. My journey shares how I have begun to develop skills as a facilitator within this role to become accredited by the Royal College of Nursing (RCN).

Jacqueline Clarke

Following qualification as a Registered General Nurse, Midwife and Health Visitor, I have worked in varying organisations throughout Northern Ireland. I have a keen interest in multidisciplinary work and team effectiveness, having facilitated team building within the Primary Care setting in my role as a Primary Care Facilitator. I completed my academic studies through the University of Ulster achieving a BSc (Hons) Professional Development in Nursing with the community option in Health Visiting, an MSc in Health Promotion, and I have received RCN accreditation for facilitation and the Postgraduate Certificate in Life Long Learning. I am currently working as a PD Facilitator in an integrated Trust in Northern Ireland. This area of work has been pivotal in driving forward strategies and policies for the trust. For me, PD is there for the ultimate benefit of patients/clients. My motivation and enthusiasm has been reinforced by the support and encouragement I receive from both my nursing colleagues and practitioners from other disciplines.

Narratives of our facilitation journeys

During our discussions about our respective journeys, we identified a number of common themes underpinning our learning and development as facilitators.

These themes, identified below, have therefore been used to present key areas in our journeys:

- Facilitation as an unconscious activity
- Becoming aware
- Developing knowledge and skills
- Building expertise

Shirley
Facilitation as an unconscious activity

I was working as a clinical educator within an acute Paediatric setting and my role involved staff support in the clinical area. This was conducted at the bedside and through formal education sessions with the learning outcomes focusing on skills and knowledge acquisition. I did not use critical questioning in my facilitation of the learning of staff. I initially saw my role as one of provider of knowledge rather than a facilitator. My role was seen as the panacea to all the issues within the clinical area; it seemed that the educator was there to 'fix' the problems. I spent my time 'putting out fires'.

Looking back now, the nursing staff took little responsibility for developing their own practice. I found it difficult to develop independent learning within the nursing staff and in engaging staff in developing practice, such as in the implementation of change or use of evidence to guide practice.

Becoming aware

I would have continued to work in this way, driving practice change and running from fire, to fire until I attended the RCN PD week-long school in 2003. This experience was rather overwhelming for me as the concepts and processes of PD were completely new to me and I came away feeling rather shell shocked. I felt challenged in my assumptions around learning and development and my role as an educator. I came to realise that my facilitation of learning and development of staff involved a 'working on' rather than a 'working together' approach. I saw the potential for my role to become more a facilitator rather than a provider of learning and returned to my workplace enthused by the possibility that PD could enable the nursing staff on the paediatric units to become more accountable for their own practice.

Encouraged by this prospect, I began to utilise questioning skills to enable staff to take ownership of their own learning and the issues identified within the clinical area. As nursing staff approached me with educational issues, I tried to develop in them some ownership and responsibility for taking action but the nursing staff were comfortable in their role as dependent learners. My new approach was met with resistance and held me up for criticism as I struggled with the concept that if I was not providing what the staff needed or felt that they needed, then maybe I was not performing in my role as a nurse educator. This internal dilemma was something that I found difficult to overcome and I sought support from a more experienced practice developer. This relationship provided me with the necessary support and challenge and together with a process of critical self-reflection I began to improve my questioning skills to become more enabling in my role as an educator.

The majority of my interactions focused on one-to-one support for junior staff in the clinical area. I still did not feel that I was achieving much in changing staff attitudes but felt that I had grown in my knowledge and skills. I was now more confident to challenge and support staff to reflect on their own practice.

Developing knowledge and skill

Co-facilitation

My own facilitation journey continued in 2004 when I was involved in the co-facilitation of action learning groups. The group members were other educators who had shown an interest in developing their own enabling skills. This model of co-facilitation was chosen as there was limited experience in facilitation within the healthcare network. The purpose of this model was to allow me to gain some skills in facilitation in a supported environment and to allow the dissemination of facilitation knowledge from the lead facilitator who was an experienced PD facilitator. The co-facilitation was evaluated after 6 months using a creative process. I have presented my personal learning through this process.

Getting started

Although I had attended PD school as a participant and had witnessed the facilitation of action learning (AL) and had a sound theoretical knowledge around AL process and the structure of running a group, I had a feeling of uncertainty. I did not feel equipped to deal with the actual facilitating of groups. It was time to test my theoretical knowledge in a real way. As a facilitator, the group members looked to me as an expert, particularly in adhering to and reviewing the process. This left me feeling quite out of my depth at times.

As I grew in my facilitation skills and knowledge, I began to develop more confidence. I utilised strategies for allowing participants to feel safe and comfortable in the group. The use of icebreakers such as 'Trauma, Trivia and Joy' (McGill & Beaty, 2001) and sharing of personal reflections at commencement of each group helped in this. I recognised the importance of high challenge/high support in balance, sometimes by trial and error, and my skills around reviewing the AL process and how to stay on track began to take shape.

Although my confidence in facilitating the groups had grown, I continued to experience the see-saw of feeling confident and then being challenged on a particular day or moment taking one back to all those feelings of uncertainty and shakiness. This became less apparent as time and experience allowed my skill level to increase. I found that adhering closely to the process within the AL group and being mindful of ensuring that processes such as ground rules are adhered to and can be referred back to if necessary allowed me as a novice to feel a sense of security in my facilitator role.

Dealing the catharsis

There were issues within the AL groups that led to outpouring of emotions. This was a huge challenge for me as a novice facilitator. Dealing with catharsis within the group felt like 'a baptism of hell'. I saw the expert facilitator role model, the use of practice domains such as graceful care and attentive listening skills as described by Titchen (2000), which allowed participants to feel valued and respected. This together with the use of ground rules, as previously described, assisted me in managing the difficult issues within the groups.

The catharsis within the group contributed very much to that see-saw effect: 'Just as you get your confidence up . . . the dealing with emotive issues seems to send you right back where you started'. I found that it was an emotional roller coaster and was often quite drained after AL sets.

Holding hands

The lead facilitator acted very much as a role model. In the initial AL groups, she role modeled her own facilitation style. I learned from observing the way she interacted with participants using high support and high challenge to enable the learning within the group to occur. I focused on my own questioning skills using Heron's Interventions (Heron, 2000) to guide me in becoming more enabling in the group. As I began to take the lead facilitation role within the group, I relied on the expert facilitator to take over when I was out of my depth. It was important that I test out my facilitation skills in the real world and be allowed to take risks, but to feel supported. Close facilitation relationships were developed between us. We used body language and eye contact to communicate and rely on one another. This developed into what was seamless co-facilitation for participants within the group.

Learning

The challenge and support provided by the lead facilitator in the meetings following each AL group allowed me to reflect on how I was growing in my own facilitation role. This provided the basis of my learning journey: 'you learn a lot from reflection . . . . at the time, you've just got to get on with it . . . later on when you think about it . . . . "okay that was handled well because of this and that wasn't because of that" and how would you do it differently?'. Schon (1983) refers to this process as reflection-in-action and reflection-on-action. I learned to 'wing it' and reflect within the group on how things were going, especially during difficult sessions, and to hope that it all went well; and then use the time after the AL set to reflect on my facilitation within the group and on my own learning.

The relationship between facilitators was one similar to critical companionship as described by Titchen (2000). I was never made to feel stupid, but my critical companion, co-facilitator, enabled me to reflect on how I was moving along the learning continuum. This allowed me to feel quite normal and to bolster my self-esteem, especially following cathartic group sessions when I was left feeling quite inadequate in facilitation skills.

I changed in my educator role from 'working on' staff to 'working with' them. The change in approach embraced a facilitative way of working alongside staff, providing challenge and support and utilising skills learned through the AL groups.

Building expertise

New challenges

As I developed as a facilitator in PD work, I took on an additional role to introduce the concept of PD to another organisation. This was a challenging role as I moved from being a learner in PD to being seen as the expert. As a relatively novice facilitator, I was now challenged to role model facilitation skills to others. I set up some critical reflection groups within the middle leadership in the hospital, utilising a co-facilitation process with the principal nurse educator similar to that experienced in my own learning journey.

I emulated the facilitation style of my lead facilitator. I recognised the need to adhere very closely to the AL process and role model questioning skills; but I found myself being more supportive than challenging as I tried to engage participants in the process. I believe that this was driven by a need to make my AL groups seem like a success in order to engage others within the organisation who were watching the progress. As I gained confidence in this role and the commitment to the group was more established, I felt more able to use challenge within the AL groups to better enable the participant learning.

I had little support in this role and found myself often out of my depth. I developed close co-facilitation relationship with the principal educator and utilised review and reflection following each AL group to move forward together in our journey of facilitation. I attended an AL set of which I am a group member to gain personal support. This enabled me to recognise that I had a toolbox of necessary skills and knowledge and although I still had a long way to go in my facilitation journey, this gave me a sense of achievement. I believe that sometimes we need to take the risk and move forward into the unknown to recognise our own abilities.

PD school revisited

In 2006, I was given the opportunity to co-facilitate at a PD school. I was exposed to a very different facilitation style with an experienced PD facilitator with whom I co-facilitated. This seemed to be a much more relaxed, calm style with group participants allowed to take control of the group processes and their own learning within the group. I observed this facilitator engaging group members, establishing relationships and using non-verbal cues to ensure that everyone felt a sense of belonging and of being important in a very enabling way. The skills of active listening, appropriate questioning and building trust were very evident. The pace was slower with more use of silence. This led me to reflect on how the facilitator seems to effortlessly guide the group to where it needs to be through gentle support and challenge in the right balance. The facilitation style allowed the group to take on the ownership of their own learning and move to become autonomous at the end of the week (Heron, 2000).

As a co-facilitator, I once again found myself out of my comfort zone and was initially left feeling less adequate in my skills and knowledge. I was challenged by the pace at which the group moved forward into independent active learning and to directing their own learning, which I felt was often out of my scope. After further reflection, I have recognised the enormous learning from this and have had to re-frame the experience to recognise that my facilitation journey has only commenced and I have a long way to go. This experience has provided me with a rich knowledge of use of self in the facilitation relationship, which I can now take with me on the journey towards developing my own unique style of facilitation.

Helen
Facilitation as an unconscious activity

I started my journey in facilitation by being a clinical support nurse predominantly working one to one with nurses at the bedside. This interaction tended to focus on enabling staff to be clinically competent with skills and knowledge necessary for intensive care nursing. Much of this work was supported by the provision of formal teaching on study days and assessment documentation.

These clinical support shifts tended to be prearranged and would concentrate on staff new to intensive care, enabling them to be assessed as clinically competent in line with our documentation. With more confident staff these shifts involved supporting them to care for a more challenging patient or develop skills with a piece of equipment that was unfamiliar to them. Although the purpose of these shifts was to develop clinical skills, this tended to be in such a manner that staff had to prove their competence and knowledge base and in this way were very task orientated. The need to ensure clinical competence is still necessary; however, I realise now that my approach was inflexible and challenging. With insight into the role of a facilitator, I recognise that in many cases this was probably not the most effective way to help individuals learn. This became apparent whilst critically reflecting on my clinical practice to achieve the Royal College of Nursing (RCN) standards for facilitator accreditation (Royal College of Nursing, 2006).

Becoming aware

On reflection with the benefit of the theory underpinning facilitation there were many aspects that I didn't consider about the relationship I was entering into with the individual staff. For example, I didn't get to know the learner very well (Titchen, 2003), identify or negotiate their learning style and although felt I offered high challenge/high support, perhaps I did not and in reality this was probably more the result of the presence of a senior colleague. It was often difficult to feel like we had achieved anything during these shifts and I always felt the learner still had a long way to go. I appreciate now that I didn't have the insight into how effective my role could be. If only I had a toolkit!

During these interactions, I recall being mindful of the type of questions I asked but these were all trying to elicit information or proof of knowledge and probably when considering Heron's six category intervention analysis (Heron, 1989b) were mainly confrontational with some being more supportive. During the formal study days when I taught alongside these shifts the skills I demonstrated were also limited to an authoritative manner with minimal participation from the learners.

Developing knowledge and skills

As my facilitation skills developed within this role, my interactions with learners became more relaxed and embraced a more personal approach. I began showing an interest in where they were with their learning and aimed to identify with them any specific needs or issues they had, as well as anything else that might have affected their work. This contact was reciprocated with self-disclosure by me as the facilitator. I began illustrating explanations with examples from my personal experiences demonstrating the use of critical companionship (Titchen, 2003). Building relationships in this way benefited me by increasing my confidence to act as a role model and work more in partnership with learners rather than be confronting and challenging.

I began to feel more competent in my role and gained more job satisfaction as I saw people developing. My relationship with colleagues became richer, some staff began being proactive in trying to arrange shifts with me and seek me out for support. These shifts became a protected resource and a valued commodity as colleagues experienced the skill mix, competence and confidence of staff improving. Furthermore, additional posts in this role were created within the intensive care unit highlighting how facilitation was being supported by a change in culture and how, within my role, I had influenced this.

Building expertise

A pivotal point in my development as a facilitator was my involvement in a trust-wide emancipatory action research project (Kemmis, 2001), facilitated by the Royal College of Nursing, London. The reasons for this are multifaceted but I feel can primarily be attributed to the experience of working closely with an experienced facilitator and being involved in an AL group (McGill & Beaty, 2001). Some of the skills I developed during this time include critical self-reflection as well as challenging myself to ask the right questions whilst avoiding being too supportive but enabling my colleagues to realise their own solutions and carry them out. Involvement with this group enabled me to feel confident to undertake an exercise to gain feedback from my colleagues about my role and performance known as 360° feedback (Ward, 1997). Although this was challenging, many of the comments were positive and gave me a great deal of confidence and insight into how others saw me and my role.

Being a practitioner–researcher (Carr & Kemmis, 1986) within the action research project enabled me to become aware of and develop many more facilitation skills. These included action planning, giving and receiving feedback and enabling others to develop facilitation knowledge and skills. As my role developed I began to manage a team of clinical support nurses, which enabled me to focus on my facilitation skills. The relationship I developed within my team fostered a culture of facilitation and two-way learning. I became very excited by the concept and its power to enable and develop others, particularly when using activities such as AL. In doing this, I embraced the opportunity to become an RCN-accredited facilitator. This process encouraged me to analyse my skills and approach, in the light of facilitation theories such as critical companionship (Titchen, 2003) and Mezirow's theory of reflectivity (Mezirow, 1981) whilst developing a portfolio of evidence.

Certainly, from having considered my practice in relation to some of the theories underpinning facilitation, I feel that I have had many 'light bulb' moments demonstrating Mezirow's perspective transformation (Mezirow, 1981). For example, when reflecting on a series of one-to-one facilitation sessions with a member of my team, for the purpose of providing evidence for my accreditation portfolio, I recognised that inadvertently I had guided the learners thinking through Mezirow's stages of perspective transformation. The outcome achieved for the learner was a change of attitude as they recognised an alternative way of dealing with a situation. For me this realisation was a light bulb moment as I recognised not only how this theory could be useful but also that I had already developed my problem solving during facilitation in a similar methodological manner.

As a practitioner–researcher I undertook aspects of the research within clinical areas, which presented me with a variety of opportunities to develop my facilitation skills further. For example, I enabled and empowered others to become stakeholders in any project work and use action planning to clearly identify how they would take these forward rather than taking on this role myself. A key part of my role was to develop and update clinical guidelines and protocols. As part of the action research project, we began looking at these with a tool. In doing this, more staff became involved in reviewing guidelines and developing action plans for revising them. Once I had introduced this tool and enabled staff to participate, they became more confident with the process and identified additional areas they wished to focus on to develop new guidelines. As a facilitator, my role was then to provide these staff with support and resources to enable them to pursue the process, rather than do it myself.

I began to be more deliberate in my approach to facilitation with my team, using more structured activities such as AL or critical companionship where appropriate. I gained great insight into the opportunities for group and personal development that AL offered and was keen to share this with my team as I was undertaking a lot of one-to-one work with them using critical companionship and much of this was duplicated. I felt strongly that this approach was invaluable, enabling the team to support each other's development as well as learn many other useful skills, as I had. However, my enthusiasm wasn't enough to convince my team that it was something they should do and I faced the challenge of selling the concept to them, justifying how it was an effective use of their time both as individuals and collectively. I achieved this by sharing information about AL and allowing them to consider the benefits and consequences of the meetings on a personal and professional level. The group felt that they needed feedback from the wider team about their performance and effectiveness so we decided to use the format of AL and 360° review to work through and share this feedback. The group was familiar with the 360° review process that I had previously used to invite them to furnish me with feedback as part of the action research project. Following assimilation of this in my AL I felt able to share with them my experience and action plans as I recognised that we shared some common issues. This proved to be effective and the group embraced the process from then.

Being a facilitator is a lifelong journey of development, which I have really only just begun, but I am constantly experiencing enlightenment as the opportunities to be a facilitator arise. In this way, I have continued to influence the culture supporting facilitation both within my clinical area and the hospital as well as further developing my own skills. I believe opportunities arise for a reason and continue to embrace the challenge of facilitation and develop my own toolkit! As the Chinese proverb says, 'when the pupil is ready the teacher will appear'.

Jacqueline

> *We must trust our feelings and risk the challenges of new experiences. Lets rededicate ourselves to provide learning communities to accomplish that goal we must step back and trust our students and ourselves, and give us all the freedom to learn.*
>
> *(Rogers & Freiberg, 1994, p. 375)*

Rogers and Freiberg's (1994) statement underpins the ethos of my facilitation journey. As I have progressed/developed I have been aware of gradual changes in my thinking and approaches to facilitation, and the importance of learning together by gaining the confidence in trusting my own experiences and intuitions, and the creation of an exploratory culture as advocated by Goleman (1996).

My reflective journey of facilitation has touched on elements where I have viewed development or a change in my attitude and practice. I have taken consideration of the Postgraduate Certificate (PG Cert) in Life Long Learning (University of Ulster). This 1-year course via the internet is based on a model of personal and professional development. It aims to encourage critical reflection and analysis of practice and promote innovative approaches to work practices within the practitioner's organisation. I have also highlighted the theories of learning and the tools that can be used in facilitation to assist in the promotion of a learning culture with the ultimate development of professional craft knowledge (Titchen, 1999).

Facilitation as an unconscious activity

Prior to commencing the PG Cert in Life Long Learning, I facilitated many groups both uni-professional and multi-professional. These groups did have aims and objectives and they did achieve outcomes. However, looking back, these aims and objectives were often my own thoughts and ideas and hence probably quite hierarchical in nature (Heron, 1989b). I know that when I would have been facilitating a group, I would have been more conscious of the task being addressed than perhaps being conscious of the process, e.g. protocol development, audit outcomes, etc. Before undertaking the PG Cert, I felt that my facilitation was satisfactory. I felt that I was achieving outcomes. Things were organised into their compartments and I was in control. I would say that there was probably little 'intentional' consideration of the process unless there was evidence that certain techniques did not work, e.g. media, written materials used, etc., to achieve the outcome. This attention to technical facilitation (Manley & McCormack, 2003) could well have been to the detriment of the individual and the group dynamics, which McCormack and Wright (2000) ascertain should be afforded equal attention. I feel now that there has been some degree of transition (Mezirow, 1991), whereby I give more consideration to the process of facilitation and in the preparation for the facilitation session.

Becoming aware

The lifelong learning PG Cert and my experiences have strongly reinforced that the means or process of facilitation is essential for sustainable professional and personal development. However, in reflecting back, this only scrapes the surface of my journey through facilitation. The real benefit for me was through the challenge of my colleagues and tutors in my statements on the on-line discussions, which really encouraged and motivated me to look more deeply at the varying aspects involved in facilitation. Throughout my own learning, the on-line discussion postings in the lifelong learning course proved to be a true support and really challenged and motivated me to reflect deeper. Positive reinforcement is a great motivator supporting Herzberg's motivational hygiene theory (Atherton, 2002).

The work of Honey and Mumford (1992) highlights the following four types of learners: 'activists' tend to have lots of experiences; 'reflectors' do lots of reviewing; 'theorists' reach lots of conclusions, and 'pragmatists' make plans. Unless we are aware of these we can misinterpret our learners. As a reflector myself (Honey & Mumford, 1992), I would often have mulled over events or experiences by myself. This would have been a very superficial type of reflection without probably reaching the final stage where a plan of action is required. However, now becoming more open and making a conscious effort for personal disclosure, I realise that few problems are new, and in the sharing of these experiences with other individuals, significant benefits can be gained (Grant, 1987).

Facilitation is not solely 'to make things easier' as in the definition of Kitson et al. (1998), but to develop the skills required for the practitioner/learner to develop and gain knowledge and understanding, which is sustainable and can be progressed. Taking Kitson et al.'s definition literally, I associated some of this to the leadership work in my personal life. To me, yes, I was making things easier but I was doing things for the learners rather than letting them develop. I would very much query the facilitation aspect. I was 'doing for', rather than facilitating. I reckon that this was due to various factors, e.g. time, age, etc. Often as facilitators we can become preoccupied with the learning outcomes/aims and objectives taking little notice of the journey in reaching these.

This elementary definition of Kitson et al. (1998) conceals an array of variables that can enhance or detract from the facilitation experience. Whilst working with practitioners in enhancing practice, the remit was identified, progress was made and action resulted. To the outsider this would appear successful, and, yes, the goal was achieved. However, I feel development of a trusting relationship, knowledge of the individual, personal disclosure, the promotion of a learning culture did not progress as much as could have been possible as the facilitation was very technical in nature.

Developing knowledge and skills

When facilitating, I felt that I was viewed as the expert. Individuals and group members often looked to me for guidance, for example, in a learning set, which was established with senior practitioners to explore and challenge routine practice with the ultimate aim of developing a strategy for their service. As such this warranted more than technical facilitation. I anticipated that the cooperative/autonomous (Heron, 1989b) mode would be most appropriate. However, feedback from these senior colleagues illustrated the view that the set should have been more structured and I should have been more directive.

Taking into consideration my new and developed insights within facilitation, this seemed to me a backward step. However, I should acknowledge that this was only the first meeting of this group and a 'new' way of working. My assumption, or what Greenwood (1993) would identify as reflection before action, prior to the set meeting would have been that the set members knew each other better than I, as they would have frequent team meetings together. However, I can now identify with much of the theory and the realism that people know each other only superficially because there may not be an environment that is conducive to open and frank discussions (McGill & Beaty, 2001).

Within the PG Cert and portfolio development, my reflections in the narratives took into consideration an awareness of my feelings and thoughts, a critical analysis of the situations and the potential for development of new perspectives (Atkins & Murphy, 1993). The use of structured models of reflection, e.g. Johns (1993) and Carper (1978) and Gibbs (1988) have enabled me to delve deeply into my own experiences and that of others. The skills of the facilitator are essential in any learning environment to enhance the relationship between the facilitator and his/her learners/colleagues. Within my reflections and mapping of RCN standards, I have tried to highlight the complexity of abilities and versatility required. These take into consideration the knowledge of the facilitator, the knowledge of the learner or practitioner and the whole context, taking cognisance of the culture within the organisation.

The utilisation of the facilitator's skills can make an immense difference to the learner. If commitment and genuineness are shown from the facilitator, it is often reciprocated and a solid relationship can be developed (Titchen, 1999). This 'realness' of the facilitator is essential, (Rogers, 1983). Disclosure on the part of the facilitator is vital. In translating some of Roger's work, those facilitators whose behaviours tend to be 'closed', the group members tend to echo the information. Conversely, where the facilitator is 'open', the members are more likely to explore and experiment (Rogers, 1969). Much of this genuineness stems from our awareness of our own internal facilitation taking into consideration 'hunches' and 'gut' feelings. Trust and honesty are essential and respect for persons needs to be reinforced (Rogers, 1983). This is evidenced in the relationship of the critical companion through mutuality and reciprocity (Titchen, 2000), strongly highlighting the importance of the humanistic aspects and being open and conscientious. I would suggest that we can show our genuineness through the giving of personal information and feeling comfortable with oneself, and the receiving of information without judgement, acknowledging limitations and denoting graceful care within the critical companionship framework.

In getting to 'know the learners', icebreakers are a useful and somewhat relaxing way of encouraging individuals to interact. It has happened to me that the group of practitioners which I thought would not be overaccepting such an approach were in fact very receptive. My intuition was very much challenged. Indeed, the set members opened up greatly and I feel that all participated much more than I had anticipated with the facilitator's role being tested to the limit in attempting to clarify, follow the flow and ensure 'turn-taking' among the participants.

Building expertise

As my facilitation journey has progressed, my confidence has grown. I would say that this has been greatly aided by the use of various tools, which are highlighted in this section, the production of a portfolio of evidence, which was submitted to the Royal College of Nursing and successfully accredited using the RCN facilitation standards and also the appointment of a secondment opportunity whereby I was the external facilitator for a variety of practice initiatives in numerous organisations throughout Northern Ireland.

In determining the significance/importance of issues for practitioners I now utilise the values clarification exercise (Warfield & Manley, 1990). This enables all members of a learning set to ascertain beliefs and values, and what really matters to them, and ensures everyone recognises alternative views to his/her own without judgment. In one particular group when using this tool, I felt that their responses were really very honest, but what I really noticed with this group was how similar and comparable they felt about their role and how they felt they had no defined remit. In fact, the majority of members felt that they were taking on roles that were the responsibility of other professionals. It powerfully struck me that this indeed would be a very challenging and risk taking group, as part of the remit was the development of a strategy for their particular service and would ultimately entail a change in working practices.

Within our Trust we have established a number of learning sets. Concerted efforts have been made to get to know one another through icebreakers and various warm-up exercises. The use of icebreakers has been a new experience to me in the facilitation setting; I suppose I felt introductions were sufficient! However, I realise that these activities do provide space for acknowledgement of emotions or other factors that may be deterrents to the learning process. They also allow for the development of interpersonal relationships, which affords practitioners the confidence and willingness to reveal 'things' that are personal and sensitive to them.

The establishment of ground rules is an essential element in any learning set and really contributes to the development of relationships within the set. They set the boundaries and thus, if crossed, individuals can challenge without the challenge being taken personally as all members have agreed to these ground rules initially. They really encourage a safe and trusting environment.

Throughout my experiences I would emphasise the importance of reflection, not just ad hoc superficial reflection, but structured with the use of models such as the 'model of structured reflection' adapted from Johns (1993) and Carper (1978), Schon's (1987) reflective practitioner or Kolb's (1984) 'Learning from Experience' cycle. It is only when we truly analyse that we actually can have insight and thus move on. In concluding, I would certainly agree with Revans (1983), 'there is no learning without action and no action without learning', even though we may not realise it at the time!

Our journeys explored

From our individual narratives, we have identified a number of themes that underpin our collective experiences.

Knowing the learners

Often as facilitators, as highlighted, we can become preoccupied with the learning outcomes/aims and objectives taking little notice of the journey in reaching these. Allowing learners to identify priorities, barriers and enablers for their learning such as learning styles and motivational drivers is essential. The literature would support various theories and styles for learning and assimilating knowledge. Brockbank et al. (2002) suggest that style, content and significance of learning will vary over time, and thus flexible learning styles are required within individuals. This flexibility has been mirrored by ourselves as we have developed to effectively enable others. Motivation is fundamental to the facilitation process. Houle (1961) has identified three motivational styles: goal orientation, activity orientation and learning orientation. However, as adults, motivation is driven by need or relevancy. It is evident from previous experience that if people are nominated onto a group rather than volunteering themselves the outcome may not be as productive. Helen has highlighted an example of how she shared the need for AL with her team so enabling them to participate voluntarily.

Facilitation is made more effective by building relationships with the learners. Titchen (1999) has emphasised this within the relationship domain of her critical companionship framework. She encourages facilitators to be physically and emotionally present to create a culture of feeling valued in promoting a trusting relationship. Our journeys each demonstrate how our experiences became richer as we became more aware of the benefits of building mutual relationships with our learners. It is important to create a culture of feeling valued and to get to know the individuals at personal and professional levels. In a learning environment, the Johari Window framework (Luft, 1984) can help in examining how open we perceive ourselves. There are some things that do not need to be shared, but the difficulty arises if the lack of openness or the disparities are detrimental to the functioning of the individual relationship or group dynamics and hence there is a view of incongruence.

Skills of the facilitator

Overreliance on the facilitation role by the learner is a potential problem and sometimes as a facilitator it is difficult to know when to let go. Heron (1989b) ascertains that the overuse of informative interventions can lead to dependence on the facilitator. This reinforces the need for facilitators to be skilled in various approaches and to identify what is important in the context/situation whilst being flexible in their approach. It is important to reinforce that each individual brings his/her own expertise and knowledge and that group members including facilitators are all equal. As novice facilitators, we have really been made aware that the process and keeping control of the group are paramount to the safety within it. As we developed confidence in our own skills to trust that control of the groups we were facilitating would not be lost, we were more capable of enabling these learners to become independent in their learning and development.

The learning style of the facilitator may inhibit the use of other learning styles to the detriment of his/her students and we need to be open to show this. It is important for the facilitator to acknowledge his/her own limitations. Sharing with others what difficulties the facilitator may have in relation to aspects of learning, for example, may be beneficial and enlightening for the learners. Consequently, the facilitator can learn from the learners as he/she reflects. This supports the work of Jack Mezirow (1991) in the aspect of perspective transformation, which may either be a sudden insight or may be transitional. This also compliments the two-way relationship. The facilitator cannot expect the student to be open if he/she is not. If commitment and genuineness are shown from the facilitator, it is often reciprocated and a solid relationship can be developed, which benefits from the mutual exchange of knowledge and experiences reinforcing the critical companionship framework (Titchen, 1999).

Supportive mechanisms

An enabler of effective facilitation common in all our journeys is the co-facilitation model. This allowed us to observe an experienced facilitator and try out the skills in a supported but challenging environment. This was evidenced in the gaining and testing out of skills in the AL sets. Acquisition of the skills necessary for facilitation such as critical reflection (Burrows, 1997) is enhanced through this experiential process, and the close adherence to the process within AL groups gives one a sense of security. To be mindful of ensuring that processes such as ground rules are adhered to and can be referred back to if necessary allows the novice facilitator to feel more competent and confident as evidenced by both Shirley and Jacqueline.

The three journeys highlight that as facilitators the support of an experienced critical companion/clinical supervisor is essential. The role of this person is to challenge and support the novice facilitator in his/her reflections. There needs to be a role modeling of expert facilitation skills. Harvey (1993) and Loftus-Hill and Harvey (2000) suggest that most facilitators develop their skills and styles of working through such experiential processes, either informal or more formally. In this way, the novice facilitator can learn by observation, practice and reflection.

Becoming independent

There is continuous learning throughout the facilitation journey. An increasing level of challenge and risk taking, together with personal reflection on performance, is required to move forward and test out new skills. Our stories demonstrate that as we developed our skills, dissemination of this knowledge is required to mentor and support others in their facilitation journey. As confidence in our own skills increased we were able to step back and facilitate the learners to become independent in their learning and development, allowing them to progress from a state of dependency on the facilitator to being autonomous in their learning and development (Heron, 1989b).

Box 12.1   Heron's six categories of questions (summarised from Heron [1989a]

Prescriptive: The supervisor explicitly directs the supervisee by giving advice or direction.

Informative: The supervisor intends to provide information, to instruct the supervisee.

Confrontative: The supervisor challenges the beliefs or behaviour of the supervisee. Such confrontation does not imply aggression, rather invites the supervisee to consider some aspect of their work or themselves that was perhaps previously taken for granted.

Cathartic: The supervisor attempts to help the supervisee move on through the expression of thoughts or emotions previously unacknowledged or unexpressed.

Catalytic: Interventions are focused on helping the supervisee become increasingly self-directed and reflective. They aim to 'bump up' the developmental level of the supervisee as a professional.

Supportive: The supervisor attempts to reinforce the confidence of the supervisee through focusing on their areas of competence, and attending to what they did well.

Facilitation is recognised as being most effective in environments where the culture offers both challenge and support. Facilitators are pivotal to enabling such environments to develop through demonstrating transformational leadership (Antrobus & Kitson, 1999). This is aided by asking the right questions. Heron (1989a) offers us six categories of questions that offer different approaches (Box 12.1). This creates a culture with two-way dynamics where colleagues are encouraged to develop and articulate ideas, whilst being supported with the necessary knowledge, information and skills.

Conclusion

Our learning and development in facilitation was derived from an exploration of the narratives described in our individual journeys. Our development within the facilitation roles continues. For the purpose of this chapter, we have summarised what we feel are the key points for anyone undertaking this journey in facilitation.

At the beginning of our journeys, we recognised that we were perceived as experts within our fields and in order to share this knowledge tended to work 'on' our learners. Reflection in and on our practice has illustrated how this approach may limit the development of others rather than enhancing it. We demonstrated that facilitation is much more about working with our learners and understanding the influences this has on learning. We identified that building a mutual, trusting relationship with our learners was vital to the success of facilitation. This enabled us to clarify what was important for the learners and any contextual priorities.

We have been supported in our development by participating in mechanisms such as AL or clinical supervision. These have enabled us to practice critical self-reflection, giving and receiving feedback and learning to ask the right questions within a safe environment of high challenge and high support. In doing this, we were able to develop our own skills and toolkits thereby increasing our flexibility and adaptability, which influences, in a positive direction, our ability to facilitate effectively. We also benefited from observing role models whilst working with expert facilitators and/or using the co-facilitation model to develop our skills.

Applying our skills to the framework for RCN facilitation standards was useful in mapping our journeys. It assisted in highlighting our experiences and linking the theory to practice. This enabled us to identify gaps in our expertise and learning as well as celebrate our strengths. As we have repeatedly illustrated, being a facilitator is a continuous two-way learning process and our journeys have really only just begun.

We have highlighted how facilitation is less preoccupied with outcome, aims or competencies but working towards the process of enabling others to explore what is important or salient and problem solve towards being guided to a solution. This approach and thinking may be seen to achieve a more sustainable move towards change. In conclusion, learning through facilitation requires an organisational culture that is receptive to challenge and creativity (Ward & McCormack, 2000) through critical reflection; indeed what Manley describes as a 'transformational' culture. As Manley states:

> *The very first step is to break the cycle of 'busyness' and create time to start these processes*
> *Manley, 1999, p. 100*

References

Antrobus, S. & Kitson, A. (1999) Nursing leadership: Influencing and shaping health policy and nursing practice. *Journal of Advanced Nursing.* **29**(3), 746–753.

Atherton, J.S. (2002) *Learning and Teaching: Motivation to Learn.* Maslow Inc., UK. Available from http://www.staff.dmu.ac.uk/~jamesa/learning/motivirn.htm.

Atkins, S. & Murphy, K. (1993) Reflection: A review of the literature. *Journal of Advanced Nursing.* **18**, 1188–1192.

Brockbank, A., Beech, N. & McGill, I. (2002) *Reflective Learning in Practice.* Gower, London.

Burrows, D.E. (1997) Facilitation: A concept analysis. *Journal of Advanced Nursing.* **25**(2), 396–404.

Carper, B. (1978) Fundamental ways of knowing in nursing. *Advanced Nursing Science.* **1**, 113–123.

Carr, W. & Kemmis, S. (1986) *Becoming Critical: Education, Knowledge and Action Research.* Falmer, London.

Gibbs, G. (1988) *Learning by Doing: A Guide to Teaching and Learning Methods.* London.

Goleman, D. (1996) *Emotional Intelligence – Why it Can Matter More Than IQ.* Bloomsbury, London.

Grant, J. (1987) Designing groupwork for professional updating. In: *Open Learning for Adults* (eds M. Thorpe & D. Grugeon). Longman Group, Harlow.

Greenwood, J. (1993) Reflective practice: A critique of Argyris and Schon. *Journal of Advanced Nursing.* **27**(5), 1183–1187.

Grundy, S. (1982) Three modes of action research. *Curriculum Perspectives.* **2**(3), 23–34.

Harvey, G. (1993) Nursing quality: An evaluation of key factors in the implementation process. Unpublished PhD Thesis, South Bank University, London.

Harvey, G., Loftus-Hills, A., Rycroft-Malone, J., Titchen, A., Kitson, A., McCormack, B. & Seers, K. (2002) Getting evidence into practice; the role and function of facilitation. *Journal of Advanced Nursing.* **37**(6), 577–588.

Heron, J. (1989a) *Six Category Intervention Analysis*, 3rd edn. Human Potential Resource Group, University of Surrey, Guildford.

Heron, J. (1989b) *The Facilitator's Handbook.* Kogan Page, London.

Heron, J. (2000) *The Facilitator's Handbook.* Kogan Page, London.

Honey, P. & Mumford, A. (1992) *The Manual of Learning Styles.* Peter Honey, Maidenhead.

Houle, C.O. (1961) *The Inquiring Mind.* University of Wisconsin Press, Madison, WI.

Johns, C.C. (1993) Professional supervision. *Journal of Nursing Management.* **1**, 9–18.

Kemmis, S. (2001) Exploring the relevance of critical theory for action research: Emancipatory action research in the footsteps of Jurgen Habermas. In: *Handbook of Action Research: Participative Inquiry and Practice* (eds P. Reason & H. Bradbury), pp. 91–102. Sage, London.

Kitson, A., Harvey, G. & McCormack, B. (1998) Enabling the implementation of evidence based practice: A conceptual framework. *Quality in Health Care.* **7**, 149–158.

Kolb, D. (1984) *Experiential Learning.* Prentice-Hall, Englewood Cliffs, NJ.

Loftus-Hill, A. & Harvey, G. (2000) *A Review of the Role of the Facilitators in Changing Professional Health Care Practice.* RCN Institute, London.

Luft, J. (1984) *Group Processes – An Introduction to Group Dynamics.* Mayfield Publishing, Palo Alto, CA.

Manley, K. (1999) Developing a culture for empowerment. *Nursing in Critical Care.* **4**(2), 57–58.

Manley, K. & McCormack, B. (2003) PD: Purpose methodology, facilitation and evaluation. *Nursing in Critical Care.* **8**(1), 22–29.

McCormack, B. & Wright, J. (2000) Achieving dignified care for older people through PD: A systematic approach. *Nursing Times Research.* **4**(5), 340–352.

McGill, I. & Beaty, L. (2001) *Action Learning: A Guide for Professional, Management and Educational Development*, 2nd edn. Kogan Page, London.

Mezirow, J. (1981) A critical theory of adult learning and education. *Adult Education.* **32**(1), 3–24.

Mezirow, J. (1991) *Transformative Dimensions of Adult Learning.* Jossey-Bass, San Francisco.

Revans, R. (1983) *The Origins and Growth of Action Learning.* Chartwell Brant, Bromley.

Rogers, C.R. (1969) *Freedom to Learn.* Charles E Merrill, Columbus, OH.

Rogers, C.R. (1983) *Freedom to Learn for the 80's.* Charles E Merrill, Columbus, OH.

Rogers, C.R. & Freiberg, H.J. (1994) *Freedom to Learn*, 3rd edn. Prentice-Hall, Englewood Cliffs, NJ.

Royal College of Nursing (2006) *RCN Facilitation Standards – Version 1.* Available from www.rcn.org.uk/resources/practicedevelopment/downloads/about-pd/RCN_Facilitation_Standards_V1.pdf.

Schon, D.A. (1983) *The Reflective Practitioner.* Temple Smith, London.

Schon, D.A. (1987) *Educating the Reflective Practitioner.* Jossey-Bass, San Francisco.

Titchen, A. (1999) A conceptual framework for facilitating learning in clinical practice. Occasional paper 2. Royal College of Nursing Institute, Radcliffe Infirmary, Oxford.

Titchen, A. (2000) Professional craft knowledge in patient-centred nursing and the facilitation of its development. In: *University of Oxford DPhil Thesis*. Ashdale Press, Oxford.

Titchen, A. (2003) Critical companionship: Part 1. *Nursing Standard*. **18**(9), 33–40.

Ward, M. & McCormack, B. (2000) Creating an adult learning culture through practice development. *Nurse Education Today*. **20**, 259–266.

Ward, P. (1997) *360 Degree Feedback*. Institute of Personnel and Development, London.

Warfield, C. & Manley, K. (1990) Developing a new philosophy in the NDU. *Nursing Standard*. **4**(41), 27–30.

13. *Leadership Support*

Annette Solman and Mary FitzGerald

Introduction

Early proponents of practice development (PD) epitomised and demonstrated the importance of a particular style of clinical leadership from positions in practice (Pearson, 1983; Manley, 1997; Binnie & Titchen, 1999). The style promoted professional practice and fostered a culture where PD was an inclusive pursuit that was a team responsibility and achievement. As the conceptualisation of PD has matured, leadership has been confirmed as a central construct that constitutes practice culture and in turn is shaped by it (Manley, 2000a, 2000b, 2004). So much so that strategic leadership development and support have become an essential consideration when engineering the introduction and sustainability of PD within an organisation. Leadership programmes in a range of guises have been around for some time now; the examples used in this chapter are drawn from a leadership programme that is an integral part of a service-wide PD strategy that used a transformational leadership framework (FitzGerald & Solman, 2003).

In this chapter, we draw on our experience in one large Australian Health Service where we looked for and adopted strategies designed to support the implementation and sustainability of PD with dual support for leadership and PD. The process is described, explained and critiqued with cross-reference to theory and experience. Our critique of this development inevitably highlights the incongruence between theory and practice in a messy world and raises questions for practice developers, and indeed senior managers, who hope to support person-centred care at both unit and organisational levels. The questions raised are designed to be constructive rather than destructive and help all parties to understand and traverse a complicated and harassed health service with marginally less angst and stress than is usually the case.

Leadership and practice development links

What attributes of leadership were evident in the movie *Gladiator*, where Maximus (Russell Crowe) was successful in bringing disparate men together as a team? In

260

this movie, men were captured and expected to fight to the death to entertain others or to be the victors of the fighting. Leadership was demonstrated by Maximus through inspiring a shared vision, using language that was meaningful to the fighters and in adopting a strategy that would maximise the fighting strength of the group. He role modeled a team approach and strategy while encouraging others to work together to achieve team goals rather than individual goals. He got to know individuals and established a relationship with them, which demonstrated interest in them as a person. The team of fighters became more successful and well known through the leadership and teamwork that was demonstrated to the extent that the *Gladiator's* attributes drew in the spectators and won over their support. The leadership attributes that were demonstrated were bringing individuals together to create a shared vision, enacting (role modeling) what was expected by all members of the fighting team, a team approach to decision-making, celebrating success, sharing and acknowledging of individuals strengths, having a strategy that was developed by the team that was focused on the team goals and a passion for what they were trying to achieve, which resulted in a self-belief of the individuals that they could do what was required to be the victors. The spectators could see that this was a team of highly skilled fighters who were working together to achieve a shared goal. They admired the leadership and sense of presence that the 'Gladiator' demonstrated, who used strategies to draw in the audience by engaging with them to create an environment of excitement and expectation.

There has been much written about the attributes of effective leaders, and leadership has been defined as 'the ability to influence a group toward the achievement of its goals' (Morrison et al., 1997). This is a reasonably vague definition, which does not prescribe a style of leadership. On the other hand, the definition of PD explicitly requires context and culture conducive to person-centred care (Garbett & McCormack, 2002). The pursuit of these elements of PD leans naturally towards a transformational leadership style with a whole host of ideal characteristics to be fostered in the aspiring leader and indeed the entire team.

Transformational leadership has been defined by many authors, and their work supports the following conclusion: '[t]ransformational leaders motivate others to do more . . . more than they felt possible. They set more challenging expectations and typically achieve higher performances' (Dunham-Taylor, 2000, p. 24). This facilitative type of leadership is congruent with professional practice and organisations with flattened hierarchies as progress is made through the contributions of the whole team of, in this case, professional nurses or health service professionals. The argument is that leadership development of facilitators and staff engaged in PD promotes the acquisition of facilitation skills and thus the sustainability of PD beyond the work of the initial leader. The promotion of a facilitative style of leadership optimises the possibility of enduring change in practice and the adoption of person-centred practice as an organisational and cultural norm (Manley et al., 2007a).

Transformational leaders are described by Barling et al. (2000) as leaders who are able to influence others towards an ideal, as well as being viewed by followers as motivational and inspirational. The leader encourages creativity and provides intellectual stimulation whilst not losing sight of individual considerations.

Inspiring a shared vision is an activity of a transformational leader and a practice developer (Manley, 1997, 2001). Typically, transformational leaders in PD work with their fellows to create a vision for work practices that are person centred. Visioning work, for example, may include values clarification (Warfield & Manley, 1990) activities that explore the identification of the beliefs and values that individual staff members hold about such things as patient care, health/illness, nursing professional practice and collegiality. This type of work can lead to an increase in and a commitment to shared understandings of workplace expectations, goals and objectives and work practices leading to a rejuvenation of the workforce with renewed commitment to the team and workplace goals. Values work assists with building trust and establishing or re-establishing working relationships with individuals and teams. The approach of the leader in initiating and facilitating others is central to the success of building the team as charisma is important and positive inspirational role modeling, which Hay (2006) describes as an indicator of a transformational leader.

Enabling others to act requires work with the team and with individuals to clearly identify work practices, roles and functions within a team, strengths and opportunities for growth in an environment that encourages challenge, support, creativity and innovation. Within PD the transformational leader may introduce a range of reflective practice strategies to support staff as individuals and as a team to grow (Manley et al., 2007b). A project focus for the team can assist with teamwork cohesion and in developing the capacity of the individual and team in problem-solving. Barling et al. (2000) suggest that this focus improves the level of work satisfaction experienced by teams.

This is all very plausible in theory and of course is given credence by the examples of transformational leadership in PD initiatives over the years. However, there has been little exploration of the extent to which these leaders can be supported to develop on a much bigger scale as opposed to appearing as they have done in the past, driven by natural or experientially learned inclination to display transformational abilities. Transformational leadership attributes align with the intent and philosophy of PD (Davidson & Davidson, 2000; Eisenbach et al., 1999). Some leaders can be challenged when their natural or preferred style of leadership is other than transformational or when their personal values do not reflect those of PD. To support change towards a transformational leadership style, we suggest that it is necessary to ensure that leaders are given access to leadership and facilitation development opportunities, and clear mandates to lead in a way that fosters professional contributions to team leadership from within their teams. While this may not transform everyone into a transformational leader, it at least requires people to reflect on their leadership style and attributes and the impact that they have on the team members and the service delivered by them.

The impact of poor leadership on teams and workplace environments

In our experience, there are clinical leaders who believe that they are effective as leaders, who work from a position of good intent and believe that they work within a framework of PD. These individuals may have little insight into their own practice and the effect their leadership practices have on the workplace culture, the work practices of the team and the experience of patients receiving care, whether those effects are positive or negative. Here we intentionally concentrate on the negative effects because of their implications for the workplace and the experience of patients receiving care. Ineffective leadership may manifest itself in many forms (Morrison et al., 1997; Murphy, 2005); in particular, a determined focus on end points, rather than on a process of inclusiveness, in decision-making to ensure 'buy in' and valuing of staff and gaining assurance of staff understandings with a commitment to change evident. Ineffective positional leadership can be seen when individuals leading a team see everything as being about them, their image, how they are perceived by those in positions of influence and authority. Ineffective leadership leads to fragmented communication, lack of teamwork, low morale, and often the focus of care may be more about the needs of healthcare providers rather than the needs of patients (Murphy, 2005).

Aversive leadership practices result in an environment that does not have in place sound strategies to enable teamwork or support for staff to undertake calculated risks with a focus on learning when a goal is not realised. Staff members may not receive the role modeling of a transformational leader and may have fewer opportunities to lead projects, to develop both professionally and personally, and to experience supportive reflective practices (Pearce & Sims, 2002).

Ineffective leaders appear to have problems maintaining professional and personal boundaries. The lack of boundaries may result in the perception by staff of 'favourites', small cliques of people who assume leadership and perhaps bullying behaviours within the workplace (McCloskey, 1990). There may be fragmented teamwork with 'game playing' evident. High-level energy is expended in activities not associated with patients; for example, game playing with other staff to get personal needs met at the expense of the team or trying to be 'invisible' so as to avoid conflict with others (Johns, 1992).

In the absence of effective leadership, staff may manifest a lack of commitment or at least ambivalence in work practices. A blame culture may be evident in the workplace with poor conflict resolution and interpersonal skills. Commencing PD without a leadership support programme for managers and leaders of PD whose leadership style is other than enabling of the team members carries an increased risk of failure of staff to flourish, as a result of PD activities (FitzGerald & Solman, 2003). It may seem incongruent to dwell on poor leadership, but it is important with respect to the amount that is currently known about noxious environments that adversely affect nursing morale and standards of care. The tendency in some organisations to accentuate the positive in order to maintain morale masks deep-seated problems that need to be identified, explored and addressed. These problems are not easily fixed and it is possibly unfair to locate them entirely in the lap of clinical leadership, but there is no doubt that if leaders are to be implicated in the problem, then the organisation has a responsibility to provide support to clinical leaders to enable constructive responses (Bennis, 1990).

Organisational approach

When we embarked on an 'organisation-wide' strategy for PD, the question we sought to answer was: *How can we, at an organisational level, support sustainable PD?* Amongst a range of strategies was to offer leadership support for clinical leaders, nurse unit managers (NUMs) and, clinical nurse consultants (CNCs) with a parallel commitment to support those who wished to engage in PD with their teams.

A stakeholder group was formed to develop a strategic plan for PD, which included a strategic approach to leadership development for senior clinical leaders in nursing as well as an evaluation strategy. A proposal was submitted for the leadership development and evaluation and was submitted to the Nurse Executive. In order to provide the context for the leadership support programme and to enable members of the executive team to experience what the programme would entail, a selection of activities were undertaken by them. There was positive support for programme commencement and indeed members of the Nursing Executive opted to join the programme as participants. The programme proposal was submitted to the larger organisation executive who endorsed funding for the programme implementation.

While senior nursing management in the organisation viewed PD and transformational leadership as preferred means of supporting person-centred care, it was deemed anti-theoretical to either movement to *dictate* adoption in clinical areas. The leadership programme was therefore open to all nursing clinical leaders. To manage the limited resources efficiently and effectively, a staged strategic approach to implementation in specific clinical areas was adopted. No preference was given to clinical areas that had already engaged in PD. However, as will be seen in the next section of this chapter, the structure and content of the leadership support programme dovetailed neatly with PD and the acquisition of facilitation and critical reflection skills.

Leadership support programme

A work needs analysis and conversations with staff revealed that leadership support was required for nursing managers and clinical nurse consultants within the healthcare organisation, a finding endorsed by consultant nurses in other settings (Manley et al., 2007b). These nurse leaders had expressed that they were experiencing challenges around the multiple and continuing changes occurring within the healthcare system, not least of which was the desire to provide a person-centered service to patients in what often appeared to be a hostile environment.

The leadership support programme (LSP) was designed to address self-identified needs to enable the individuals to move forward and meet the requirements of their positions within a contemporary healthcare context. The emphasis of the training and development activities was on self-managed learning, as individuals and collectively, through self-assessment of development needs. In addition, opportunities for learning from peers, coaching and mentoring formed part of the LSP approach to training.

Experience has shown that one of the best resources for development exists within the group being developed. This programme sought to capitalise on the availability of this resource. Additionally, staff within and external to the organisation have the expectation that the NUM[1] and CNC[2] would be cognisant of their obligations and have the necessary information and skills to execute their responsibilities effectively.

Finally, the approach recognises that there are competing demands on NUMs and CNCs in an increasingly complex and demanding environment. The number of competing priorities and development opportunities are sometimes not realised. The LSP aimed to promote and facilitate a supportive environment for maximising development.

Principles on which this programme was structured include the following:

- The effectiveness of a self-managed approach to learning.
- The commitment of the organisation in finding creative ways of addressing these needs once identified.
- People having the opportunity to learn from the day-to-day challenges presented in the workplace rather than viewing them as an inconvenience.

Support was given to assist participants in this environment. The programme was not prescriptive and offered a menu of options for participants, which included the following:

- Participate in an action learning set.
- Individual coaching.
- Project management and leading a change project.
- Support with team building and the development of workplace values, visioning and workplace culture analysis.

The programme was offered with a view to enhance not only individual leadership development but also teamwork. Some NUMs and CNCs maximised the

---

[1] In New South Wales the NUM is the clinical leader with responsibility for and authority to provide high standards of nursing care.
[2] In New South Wales the CNCs are specialists with consultation responsibilities; they provide specialist support and education to clinicians and patients.

opportunities that the programme offered whereas others selected from the menu options what they believed matched their own needs or the needs of the team.

Some participants chose individual coaching and selected teamwork activities to support their understanding of PD and in moving their leadership practices towards a transformational style. Others used the programme to support them in major capital work projects that they were responsible for leading, as many parts of the organisation were experiencing re-development of facilities, an area that was new to them. Project work became a large focus of this leadership initiative; these projects included strategic planning for specific areas of the organisation, reviewing models of care, exploring existing patient care work practices, team building and introducing evidence-based practice. Action learning sets, coaching, supportive workplace development with the clinical leader and their team by facilitators enabled leadership enhancement and team development opportunities within the context of the clinical environment.

In its developmental stages the programme was positively evaluated. There have been over 100 nurses in the programme within the organisation. A self-reporting questionnaire and focus group method of evaluation were employed, capitalising on the participant's interactions with each other and assisting with exploring and clarifying individual views (Sim, 1998; Morgan, 1988). Data were analysed using thematic analysis and reviewed by an independent reviewer to reduce bias.

Participants reported that the programme created an environment where trust was built and contributed to self-discipline, providing safety through familiarity. Enabling questions contributed to participants moving away from telling people what to do, to being more facilitative. This reinforced the concept of facilitation by

- assisting staff within the teams to make decisions for themselves, and
- transferability of action learning for exploring challenges experienced within the workplace.

Action learning sets contributed to a planned approach to change and decision-making, encouraging reflection and consideration of the process rather than just the end point of change. Participants identified that they had clarity of

- each other's work;
- the direction they were heading in; and
- the challenges people were experiencing and overcoming in order to enhance teamwork.

The time invested by the participants created energy when there was difficulty within the workplace and was a constructive and productive form of staff support. These positive comments represent a very real movement forward for these leaders and their teams and they were seen by senior management as a justification for the continuance of the programme.

Since the inception and introduction of this leadership initiative there has been major restructure of healthcare systems and processes within the organisation locally and at a state level. The direction of leadership development at a state level is one of a multidisciplinary approach, although at a local level PD is seen mainly within nursing and more recently a greater interest from allied health professionals in PD approaches.

A statewide Clinical Leadership Programme was offered in New South Wales during 2004 as a nursing initiative. The programme was developed by the Royal College of Nursing in the United Kingdom. It focused on the development of the individual as a clinical leader. The activities of the programme were centered on self-awareness of leadership attributes within the workplace and the development of a leadership style that was inclusive of others and reflected the work of Kouzes and Posner (2003) leadership attributes. Kouzes and Posner's (2003) leadership framework identifies the attributes of transformational leadership. These are inspiring a shared vision, enabling others to act, modeling the way, challenging the process and encouraging the heart. This programme was a first step towards developing a statewide strategy for nursing leadership development with the inclusion of a small number of allied health professionals.

Revisions

There is now a statewide initiative for multidisciplinary clinical leadership development in NSW. The Clinical Excellence Commission is supporting the implementation of a Clinical Leadership Programme that builds on this early leadership development approach. The Clinical Excellence Commission (CEC) of NSW (Australia) was created in August 2004 to build confidence in healthcare within NSW, by making it demonstrability better and safer for patients and a more rewarding workplace.

The local organisation chose to adopt a strategic approach for the implementation of the CEC Statewide Clinical Leadership Programme and identified key areas that the programme would be offered in the first year of implementation. The programme aims to support leadership development of staff and build sustainability into clinical leadership within organisations and by those who engage in PD work. The programme supports the development of safe and effective patient care, reflective practice skills, problem-solving capability, team building, professional practice, personal effectiveness and clinical governance in participants of the programme. This enables the leaders of clinical teams to move further towards a transformational leadership style that is required to lead and support PD.

The implementation strategy includes the professional development of the facilitators of the programme to enhance their facilitation style and understanding of transformational leadership within contemporary healthcare environments. Ongoing development of participants is supported by these facilitators, who engage with them and their clinical team. There are 21 facilitators and approximately 200 participants in the first cohort of this 11-month programme. The programme has participants from Allied Health, Nursing, Midwifery and Medicine, which mirrors the healthcare worker mix generally involved in working together within the clinical practice environment. The work-based learning approach encourages the exploration of real-time clinical challenges and opportunities within the context of patient quality care and safety. There are a series of workshops that introduce leadership concepts and promote the sharing of experiences and ideas. The participants build upon their leadership attributes and team building capacity whilst working in a person-centred way. The evaluation and outcomes from this work will be published as it becomes available.

Critical framework

There are reasonable justifications for promoting the work that has been done in these leadership programmes, mainly in order to defend it from protractors and make reasonable excuses for weakness, in order to ensure continued support and progress for the leadership programme. When all is said and done some progress is a lot better than no progress, and cultural change of this nature is more likely to evolve over years rather than months. There is much mileage in the argument that bureaucrats and traditional scientists who call for quick outcome measures to signify success do not understand the PD perspective that evaluation is as much to do with processes as with outcomes (Manley & McCormack, 2003) and that premature evaluation with an emphasis on outcome measurement can be destructive (Conway & FitzGerald, 2004).

While the above evaluation strategies may stave off detractors and satisfy proponents of PD, it is not a particularly enlightening exercise for the participants of leadership programmes. Evaluation should have an automatic feedback loop to participants to stimulate the type of critical reflection that is the heart of emancipatory PD. In order to promote a new view of our work and to stimulate a challenge for ourselves, we return to the works of action researchers such as Kemmis and McTaggart (2000) to explain the type of processes that support and sustain social change.

Emancipatory practice developers like emancipatory action researchers aim 'not only at improving outcomes, and improving the self-understandings of practitioners, but also at assisting practitioners to arrive at a critique of their social or education [nursing] work and work settings' (Kemmis, 2001, p. 94). As Kemmis and McTaggart portray, we are equally interested in 'work, the worker and the workplace' (2000), an understanding of which draws the practice developer out of an individualistic perspective and into social and cultural perspectives of practice within systems or institutions with incumbent economic, bureaucratic and political undercurrents.

Kemmis and McTaggart (2000) and later Kemmis (2001) write regarding the relevance of critical theory to emancipatory action research. In this chapter, we relate the earlier work specifically to PD and the leadership programme. Kemmis writes in response to the postmodern criticism of critical social theory and in particular the pursuit of an 'ideal form of reason capable of sustaining the critical and emancipatory aspirations of critical theory' (2001p. 96). He does this in a positive way, confident about the continuing relevance of critical perspectives by referring to Habermas' writing in *The Theory of Communicative Action* (1981) and *The Philosophical Discourse of Modernity* (1987).

Taking the Habermasian ideas of 'lifeworld' and 'system' Kemmis (2001) explains the apparent dilemma of working as an individual or group or culture[3] in a system[4] or institution if traditional scientific or even social scientific perspectives are adopted. This is because the various perspectives create 'either–or' situations where objective and subjective and individual and group are each taken to be 'right' and incompatible with each other – an uncoupling of 'lifeworld' and 'system'. Institutions appear to have systems, rules and regulations that are 'indifferent to the unique personalities and interests of the individuals' practicing within them. These myopic perspectives abound in the health service from a range of personnel – shroud waving medics advocating for a small number of patients to economic rationalist managers determined to contain spending to nurses who are focused exclusively on delivery of nursing services.

In our critique of the leadership programme, we review and critically reflect on the 'lifeworld' in connection with the 'system' involved in the working sphere of the leaders who are involved with the programme. The work setting is 'constituted and reconstituted' through the following processes described by Kemmis (2001, p. 101):

- The process of *individuation–socialisation* (by which practitioners' own identities and capacities are formed and developed).
- The process of *social integration* (by which legitimately ordered social relations among people as co-participants in a setting are formed and developed).
- The process of *cultural reproduction and transformation* (by which shared cultures and discourses are formed and developed) (see Chapter 3).

The questions that we reflect on are related to these processes:

1. How well do the participants in the leadership programme understand their role as leader and their ability to take a transformational stance?
2. To what extent are the team members drawing together to work as practice developers?
3. Is the facilitative style of leadership and PD becoming a cultural norm in this health service?

The answers to these questions are sought discursively in light of both objective and subjective evidence. The insight of the participants regarding their own practice or actions is crucial but of course concrete evidence from other sources is enlightening. The later two questions lead away from the personal or individualistic frame of reference and are more dependent on the ways that leaders interact with team members and the institution. These are typically the sort of reflections that are drawn out in action learning sets, but unless they are recognised as evaluation data they are seldom utilised for the purpose of evaluation with of course some notable exceptions (Wilson et al., 2003).

---

[3] 'Lifeworld' is constituted of personal, social and cultural processes.
[4] 'System' orientated to functionality and outcomes.

269

Critique

Over decades, there has been an accumulation of evidence that confirms the common-sense notion that it is clinical leaders in nursing who have most influence on standards of care delivery in health service organisations (McNeese-Smith, 1997); influence over such things, for example, morale, learning environments, standards of care. Despite this recognition the authors' observation is that it is still the case that most clinical leaders find themselves in a situation that is not conducive to transformational leadership practice. Further to this they are in the middle of a large organisation with strictures, structures and systems that hardly encourage entrepreneurs; no matter what the rhetoric is from above to innovate and take risks.

The programme we describe has had positive success in supporting able people to reach further and achieve more and it has challenged people who have previously resisted critical reflection of their own work. However, in terms of an impact on the delivery of higher standards of care in a team environment the jury is still out. At its least the programme offers the type of support and mentoring that leaders in industry have received as a matter of course for a long time. It has enabled the programme leaders to showcase the area and influence other associated developments in the state. But to what extent has the programme had an effect on the working culture in the Health Authority. Anecdotally, we can present examples of nurses working in facilitative ways amongst themselves and in multidisciplinary forums. However, these examples do not represent the norm.

Conclusion

Ironically, the success of leadership development in the health service appears to create as many problems as it addresses, for it has become a norm for people displaying transformational leadership abilities to be offered new and exciting jobs before there has been time to ensure succession with a similarly inclined leader. While a focus on the development of transformational leadership attributes is a reasonable course for organisations that want to support PD on a large scale, the addition of succession planning and the development of future leaders in the plan is a prudent move.

References

Barling, J., Slater, F. & Kelloway, E. (2000) Transformational leadership and emotional intelligence: An exploratory study. *Leadership & Organization Development Journal.* **21**(3), 157–161.

Bennis, W. (1990) *Why Leaders Can't Lead*. Jossey-Bass, San Francisco.

Binnie, A. & Titchen, A. (1999) *Freedom to Practise: The Development of Patient-Centred Nursing* (ed J. Lathlean). Butterworth-Heinemann, Oxford.

Clinical Excellence Commission (CEC) of NSW (Australia) (2004) www.cec.health. nsw.gov.au.

Conway, J. & FitzGerald, M. (2004) Processes, outcomes and evaluation: Challenges to practice development in gerontological nursing. *International Journal of Older People Nursing.* **13**(6b), 112–120.

Davidson, J.U. & Davidson, J.C. (2000) Fundamentals of restructuring: How to accomplish transformational change via transformational leadership. *Kansas Nurse.* **75**(4), 1–3.

Dunham-Taylor, J. (2000) Nurse executive transformational leadership found in participative organisations. *Journal of Nursing Administration.* **30**(5), 241–250.

Eisenbach, R., Watson, K. & Pillai, R. (1999) Transformational leadership in the context of organizational change. *Journal of Organizational Change Management.* **12**(2), 80–88.

FitzGerald, M. & Solman, A. (2003) Clinical practice development in central coast health. *Collegian.* **10**(3), 8–12.

Garbett, R. & McCormack, B. (2002) A concept analysis of practice development. *Nursing Times Research.* **7**(2), 87–100.

Habermas, J. (1981)*The Theory of Communicative Action.* Beacon, London.

Haberman, J. (1987) *The Philosophical Discourse of Modernity* (Trans. Frederick Lawrence). MIT Press, Cambridge, MA.

Hay, I. (2006) Available from http:/www.weleadinlearning.org/transformational-leadership.htm [accessed 07/12/2006].

Johns, C. (1992) Ownership and the harmonious team: Barriers to developing the therapeutic nursing team in primary nursing. *Journal of Clinical Nursing.* **1**, 89–94.

Kemmis, S. (2001) Exploring the relevance of critical theory for action research: Emancipatory action research in the footsteps of Jurgen Habermas. In: *Handbook of Action Research* (eds P. Reason & H. Bradbury), pp. 94–105. Sage, Thousand Oaks, CA.

Kemmis, S. & McTaggart, R. (2000) Participatory action research. In: *Handbook of Qualitative Research* (eds N. Denzin & Y. Lincoln), 2nd edn, pp. 567–607. Sage, Thousand Oaks, CA.

Kouzes, J. & Posner, B. (2003) *The Leadership Challenge*, 3rd edn. Jossey-Bass, San Francisco.

Manley, K. (1997) A conceptual framework for advanced practice: An action research project operationalising: An advanced practitioner/consultant nurse role. *Journal of Clinical Nursing.* **6**(3), 179–190.

Manley, K. (2000a) Organisational culture and consultant nurse outcomes: Part 1 organisational culture. *Nursing Standard.* **14**(36), 34–38.

Manley, K. (2000b) Organisational culture and consultant nurse outcomes: Part 2 consultant nurse outcomes. *Nursing Standard.* **14**(37), 34–39.

Manley, K. (2001) Consultant nurse: Concept, process and outcomes. Unpublished PhD Thesis, University of Manchester/RCN Institute, London.

Manley, K. (2004) Transformational culture: A culture of effectiveness. In: *Practice Development in Nursing* (eds B. McCormack, K. Manley & R. Garbett), pp. 51–83. Blackwell, Oxford.

Manley, K. & McCormack, B. (2003) Practice development: Purpose, methodology, facilitation and evaluation. *Nursing in Critical Care.* **8**(1), 22–29.

Manley, K., Sanders, K., Cardiff, S., Garbarino, L. & Davren, M. (2007a) Effective workplace culture: draft concept analysis. In: *Royal College of Nursing, Workplace Resources for Practice Development*, pp. 6–10. RCN Institute, London.

271

Manley, K., Webster, J., Hale, N., Hayes, N. & Minardi, H. (2007b) Leadership role of consultant nurses working with older people: A co-operative inquiry. *Journal of Nursing Management.* (In press)

McCloskey, J. (1990) Two requirements for job contentment: Autonomy and social integration. *Image: Journal of Nursing Scholarship.* **22**, 140–143.

McNeese-Smith, D. (1997) The influence of manager behaviour on nurses' job satisfaction, productivity and commitment. *Journal of Nursing Administration.* **27**, 47–55.

Morgan, D.L. (1988) *Focus Groups as Qualitative Research.* Sage, Newbury Park, CA.

Morrison, R.S. Jones, L. & Fuller, B. (1997) The relation between leadership style and empowerment on job satisfaction of nurses. *Journal of Nursing Administration.* **27**(5), 27–34.

Murphy, L. (2005) Transformational leadership a cascading chain reaction. *Journal of Nursing Management.* **13**, 128–136.

Pearce, C. & Sims, H. (2002) Vertical versus shared leadership as predictors of effectiveness of change management teams: An examination of aversive, directive, transactional, transformational and empowering leader behaviours. *Group Dynamics: Theory, Research, and Practice.* **6**(2), 172–197.

Pearson, A. (1983) *The Clinical Nursing Unit.* Heinemann, London.

Sim, J. (1998) Collecting and analyzing qualitative data: Issues raised by the focus group. *Journal of Advanced Nursing.* **28**(2), 345–352.

Warfield, C. & Manley, K. (1990) Developing a new philosophy in the NDU. *Nursing Standard.* **4**(41), 27–30.

Wilson, V., Keachie, P. & Engelsmann, M. (2003) Putting the action into learning: The experience of an action learning set. *Collegian.* **10**(3), 22–26.

14. Becoming and Being Active Learners and Creating Active Learning Workplaces: The Value of Active Learning in Practice Development

Jan Dewing[1]

Introduction

A popular definition of practice development (PD) advocates the advancement of knowledge and skills as a necessary part of achieving the transformation in workplace cultures (Garbett & McCormack, 2004). This is not simply a technical acquisition of knowledge, nor is it a linear or simple process. Earlier in this book (Chapter 6), Clarke & Wilson suggest that learning, by individuals and by organisations, is at the very heart of PD activity. In addition, the place of work-based learning (Hardy et al., 2007) and critical reflection (Kim, 1999; McCormack et al., 2002; Dewing & Wright, 2003) in contributing to the ultimate purpose(s) of PD is also now being highlighted. Dewing et al. (2006) have added to this, suggesting that work-based learning needs to be 'active'. By 'active' the author of this chapter means, learning in PD work revolves around reflection, dialogue with self and others and engaging in learning activities in the workplace that make use of the senses, multiple intelligences and doing things (i.e. workplace learning activities) together with colleagues and others.

Thus, in this chapter, I propose that one of the central tenets and processes in PD is systematic active learning. Consequently, facilitation of active learning needs to be recognised as a core responsibility of practice developers and needs to be enabled within organisations. Practice developers then must have the means to

---

[1] With a contribution from Irmajean Bajnok.

assess and evaluate their interventions to ensure that they maximise opportunities for active learning for individuals and groups (McCormack et al., 2002; Dewing et al., 2004). Since every encounter in PD is a learning opportunity, there are many ways active learning can be a part of PD. This chapter offers you a selection of ways in which active learning can be facilitated, so you first have a sense of how it can be 'made real' and secondly you can actively reflect, on your own or with others, on the methods and consider what they mean for your practice and your workplace.

You will note that in this chapter the terms facilitator and 'co-learner' are used. This is because, as McCormack and Garbett (2003) amongst others indicate, practice developers essentially operate through being skilled facilitators of practitioners and other stakeholders in PD and simultaneously along with those they are facilitating, and are also learners – active learners I hope. This makes for more effective learning, and, as I suggest in this chapter, the more engaging and active the learning is, the more effective it is. It is this type of effectiveness that contributes to the sustainability of the philosophy, approaches and methods of PD.

There are four aims for this chapter, all at the heart of developing an increased appreciation for active learning and its contribution in PD. However, you might like to consider, for a moment, a couple of points. First, what feelings and thoughts do you have about active learning as you are about to engage with this chapter? Second, what questions do you have on active learning that you hope this chapter will cover?

Aims of the chapter
1. To set out key principles of active learning and provide examples of active learning from different PD work.
2. To discuss the theoretical underpinnings of active learning.
3. To reflect on the usefulness of active learning with regard to the purposes of PD.
4. To discuss some of the key challenges for active learning in PD.

What is active learning? A model to illustrate and explain
As way of general introduction, active learning can be seen as an approach or methodology for learning that draws on, integrates and creatively synthesises numerous learning methods. It is important to acknowledge the principles embraced by active learning before rushing to consider specific methods. Once practice developers have clarified their values and beliefs about learning and have a shared or common vision about learning within PD, agreed upon principles can then be used to guide the choice of methods and evaluate their effectiveness. Critical dialogue with others may be preceded by visioning or another imagery activity, about what is meant by learning and what it looks like in a workplace that has effective PD. This can be a useful starting point to identify and discuss assumptions about learning in the transformational workplace. For example, it is not unusual to find teams that may commit to developing person-centred workplaces yet still believe learning is something that takes place away from the workplace and is 'taught' mainly through study days and formal teaching methods.

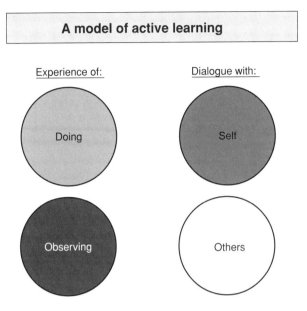

Figure 14.1 A model of active learning.

At its simplest, the central principles in active learning usually involve making multiple uses of the senses, and dialogue with self and others. Fink (1999) offers a fourfold conceptual model of active learning (Figure 14.1) that shows these core principles, which are explained in the following way.

Active learning involves engagement with all our senses (hearing, seeing, feeling, etc.), an internal dialogue with our 'self' such as critical reflection and interacting with other people and objects in the environment. This stimulates both sides of the brain and multiple areas therein and related multiple intelligences to act to their potential. Additionally, it is more likely to lead to a desire for action. In active learning, like other approaches to learning, there is an emphasis on looking for evidence that learning has taken place through the ways in which co-learners respond in terms of thoughts, feelings and actions.

To get us going, Finks simplified model is explained in words below, and I include an example of how each principle can be realised through a specific method.

Dialogue with self. Creatively imaging and thinking about an aspect of practice and critically reflecting on how the practice took place/could take place, the desired or actual outcomes, and its meaning.

Example. *Following a visioning or imagination activity based on the prompt 'imagine you are walking through your workplace where PD is embedded in the culture. You talk yourself through the following cues: what might you see, hear, feel and generally notice as you go on your walk?'*

Dialogue with others. One-to-one or group dialogue between practitioners about a practice topic or activity with the purpose of eliciting ideas and reflections about the practice, its outcomes and its meaning.

Example. *A dyad activity where each co-learner takes a turn at listening to a short reflection on 'my experience of a patient saying they feel sad'. After each co-learner has talked they share their learning both from their own practice account and also their learning on the process they have just experienced within the dyad.*

Observing. Occurs whenever practitioners watch or listen to someone else doing something that is related to what they are learning and is most effective when linked to dialogue with self. However, the observation must be set up with the intent of learning.

Examples. *Sitting in a patient's chair by their bed, in a waiting area or day room/lounge.*

An observation of practice activity in the workplace where co-learners are asked to observe what goes on either directly or indirectly with an aspect(s) of patient care. This activity as with all active learning activities is adapted according to the confidence and skills of the facilitators and co-learners.

Doing. May be direct or indirect. Case studies, role-playing and simulation activities (plus many other methods) offer ways of vicariously engaging co-learners in the doing process and can be combined with dialogue with self and others.

Example. *Co-learners are invited to role-play an incident from practice.*

In PD, the primary place for active learning is the workplace. Workshops and other similar events are preparation ground for taking activities into the workplace. The skilled facilitator always looks at how a learning activity can be transferred to the workplace. Transferring active learning to the workplace in relation to doing, as shown in the last example, would mean focusing on role-playing a scenario based on a real practice incident in which the learners had been involved. Similarly, the examples included with the dyad and observation activities above could be transferred to the workplace. PD groups and other PD encounters such as workshops and project days are a rehearsal ground for taking active learning into the learners' workplaces. Active learning is not complete until it is being transferred into the workplace.

Building up active learning

Introducing active learning activities starts early in any PD work with relatively uncomplicated and low-level threat activities and builds up to achieve more complex learning activities and outcomes with work colleagues, patients/service users and other stakeholders. Providing information on what active learning is about can enable co-learners to more easily grasp the purpose of learning and the reasons why it might entail a different sort of learning experience to ones previously encountered in more traditional courses or development programmes. Building up the level also takes into account workplace culture, which often may not, particularly at the start of PD work, reflect a learning or an active learning culture.

Example of an active learning activity at different levels

> **Beginners.** *Carry out a 15-minute observation in your workplace on the care environment. Notice what you see, hear, smell, touch and feel. Make notes for the next project day so that you can share your feelings and thoughts.*

With this activity, it is the place that is being observed rather than the direct giving of care. (This makes the activity less threatening in places where peer observation of care is not yet usual.)

> **Intermediate.** *Would be similar to the above with up to three observations of care with a different team member on each occasion. At the end of each observation the co-learner facilitates a dialogue with the team member about the activity and what they have experienced in terms of care that could be celebrated and care that needs to be addressed. Areas to be addressed may be discussed and the co-learner and team member share their personal learning from the experience.*

At this level, the activity has moved to observing direct care giving, includes other team members and enables use of feedback, facilitating a dialogue and introducing the idea of taking action.

> **Advanced.** *Similar to above or use (a) specific instrument(s) for the observation of care, include service users/patients, and it can be carried out for longer periods. Feedback is given to the whole team and there is a written action plan to be worked with. There is also a discussion about learning that has occurred form undertaking the activity and how it relates to PD.*

At this level, the activity has become formalised. However, the core principles of active learning, the engagement with sense, reflection and dialogue are evident. In addition, processing and evaluation of learning from the experience are an evident part of the learning. Thus, in many workplace cultures it is easy to see how opportunities for active learning may be lost when staff external to the immediate workplace or consultants external to the whole organisation come in to carry out audit or research activities, unless active learning principles are specifically built into such activities.

Fink's simple diagram, albeit effective in illustrating the essentials of active learning, does not do justice to the dynamics between and among all of the four aspects within the model as it is applied in complex PD work within healthcare organisations. Each of the four modes of learning in the model has its own distinct value. By using more than one mode, variety is added to learning experiences adding more interest for co-learners and facilitators, and increasing the effectiveness. The model does not depict the continuous loop of active learning where feedback, reflection and evaluation related to the learning experience as a whole is built in and becomes a part of the conceptual PD framework. This critique is offered to inspire you to redraw the diagram for yourself and construct your own dynamic model of active learning.

Now, let us turn our attention to further building our understanding of active learning as it can apply to PD. To achieve its purpose, active learning must take on many shapes or guises, including talking, writing, reading, discussing, debating, music, walking, acting, role-playing, games, journaling, interviewing, making displays and posters, building sculptures, many forms of creativity, imagining, visioning, theatre, and the list continues. You may want to add some of your own ideas here. Because it takes on so many forms and is accomplished through numerous and varied methods, only a few can be shown here.

Taking it into the workplace: achieving transformations

Place and context are important and often powerful catalysts in learning and creation of meaning. As indicated previously, learning is not active learning unless at some point it is transferred or takes place in the real workplace setting. Although, it can be challenging to set up opportunities in the workplace, practitioners benefit most from such opportunities and can often assist in identifying the best times and places. Initial experiences with active learning can of course take place away from the workplace setting in what is often referred to as a safe environment. This initial protection is an important part of the learning journey. However, co-learners need to move from feeling overly safe in a non-real setting to feeling safe in their workplaces and to contributing to facilitating creation of a learning community at work.

> **Example.** *Within a 1-day workshop as part of a 2-year PD project, a 1-hour session of mini scenarios and role-plays looking at how co-learners would offer challenge for poor practice in regard to privacy and dignity in patient care as it occurs. This was carried out in a patient care area in a room where there were two beds and a shared toilet. Being in the workplace really brings home to the senses what poor practice is and how it might be for patients to experience this. Carrying out the activity in the workplace meant preparation of patients, staff and visitors and created a 'buzz' about what was going on, the purpose, and why all the team were not involved. This created an opportunity for the co-learners (who were facilitating development of a person-centred culture in their workplaces) to invite team members to experience the session at a later date and to seek permission to demonstrate their learning as and when issues about poor practice arose. The co-learners did not feel that they could run formal sessions in the workplace as the teams would find this too threatening and until recently learning did not take place in the care setting but in seminar rooms. They did feel that they could run a 'mini session' of about 15–30 minutes and agreed to try it in pairs, reflect on how it went and discuss it at the next project day. The facilitator that suggested doing this in the workplace could enable co-learners to really feel what it would be like to facilitate learning with team members in their day-to-day work as this would help them identify what skills they needed to develop.*

Active learning seeks to achieve a high level of learning, resulting in improved retention and transfer of knowledge and skills into practice for the benefit of the workplace culture, themselves, colleagues and ultimately for patient care/services.

Maximum learning seems to occur most efficiently through concrete activity-based experiences. It is claimed by advocates that active learning increases the effectiveness and efficiency of teaching, facilitation and learning processes (e.g. Bonwell & Eison, 1991; Raux & College, 2004). In PD work, facilitators want co-learners to discover new knowledge and connect more fully with or rediscover existing knowledge, enhance current skills, and expand their potential for problematising and finding or creating solutions to problems. Then, facilitators want those same co-learners to retain the learning and apply it to new situations, building upon that learning to develop new perspectives. Finally, facilitators aim to have co-learners understand how they learned and continue the learning process for themselves while at the same time facilitating other co-learners in their workplaces to experience a similar journey. This replicated and ever broadening cyclical process is essential for wide-scale transformation in the workplace and for sustainability in both practitioners themselves and with PD. Active learning then needs to be embedded in strategic PD to be fully effective in the longer term. It may also be that as well as transformation of workplace culture and consequently more effective patient care and service, for some co-learners there is a deeper, more spiritual type of transformation taking place. Some facilitators such as Heron (1989) and Hanson and Hanson (2001) suggest that deeper levels of exploration and learning about one's own effectiveness will lead to spiritual enlightenment. This and the associated ethics are to date not much discussed in PD literature. I touch on it again when we look at John Heron's work later in the chapter.

It may be you can relate several methods described already in this chapter to the principles of active learning already discussed. This may be particularly apparent if you have experienced learning approaches such as problem-based learning, inquiry-based learning, learning circles, action learning, and some approaches to supervision such as critical companionship (Titchen, 2004). Each of these approaches has an inbuilt capacity for active learning. Whether this capacity is realised or not is another matter. You may have experienced these approaches yet not be able to say that active learning was something you can relate to.

Active learning and learning preferences

To recap, I have aimed to establish that the central principle for active learning, generally, is multiple uses of the senses and intelligences; however, it is more complex than this. Active learning needs to be considered alongside other ideas about how adults learn, such as preferred learning styles. (See Table 14.1 for an outline of one model on learning styles.) Learning styles inventories are useful in aiding co-learners and facilitators to identify predominant and preferred ways of learning. However, they should not be used to label or characterise people, since all learners are capable of using more than one style to learn, and of developing skills in all styles. Honey and Mumford (1982) in their learning styles inventory identify four main learning style preferences: activists, reflectors, theorists and pragmatists. Activists like to be involved and learn best by doing. They are keen to take risks and take on new tasks and learn as they go. Reflectors learn best by observing others,

Table 14.1   Preferred learning styles (Honey & Mumford, 1986)

Activists like to be involved in new experiences. They are open minded and enthusiastic about new ideas but get bored with implementation. They enjoy doing things and tend to act first and consider the implications afterwards. They like working with others but tend to hog the limelight.

Activists learn best when	Activists learn less when
<ul><li>involved in new experiences, problems and opportunities</li><li>working with others in business games, team tasks, role-playing</li><li>being thrown in the deep end with a difficult task</li><li>chairing meetings, leading discussions</li></ul>	<ul><li>listening to lectures or long explanations</li><li>reading, writing or thinking on their own</li><li>absorbing and understanding data</li><li>following precise instruction to the letter</li></ul>

Reflectors like to stand back and look at a situation from different perspectives. They like to collect data and think about it carefully before coming to any conclusions. They enjoy observing others and will listen to their views before offering their own.

Reflectors learn best when	Reflectors learn less when
<ul><li>observing individuals or groups at work</li><li>they have the opportunity to review what has happened and think about what they have learned</li><li>producing analyses and reports doing tasks without tight deadlines</li></ul>	<ul><li>acting as leader or role-playing in front of others</li><li>doing things with no time to prepare</li><li>being thrown in at the deep end</li><li>being rushed or worried by deadlines</li></ul>

Theorists adapt and integrate observations into complex and logically sound theories. They think problems through in a step-by-step way. They tend to be perfectionists who like to fit things into a rational scheme. They tend to be detached and analytical rather than subjective or emotive in their thinking.

Theorists learn best when	Theorists learn less when
<ul><li>they are put in complex situations where they have to use their skills and knowledge</li><li>they are in structured situations with clear purpose</li><li>they are offered interesting ideas or concepts even though they are not immediately relevant</li><li>they have the chance to question and probe ideas behind things</li></ul>	<ul><li>they have to participate in situations that emphasise emotion and feelings</li><li>the activity is unstructured or briefing is poor</li><li>they have to do things without knowing the principles or concepts involved</li><li>they feel they are out of tune with the other participants, e.g. with people of very different learning styles</li></ul>

Pragmatists are keen to try things out. They want concepts that can be applied to their job. They tend to be impatient with lengthy discussions and are practical and down to earth.

Pragmatists learn best when	Pragmatists learn less when
<ul><li>there is an obvious link between the topic and job</li><li>they have the chance to try out techniques with feedback, e.g. role-play</li><li>they are shown techniques with obvious advantages, e.g. saving time</li><li>they are shown a model they can copy, e.g. a film or a respected boss</li></ul>	<ul><li>there is no obvious or immediate benefit that they can recognise</li><li>there is no practice or guidelines on how to do it</li><li>there is no apparent pay back to the learning, e.g. shorter meetings</li><li>the event or learning is 'all theory'</li></ul>

and like a lot of time to learn and achieve goals. They are comfortable collecting information about a situation, listening to others and making the links to their own situation. They enjoy games to learn. Theorists like to know how what they are doing relates to an overall concept or set of concepts. They are more rational in their analysis and learn best when they can link their observations to a theoretical framework and related theories. Pragmatists like their learning to be practical and like to learn on the job. They work best when they can receive practical information, use it in a situation and receive feedback.

Honey and Mumford incorporated their theory into an 80-item learning styles inventory developed in 1982 and adapted over the years with the latest version in 2006. The adaptations have also included development of an abbreviated 40-item inventory. Similarly, Kolb (1984) has authored a learning style inventory that reflects the two dimensions of tasks and thought and emotional processes. Each dimension is viewed along a continuum with tasks varying from doing to observing, and emotions and thoughts varying from feeling to thinking. Kolb's inventory includes four styles identified as concrete experience, reflective observation, abstract generalisation and active experimentation.

Other ways of identifying one's learning preference is through the Visual–Auditory–Kinesthetic (VAK) learning style assessment (http://www.nwlink.com/~donclark/hrd/styles.html; accessed 17/11/2006). VAK assesses perceptual modalities and determines primary ways learners take in information whether it be through vision, auditory or kinesthetic means. While learners use all three styles to receive information, as with the inventories of Honey and Mumford, and Kolb, one or more of the receiving styles are usually more prominent. This prominent style reflects the best way for a person to learn. The style may differ from situation to situation depending on the task to be learned.

In active learning and PD, it is important to use variety, recognising that some learners may learn best from one particular receiving style, sense or type of intelligence. In addition when learners experience their prominent style, it helps them to learn faster or smarter. However, providing opportunity for experiencing a variety of styles can promote flexibility and offer a new and welcome challenge, when in a supportive context. Another way to look at how learning activities are introduced in groups is to consider intelligences. Gardner (1983, 1993) suggests that there are nine intelligences (See Table 14.2), including reflection, doing and interacting with others, that are part of being an active creator in the world. Gardner identified the first seven intelligences in his book 'Frames of Mind' (1983) and has since added another two. The example below shows eight intelligences (the ninth or existential intelligence is not included).

Example. *If a group member has the profile shown below (Figure 14.2) they are likely to prefer being physically active and learn through using their bodies, they also learn well when learning is related to the natural world and to pictures and images. This does not mean they will find all types of active learning using their bodies easy or as equally enjoyable. They have a good sense of self-awareness and like to learn in a group setting, but not all the time. It is tempting to say they will not like using numbers or music very*

Table 14.2   Key elements of multiple intelligence theory (Gardner, 1983, 1993)

Verbal/linguistic: Thinking in words; co-learner prefers to read and write; like stories and to play word games

Logical/mathematical: See patterns easily; likes abstract ideas, strategy games and logical puzzles; can work out sums easily in their head

Visual/spatial: Thinks in images and pictures; easily remembers where things have been put; like drawing, designing, building, daydreaming; reads maps and diagrams easily

Musical/rhythmic-auditory: Often sings, hums, whistles to self; remembers melodies; have a good sense of rhythm; may play an instrument; likes music on when studying or reading

Bodily/Kinaesthetic: Remembers through bodily sensations; finds it difficult to sit still for long; is good at sports or dance or acting or mime; has good body coordination; communicates well through gestures; learns best through physical activity, simulation and active play

Interpersonal: Understands people well; learns best by interacting and cooperating with others; good at leading and organising; picks up on other people's feelings easily; enjoys playing group and social games

Similar to emotional intelligence

Intrapersonal/reflective: Likes to work alone; is self-motivated; is intuitive; is self-confident; is aware of own personal strengths and weaknesses

Naturalistic: Makes distinctions and recognises patterns in the natural world; is curious about plants and animals; is concerned for the ecology/environment

Existential: Reflects on the meaning of life; asks questions about death; thinks about how we got here and what will happen to the world in the future

---

much for learning, but it might be more helpful to say learning activities using music and numbers need to be fewer, introduced carefully to ensure that the purpose and learning outcomes are clear and skillfully facilitated and the learning experience evaluated.

Thus planning learning experiences within PD work whether in the seminar type of setting or in the workplace is complex. Learning activities are not selected at random but with consideration of several factors such as knowing more about co-learners as persons and learners, the workplace culture, strategic aims and intentions and conceptual and philosophical principles. The probability is that in any large group there will be practitioners with a range of learning styles to accommodate and to introduce to new ways of learning.

The general principles of active learning have now been introduced with several examples. I have proposed that when blended in with other PD methods and processes, active learning can enhance PD aims and outcomes. Now the theoretical bases for active learning will be discussed in order to identify its foundations. This is included because an obvious question is 'where do the ideas for active

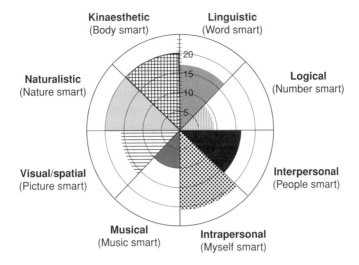

Figure 14.2   An example (Multiple Intelligences Gardner, 1993).

learning come from?' Chapter 4 makes a useful background to reading to this next section.

Theoretical underpinnings of active learning

Chapter 6 has already set out several learning theories and processes essential to the development of practice and outlines some of the key issues and approaches that may be used to promote learning, particularly approaches building on critical reflectivity and problem-solving. In this section of the chapter, we turn our attention to the work of John Heron.

John Heron's model of holistic learning

Given that active learning includes a meaningful engagement with one's self, the principles of active learning mean it can be situated within a holistic learning framework, wherein the learner is fully engaged in a significant sensual and emotional experience that enables deeply authentic (i.e. value based) and visible behavioural changes. The term 'holistic learning' signifies an approach to learning that is 'whole person' centred. John Heron defines a whole person-centred model as one that seeks to fully engage all aspects of the learner – mind, body and spirit. The underlying principle is that a complex organism such as a human being functions most effectively when all its component parts are themselves active and cooperating effectively. This idea relates very closely to the concept of synergy with the whole being greater than the sum of its parts. A 'whole person' approach to learning is much more likely to be observed within sensory-rich and creative settings. Thus there may be challenges for PD facilitators associated with creating these sorts of settings.

John Heron's framework presents learning as an interaction between four distinct modes of psychological being: feeling, imaginal, thinking and practical. Further, Heron believes that all learning is rooted in feeling. These four modes are normally represented in the form of a pyramid with feeling at the base and practical at the top. What is especially unusual about the model is that feeling is presented as our fundamental mode of experiencing and being in the world, rather than thinking. This contrasts sharply with much of traditional education, where cognitive thinking and the pursuit of intellectual competence are accorded superiority. The significance of Heron's work for PD is that the crucial requirement for each co-learner is to establish a relationship with their total learning situation in feeling mode, which is intimate, resonant and positive. Only when this is firmly in place is it considered that the co-learner will be free to access and fully engage in the other three modes of learning (imaginal, thinking and practical). Thus in PD work, active learning starts from the premise of engaging feeling. Achieving this can maximise overall learning potential. There are consequences for facilitators in terms of how they construct active learning experiences and how they facilitate individual and group processing of learning experiences so that the feeling domain is kept central. Achieving this mode of engagement with co-learners is indeed skilled facilitation work as many workplace cultures discourage the feeling domain in practitioners. Reawakening and reconnecting with the feeling domain cannot be carried out by unskilled facilitators causing practitioners to become unduly unsettled or disturbed. Facilitators need to feel comfortable working in this way and to find strategies to increase their skill and comfort level in this area of PD (Coats et al., 2006). Additionally, facilitators may need to be prepared for dealing with anxieties, queries and barriers from co-learners that active learning is too 'personal' or 'too much like therapy'. Facilitators who are lacking in confidence about working with the feeling domain of learning will need to look at their own learning and skills development needs.

An example of Heron's theory in use in the context of PD work is in situations where storytelling might be used to engage learners at the feeling level to understand the views of patients (or colleagues) in healthcare situations. Debriefing from such narratives and stories can help the co-learner empathise with the patient, perhaps imagine themselves or their loved ones as a patient, and help the co-learner begin to think about how they might act as a professional in a similar situation. At this stage, dialogue about specific professional attributes or behaviours that support patient-centred care can be introduced with opportunities for role-play or follow-up practical application. All this is possible only after the learner is engaged at the feeling level. Heron's model is also extremely useful because of the action or practical element included, which is congruent with active learning and the transformational goals of PD.

Heron's model of cooperative inquiry

Cooperative inquiry is a systematic approach to both understanding (learning) and action (application) and is another aspect of Heron's work (http://www.human-inquiry.com/cishortg.htm). It offers an approach to realising emancipatory conceptual models of PD. In this theory, learners and facilitators who are usually acting in a researcher role become one together. Cooperative inquiry is carried out in groups where all the work, including the direction, aim, processes, methods, evaluation and decision-making are agreed upon cooperatively within the group. The group engages in cycles of reflection and action and can be thought of as an advanced form of emancipatory action research that attends rigorously to whole person learning in a social context. Cooperative inquiry results in new learning that has become possible from the blending of feelings, ideas, research and action involving a group of people interested in exploring the same phenomenon, puzzle or issue about their practice. In PD, cooperative inquiry is very appropriate as a learning strategy since practitioners, usually in their naturally occurring workplace teams, strive to transform their practice by first trying to make sense of their world then to develop innovative strategies to reframe their experiences. Inclusive to this activity, practitioners aim to draw on a range of knowledge including evidence-based knowledge to maximise patient and practitioner satisfaction and effect positive health outcomes. Heron (http://www.human-inquiry.com) has identified specific procedures that can be utilised in establishing and maintaining an effective cooperative inquiry group. However, given that many PD projects or strategies are already partially set out before practitioners become fully involved and given that genuine full involvement takes time, cooperative inquiry can be seen as being idealistic in this respect.

A variation of Heron's cooperative inquiry, peer learning, or cooperative learning, is becoming an increasingly important part of PD work. In this type of learning, co-learners work in teams on problems and projects under conditions that assure both positive interdependence and individual accountability (Boud, 2001 p. 3). This variation focuses less on research, and more on learning from peers in a team situation. Thus some effective learning circles and action learning sets can resemble cooperative learning. It has been demonstrated that co-learners learn a great deal by explaining their ideas to others and by participating in activities in which they can learn from their peers. Amongst others, they develop skills in organising and planning learning activities, working collaboratively with others, giving and receiving feedback and evaluating their own learning.

Communities of practice

Lave and Wenger set out an elaborate form of cooperative learning through their ideas on *communities of practice* (Smith, 2003). Lave and Wenger (1991) purport communities of practice are in all settings – work, school, home and recreational pursuits and result in collective learning that is ongoing. Much of this thinking derives from Wenger's (1998) work that discusses learning as a social activity based in our life experiences, rather than as something we do that is university or teacher directed and quite separate from our daily interactions.

In a community of practice, members come together around a common activity and by 'what they have learned through their mutual engagement in these activities' (Wenger, 1998, 45). Wenger (1998) further defines communities of practice as being joint enterprises, involving mutual engagement that produces a shared repertoire of common resources developed by the members. This is very consistent with PD work that may, for example, involve a team that agrees to come together to transform clinical practice to be more patient centered. In the process the team develops new ways of talking about, engaging with, and caring for patients, and in addition creates resources that will support these new ways of being. Wenger intends that communities of practice are organisational wide. A community of practice then is not just a work group that comes together to complete a task. According to Wenger it involves building relationships, sharing a commitment, ideas, and memories, and developing resources that reflect the knowledge cumulated through the work of the co-participants, all of which is related to the wider organisation. Learning outcomes are then reflected in new ways of working and future strategic planning. The use of communities of practice cause practice developers to reflect on the kinds of social situations that will best facilitate learning rather than to narrowly focus on the cognitive processes and conceptual frameworks involved (Smith, 2003). Further, communities of practice theory prompts facilitators of PD to be strategic about how learning, including active learning, in the workplace can be established across the entire organisation. Learning needs to be situated in a social context, embedded in groups in the workplace and across the entire organisation.

PD based on a community of practice philosophy promotes informed and committed practice, within the practice setting. Communities of practice can be an ideal approach to leaning for PD, since the goal of PD is transformation of workplace culture and practice, resulting in new ways of being as a practitioner. Paraphrasing a comment from Lave and Wenger (1991) PD is not so much about having practitioners learn *from* talk, but rather having practitioners learn *to* talk differently for themselves as they become active participants in a community of practice. The other key strength of communities of practice theory as it relates to PD is the strong link it presents between knowledge and learning, within the specific context of the workplace, from real problems or issues.

In summary, traditional learning theories tended to emphasise teacher- or facilitator-centred instructional methods based on giving new knowledge to learners. Such theories tended to focus on covering a curriculum or pre-designated materials often excluding learner's needs or preferences. Contrary to this approach, holistic learning frameworks, and cooperative inquiry or learning, reinforce that adults already have knowledge and may need to rediscover and reconnect with it, or acquire knowledge and develop skills through full involvement (Heron, 1996a, 1996b; Silver et al., 2000; Yang, 2004; Mason, 2006). Such full involvement needs to begin with the feeling level and include a combination of dialogue and engagement, and social interaction within a learning community. As we already know, adults learn less by watching and listening to someone else showing and telling them what to do, and even less by being instructed (Dale, 1969). Dale's ideas, sometimes referred to as 'The Cone of Experience', focus mostly on the value of action, whether it be communicating about the phenomenon or applying it in an activity. This theory, while consistent with some of the cooperative enquiry theories, reflecting the power of learning from active involvement, does not appear to stress the importance of feeling, so critical in Heron's work. However, one could argue that

Box 14.1 Example 1

Timing	Key learning activity	Comments
10:30–12:30	Facilitating meetings with the team	Key question to ask:
	Small groups use either claims concerns and issues or record key aspects from recent critical incidents; one person per group to feedback	How effectively do we run our team meetings?
	Short presentation on attributes of effective meetings	
	Questions and answers/discussion	
	Action planning in small groups	

as the co-learner engages with the knowledge in teaching or implementing the new learning there is a feeling level attached. PD that focuses on adult professionals in active clinical practice can embrace holistic learning frameworks and cooperative inquiry or learning to better facilitate development of evidence-based innovative practices in an environment of patient-centred care.

More on active learning methods

Ensuring that learning activities within any single learning encounter and over several encounters address observing, doing, interactions with self and others, and take into account feeling as the basis for learning and acknowledge co-learners intelligences provides a starting point. There are a vast range of practical methods that can be used to maximise active learning. Using a variety of active learning strategies or methods and avoiding patterns that become routinised, such as repeating the same activity with regularity, are important.

In PD work, the emphasis often needs to be on *uncovering* topics and what practitioners already know about them in relation to their practice, rather than covering new topics in the form of teaching. Facilitation of learning may often be about supporting co-learners to reconnect with their feelings through uncovering or unconcealing them so the feeling domain becomes accessible as learning material. By doing this, the facilitator is starting where the co-learner is and working with the co-learner's previous experience and established values and beliefs. Where co-learners imagine/draw/write their own feelings/thoughts on a topic (dialogue with self) *before* they engage in small group discussion (dialogue with others), the group discussion should be richer and more engaging.

Consider the two examples in Boxes 14.1 and 14.2. The first one is from a more traditional yet still learner-centred session in a PD workshop. The second one shows how the same session is facilitated using active learning methods.

Asking effective questions is a key skill in being an effective facilitator of active learning in PD in general and within any active learning activity many facilitation interventions will come through the use of questions. Questions are

Box 14.2 Example 2

Timing	Key learning activity	Comments
10:30–12:30	Facilitating meetings with the team	Key question for facilitators to consider:
	Introduction – ask participants to look at why we are looking at this topic using examples from workplace and PD vision; 10 min	How effectively do we run our team meetings?
	Ask participants to generate list of their own questions on this topic; all participants to post their questions on flipchart/board (questions can go back to workplace for staff to read and add to); 10 min	
	Invite participants to choose a question or questions that interest them; go for a reflective walk (inside or outside) for 10–15 min and consider question(s); participants asked to bring back an object they find that speaks to them/is symbolic of team meetings	
	Viewing of objects	
	Focused discussion in small groups (2–6); 15 min	
	Groups to identify key attributes of an effective team meeting; rotate work of each group around other groups for written feedback and critique; 15 min	
	Groups collate into one set of attributes; 15 min (offer to observe process and give feedback – or a participant may offer)	
	Group invited to plan how they intend to share this learning activity with their teams and how they can facilitate teams to develop ownership for improving effective of meetings	

aimed at unconcealing and reconnecting feelings, enhancing observation skills, promoting reflection (interaction with self), focused discussion (interaction with others) and promoting action particularly in the workplace. In active learning, the goal of using questions is to promote internal reflection and discussion with others, not just getting an answer from those that speak up (Felder & Brent, 2003). Thus, coming up with good questions is only half the challenge for facilitators. The other half is asking them in a way that has the greatest positive impact on the co-learners and contributes to achieving the ultimate purpose of PD work. Imagine, in the traditional class/seminar scenario on a study day, the teacher/facilitator asks a question to the group and waits for someone to volunteer an answer whilst other co-learners remain silent (e.g. 'who has a question about'). Silent group members may of course be reflecting, but that is not usually known. A more effective and active way is to invite co-learners to develop the questions for themselves and then work out responses or solutions individually and or in groups and then work in pairs or groups to reach consensus.

In this example there are 20 participants:

Facilitator. *You have been discussing carrying out an observation of practice in your own workplaces – what comes to mind for you? Can you all reflect for a few moments with the aim of constructing between one and three key questions. I will then invite you to share your questions with someone else in the group and for each pair to refine the questions to three in total.*

After 10 minutes:

Facilitator. *Each pair (i.e. 10 pairs) will now have up to three questions. Let's see what you have all come up with. Can each pair write up their questions, one per sheet? Let's theme the questions and look at how you can address each theme.*

Once the themes are organised, the facilitator invites the participants to choose themes and develop responses that they share with the group and the group gives feedback on how helpful they find the responses.

Other examples of methods:

Being as creative as you would like, define the concept of [   ] in your own words.

If co-learners can be involved in both of these activities and then observe the situation in practice or in fact have previously observed the phenomena or action (observation), the dialogue should be richer and again more engaging. If this is followed by having the co-learners engage in the action itself (doing and doing differently), they will have a better sense of what they need to do and what they need to learn during doing. Finally if, after doing, co-learners process this experience by writing about it (return to dialogue with self) and/or discussing it with others (dialogue with others), this will add further insight. Such a sequence of learning activities will give the facilitator and learners powerful learning experiences both individually and as a learning community.

Significance of active learning in PD

It would be useful for you to develop responses to the question implied in the title to this section yourself, based on your experiences and what you are reading in this chapter (and book). Throughout the chapter, reference to the significance of active learning in PD methods and methodologies has been reinforced. Active learning related to PD is clearly more than simply learning by doing. Over time, it connects use of all the senses grounded in feeling and multiple intelligences, blends self-learning and learning from and with others, and embeds learning in the world of practice as it actually is and as it is envisioned. The approach enables practitioners to construct broader theoretical understandings in its widest sense, through reflection on practical activities and to prepare for addressing the realities of engaging in PD as facilitators. Active learning develops practitioners who are more highly connected with becoming and being a work-based learner and with taking ownership of PD because the active learning activities they try out and facilitate in the workplace *is* the development of practice.

Challenges for PD

Active learning requires greater commitment and increased attention to planning and delivering learning experiences within PD programmes. It demands that learning activities take place in the workplace and thus requires management support. Whilst the literature shows that PD usually focuses on the clinical/care practice arena, it must not ignore active learning in regard to corporate practices – another challenge for practice developers. Graham et al. (2006) have highlighted that nurses, particularly at and above the specialist level, need to learn about the corporate, political and business aspects of healthcare. The PD literature recognises the challenge associated with embedding PD processes and outcomes in organisations and sustaining them beyond the life of particular project timeframes. Although, attention in PD is currently directed on workplace cultures rather than corporate cultures, embedding PD activities in corporate learning strategies is one way of addressing this gap. Reflective learning strategies and in particular 'action learning' clearly have something to offer to the sustainability of PD. However, there is a need to evaluate action learning as a 'method'. Likewise, should active learning become more popular, its methods also require robust evaluation so we know what works best in workplace settings.

Active learning, of course, can be delivered in isolation from PD but it will not achieve its potential. It is better envisioned as one part of an integrated approach to realising the concepts of PD. When active learning is planned in conjunction with the principles and aims of PD, it reinforces the deep connection between the PD concepts, vision and strategic intentions, skilled facilitation and developing a learning culture. The various learning activities can then have an impact that is more than additive or cumulative thus becoming greater than the sum of their parts. The relationship between practical knowledge and so-called higher knowledge is not well understood according to Cope et al. (2003, p. 351) and traditionally this area has been the domain of educators. Despite challenges, therefore, practice developers must learn to develop necessary knowledge and skills in becoming facilitators of active learning and to develop partnerships with educators.

The NHS Education for Scotland Project synthesising the evidence relating to PD (NES Project) (McCormack et al., 2006) suggests that there are challenges about the approaches used to ensure that knowledge gained will effectively bring about action/change and support learning in PD. In particular, the project asks 'how do approaches taken to support learning within PD have an impact on outcomes?' This will continue to be an important question for some time as there is, at present, little evidence in the literature of a direct relationship between learning approaches and methods utilised and the PD outcomes achieved. The most commonly reported outcome in regard to learning approaches is that of 'increased confidence' among participants. Although, the NES Project that suggests there is already evidence of 'active learning' taking place within PD, it should be noted that this tends to be limited to 'reflective learning' and more broadly to adult learning theories. The dominant approach reported is action learning. However, as yet, there are very few studies of the effectiveness of action learning within PD.

In recent years, universities and other institutions of higher education in many countries have had to consider their place within the spectrum of lifelong learning. Candy (2000) broadly sets out two approaches that universities and other institutions might take. They produce lifelong learners themselves in a traditional way. Alternately, they can both administratively and pedagogically support and encourage lifelong learning itself through more 'sideways' support to learning that occurs in the home, workplace or community, and 'forwards' to embrace students' post-graduation learning experiences, including their participation in further formal study. The role for higher education institutions (HEIs) and other organisations providing nursing education and development has been recognised by NES Project (McCormack et al., 2006). The report comments that collaborative relationships with HEIs can provide knowledge on how practice developers create systematic and rigorous processes in PD work. However, there is still much to do in terms of HEIs offering programmes of learning and ones situated in the workplace rather than formal education modules and pathways that are specific to the needs and purposes of both transforming practitioners and workplaces and thus for PD. Additionally, practice developers venturing into provision of active learning must appreciate learning theories, learning styles and processes.

Given that higher order learning does not necessarily lead to competence in practice and being more knowledgeable does not in itself ensure expertise in practice, here are challenges associated with measuring how personal transformation creates increased effectiveness as a practitioner. The claim here is that active learning within a safe learning community makes a significant contribution to personal transformation. Personal transformation is a prerequisite to sustained collective transformation in the workplace, the ultimate purpose of PD. However, wide-scale evidence is needed in supporting such claims. Thus there is a challenge for facilitators committed to transformational working and that is to continue to attend to one's own holistic development (which is greater than professional development) and sustain passion for contributing to transformational working and being and ultimately to quality patient care, whilst seemingly doing very similar PD work over and over.

For facilitators, engaging in self-growth and becoming a co-learner takes courage, commitment and consistency. It requires that the facilitator engages in perspective transformation whereby they see a fundamental shift in power away from themselves and towards the co-learners (even if other co-learners do not share the same perspective at that time). This is achieved by moving beyond the usual tools and techniques associated with facilitation to making participatory and emancipatory theories and methods transparent to others. The ability for the facilitator to transform themselves along with the co-learners with whom facilitators are working requires holistic and critical reflection upon the values and beliefs held, as well as the foundational philosophical and theoretical paradigms resulting in exposure of contradictions, un-learning and re-learning. Some experienced facilitators seek to rediscover the spiritual dimensions of facilitation (Heron, 1996c; Hanson & Hanson, 2001). The boundaries between work and the personal and indeed the private self become increasingly blurred here as do the boundaries between learning and therapy, thus being clear about intent is vital. The ongoing challenge for practice developers is to continuously clarify just how much and what level of transformation is needed and probably to recognise that not everyone wants to engage in extreme levels of personal transformation in order to be a competent practitioner. I suggest that there can be problems associated with co-dependency between facilitators and participants in PD work. Ensuring that active learning is in place and that it covers exploration of the co-facilitation relationship may go some way in preventing or reducing concerns and issues around co-dependency.

Concluding comments

I have addressed the key principles of active learning, demonstrated how active learning fits with adult and holistic learning theories, and provided examples of active learning from different PD work. It is hoped that the examples in particular inspire you to be creative with active learning in your workplace or within your PD facilitation. The intension here, has been to demonstrate how active learning contributes to the purposes of PD, although it is acknowledged that further evidence is needed to strengthen the beliefs espoused and claims made in this chapter.

In essence, active learning is concerned with providing holistic learning opportunities rather than with teaching of PD. It is based on multiple uses of the senses, reflection and dialogue with others and is grounded in feeling. In part, it is achieved through a skilled facilitation relationship that aims to make effective use of and maximise learning opportunities in the workplace. The purpose of this can be multifocal. Primarily it is done to contribute to transformation of the workplace and patient care. It can also act as a catalyst to personal transformation(s) in practitioners whereby practitioners reconnect or become fully engaged in a holistic way with developing knowledge and their way of being as a person. A debate is needed over whether these added benefits in terms of personal discovery, transformation and overall growth as a person are necessary or not and, if they are, to what degree.

Active learning may indeed have a lasting impact on personal life philosophy – but this is necessary for PD?

> *The secret of wisdom is to be curious – to take the time to look closely, to use all of your senses to see and touch and taste and smell and hear; to keep wandering and wondering.*
> Merriam, 1991

References

Bonwell, C.C. & Eison, J.A. (1991) *Active Learning: Creating Excitement in the Classroom*. ASHE-ERIC Higher Education Report No. 1. The George Washington University, School of Education and Human Development, Washington DC.

Boud, D. (2001) Introduction: Making the move to peer learning. In: *Peer Learning in Higher Education* (eds D. Boud, R. Cohen & J. Sampson), p. 3. Kogan Page, London.

Candy, P.C. (2000) Reaffirming a proud tradition Universities and lifelong learning. *Active Learning in Higher Education*. **1**(2), 101–125.

Coats, E., Dewing, J. & Titchen, A. (2006) *Opening Doors on Creativity: Resources to Awaken Creative Working*. RCN Institute, London.

Cope, P., Cuthbertson, P. & Staddart, B. (2003) Situated learning in the practice placement. In: *Mentoring in Practice: A reader* (eds C. Downie & P. Basford), pp. 351–361. University of Greenwich, London.

Dale, E. (1969) *Audiovisual Methods in Teaching*. Holt, Rinehart and Winston, New York.

Dewing, J., Brooks, J. & Riddaway, L. (2006) Involving older people in practice development. *Practice Development in Health Care Journal*. **5**(3), 156–174.

Dewing, J., Hancock, S., Brooks, J., Pedder, L., Riddaway, L., Adams, L., Uglow, J. & O'Connor, P. (2004) An account of 360 degree review as part of a practice development strategy. *Practice Development in Health Care*. **3**(4), 193–209.

Dewing, J. & Wright, J. (2003) A practice development project for nurses working with older people. *Practice Development in Health Care*. **2**(1), 13–28.

Felder, R.M. & Brent, R. (2003) Learning by doing. The philosophy and strategies of active learning chemical engineering. *Education*. **37**(4), 282–283.

Fink, D.L. (1999) *Active Learning*. Available from http://honolulu.hawaii.edu/intranet/committees/FacDevCom/guidebk/teachtip/active.htm [accessed 12/08/2006].

Garbett, R. & McCormack, B. (2004) A concept analysis of practice development. In: *Practice Development in Nursing* (eds B. McCormack, K. Manley & R. Garbett). Blackwell, Oxford.

Gardner, H. (1983) *Frames of Mind: The Theory of Multiple Intelligences*, 10th Anniversary edn. Basic Books, New York.

Gardner, H. (1993) *Multiple Intelligences: The Theory in Practice*. Basic Books, New York.

Graham, I., Fielding, C., Rooke, D. & Keen, S. (2006) Practice development 'without walls' and the quandary of corporate practice. *Journal of Clinical Nursing*. **15**, 980–988.

Hanson, L. & Hanson, C. (2001) *Transforming Participatory Facilitation: Reflections from Practice. PLA Notes*. Available from http://www.iied.org/NR/agbioliv/pla_notes/documents/plan_04107.pdf [accessed 04/01/07].

Heron, J. (1989) *The Facilitators Handbook*. Kogan Page, London.

Heron, J. (1996a) Working with experience: Animating learning. In: *Working with Experience* (eds D. Boud & N. Miller). Routledge, London.

Heron, J. (1996b) *Cooperative Inquiry: Research into the Human Condition*. Sage, London. Available from http://www.human-inquiry.com/cishortg.htm [accessed 17/11/2006].

Heron, J. (1996c) Helping whole people learn. In: *Working with Experience: Animating Learning* (eds D. Boud & N. Miller). Routledge, London.

Honey, P. & Mumford, A. (1982) Available from http://www2.le.ac.uk/institution/merlin/HoneyAndMumford [accessed 15/11/2006].

Honey, P. & Mumford, A. (1986) *The Manual of Learning Styles*, 2nd edn. Peter Honey, Maidenhead.

Kim, H.S. (1999) Critical reflective inquiry for knowledge development in nursing practice. *Journal of Advanced Nursing*. **29**(5), 1205–1212.

Kolb, D.A. (1984) *Experiential Learning: Experience as the Source of Learning and Development*. Prentice-Hall, Englewood Cliffs, NJ.

Lave, J. & Wenger, E. (1991) *Situated Learning: Legitimate Peripheral Participation*. Cambridge University Press, Cambridge.

Hardy, S., Garbarino, L., Titchen, A., & Manley, K. (2006) A framework for work-based learning. In: Royal College of Nursing *Workplace Resources for Practice Development*, pp. 8–56. RCN, London.

Mason, R. (2006) Holistic course design using learning objects. *International Journal of Learning Technology*. **2**(2–3), 203–215.

McCormack, B., Dewar, B., Wright, J., Garbett, R., Harvey, G. & Ballantine, K. (2006) *A Realist Synthesis of Evidence realting to Practice Development*. NHS Scotland, Edinburgh.

McCormack, B. & Garbett, R. (2003) The characteristics, qualities and skills of practice developers. *Journal of Clinical Nursing*. **12**, 317–325.

McCormack, B., Illman, A., Culling, A., Ryan, A. & O'Neill, S. (2002) 'Removing the chaos from the narrative': Preparing clinical leaders for practice development. *Education Action Research*. **10**(3), 335–352.

Merriam, E. (1991) *The Wise Woman and Her Secrets*. Simon & Schuster, New York.

Raux, D.J. & College, S. (2004) Implementing active learning in college. *Explorations in Teaching and Learning*. **2**(1), 2–4.

Silver, H.F., Strong, R.W. & Perini, M.J. (2000) *So Each May Learn: Integrating Learning Styles and Multiple Intelligences*. Association for Supervision and Curriculum Development, Alexandria, Vancouver.

Smith, M.K. (2003) *Communities of Practice, The Encyclopedia of Informal Education*. Available from www.infed.org/biblio/communities_of_practice.htm. Last updated: 21 June 2006 [accessed 17/11/2006].

Titchen, A. (2004) Critical companionship Part 1. *Nursing Standard*. **18**(9), 33–40.

Wenger, E. (1998) *Communities of Practice: Learning, Meaning, and Identity*. Cambridge University Press, Cambridge.

Yang, B. (2004) Holistic learning theory and implications for human resource development. *Advances in Developing Human Resources*. **6**(2), 241–262.

15. *Evidence Use in Practice Development*

Rob McSherry and Karen Cox

Introduction

Despite the rise of the evidence-based movement across the globe and the reported strengths and difficulties of using evidence within medicine, nursing and allied healthcare practice, the application of evidence into practice remains challenging and problematic for some healthcare professionals (see Chapter 5). A combination of individual and organisational factors seems to mitigate this problem, for example a lack of confidence or time to engage with the evidence or insufficient support from peers, managers and the organisation to name but a few. Practice development (PD) is an untapped resource when it comes to promoting evidence-based practice offering new horizons in resolving this problem. This is because of its facilitative, supportive and communicative approach to empowering, engaging, encouraging, and enlightening individuals and teams to innovate and change. PD focuses direct and indirect attention on the individual and organisation to take a leading role and responsibility for engaging with and applying evidence into practice through a range of frameworks.

The purpose of this chapter is to provide a practical guide to the generation and use of evidence, outline the infrastructure challenges in doing so and identify how PD can help support individuals and organisations to achieve this goal. This will be achieved by providing definitions of evidence-based practice and PD and outlining why and how PD is ideal in facilitating evidence into practice. The chapter will also offer other useful practical tools and techniques for promoting evidence-based practice along with using case studies to illustrate the reality of achieving this in practice. The chapter concludes with a summary critique about the relative challenges and difficulties of using PD in promoting evidence-based practice at an individual and organisational level.

Changes in social and political structures across the globe are such that they are driving all healthcare professionals to practice using an evidence base (Nursing Midwifery Council, 2004; Health Professions Council, 2003; General Medical Council, 2001; American Nurses Association, 2002; Australian Nursing and

Table 15.1 Factors driving forward quality in healthcare

- Rising patient/client, carer expectation
- Increased dependency of those accessing services
- Technological advances
- Demographic changes in society
- Changes in care delivery systems
- Lack of public confidence in healthcare services
- Threat of litigation
- Demands for greater access to information
- Rising expectation from professional bodies that decision-making will be underpinned with best evidenced

Midwifery Council, 2003; Ministerie van Volksgezondheid Welzijn en Sport, 2006). The rationale for the development of evidence-based practice according to Pickering and Thompson (2003) is attributed to a perceived decline in the standards and quality of care provision. A point confirmed by McSherry and Pearce (2007), who argue that the origins for developing quality services arise from a combination of societal, political and professional factors such as highlighted in Table 15.1.

More importantly, there has been a growing awareness of the fragility of the knowledge base of the profession; this is predominately because of a lack of available robust evidence to substantiate decision-making and action in practice. This fragility of the knowledge base has led to the development of evidence-based practice being positioned at the centre of clinical governance and best value in the overarching quest for quality enhancements (McSherry & Taylor, 2003). Yet, despite the plethora of evidence-based literature (Rycroft-Malone et al., 2004b) and numerous models (Stetler, 1994; Kitson et al., 1996; Rosswurm & Larrbee, 1999; Snares & Heliker, 2002; Rycroft-Malone et al., 2002; Hogan & Logan, 2004) and frameworks (Funk et al., 1991; Ward et al., 1998; Thompson, 1999; Mohide & King, 2003; Clarke et al., 2004; Newhouse et al., 2005) designed to facilitate and develop such important skills, getting evidence into practice remains problematic.

The purpose of this chapter is to provide a practical guide to the generation and use of evidence. However, the chapter will primarily focus on 'evidence use' and the infrastructure challenges involved in doing so. How PD can help to support individuals and organisations to achieve this goal will be emphasised. This will be achieved by

- defining evidence-based practice and PD;
- outlining why PD is ideal for facilitating evidence-based practice;
- using the PARIHS framework of context and facilitation as an overarching framework for promoting evidence-based practice;
- providing practical frameworks and case studies for the reader to use in the quest for evidence-based practice.

The case of need for practice development and evidence-based practice

PD and evidence-based practice play an important role within contemporary healthcare settings in supporting innovation and change, which is crucial if a health and or social care service is to modernise (McCormack et al., 2006). Modernisation within the context of PD and evidence-based practice is associated with the provision of continuous quality improvement and achievement of excellence in practice (see Page & Hamer 2002 and Chapter 2 of this book). However, the latter is difficult to realise because modernisation means different things to different individuals (clinical and non-clinical) and professional disciplines working within the service. The reasons for varied views of modernisation could be attributed to the fact that healthcare services such as the National Health Service (NHS) in the United Kingdom are complex establishments incorporating (yet often viewed as being separate) a multitude of diverse healthcare organisations and personnel covering a whole range of settings/specialities across and between community, primary and acute sectors. The consequence of being such an enormous and diverse establishment provides a challenge to ensure that changes occurring as a direct result of modernisation maintain equity, equality, efficiency and effectiveness of services locally, regionally, nationally and internationally. PD provides a framework to address the misconceptions surrounding what modernisation means in terms of service improvement, healthcare improvement or health service reform by ensuring that responding to and engaging with change becomes part of everyone's role and responsibility (regardless of how big or small the contribution) through their job description. By taking an inclusive or collective approach to change rather than a singular or isolative view, the possibilities of advancing and evaluating practice or services are enhanced. This is because PD focuses on nurturing the whole system approach to advancing and evaluating practice; that is to say, informing, involving and engaging where possible and appropriately the entire multi-disciplinary team with the change, innovation or evaluation processes (Rycroft-Malone et al., 2004a; Kitson et al., 1996). This approach is more likely to create a working environment and culture in which excellence can flourish (McSherry, 2004).

McCormack et al. (2006), Simmons (2004) and Harvey et al. (2002) argue that PD is about promoting and or facilitating advances and/or evaluations in practice through the utilisation of a cyclical set of systems and processes within the context of individual and/or professional practice. The foundation can be utilised to advance and evaluate practice at both an individual and/or organisational level, usually simultaneously. The primary role and function of PD is therefore the promotion and facilitation of person-centred care, services and/or organisation. Person centredness is dependent upon the establishment and delivery of efficient and effective channels of communication, collaboration and partnerships and creating an effective organisational culture and working environment. The creation of person centredness through PD involves the identification and management of risks, the auditing of standards/practices, the continued professional development of staff and the sharing and circulating of practices.

PD promotes evidence-based practice through the integration of clinical expertise with the best available external evidence from systematic research, following an evaluation of existing or newly devised standards for practice. It should therefore be argued that PD is an ideal model in promoting best practice within the context of clinical governance because it is pertinent to all healthcare professionals, teams and organisations (McSherry, 2004). Yet, despite the growing evidence that both PD and evidence-based practice are associated with promoting innovation and change, enhancing the quality agenda and ensuring evidence-informed person-centred care (McCormack et al., 2006), healthcare professionals continue to struggle to define and associate with the terms. To achieve evidence-informed person-centred care as advocated by McCormack et al. (2006), it is imperative to involve and engage the patient and public as part of the change process or innovation in practice.

Patient involvement

Patient involvement, according to the Department of Health (UK) (2005, p. 3), is about, 'changing the whole system so that there is more choice, more personalised care, real empowerment of people to improve their health'. Patient involvement is not optional, but a necessity, because involvement entails direct patient participation in their care. More significant, however, is the fact that patient preference infers that involvement is also about offering choice (DiCenso et al., 1998; French, 1999; Ingersoll, 2000; Ferguson & Day, 2005). Patient preference is important within the context of evidence-based practice using a PD model, because it relates, directly, to engaging the patient, evident through the use of participative phrases, for example, considering the views of the patients, ensuring the benefit of a well-defined client/patient group, consideration of individual needs or preferences and the promotion of optimal patient outcomes. A weakness of existing evidence-based practice definitions concerning the inclusion of patient involvement is in deciphering whether this means active participation in the care process or being a passive recipient of care. Patients no longer and indeed should not be regarded as passive recipients of care but expected to be involved in and informed about decisions regarding them, their family or significant others. Patients today want to work in partnership with the professional to bring about the best possible outcome (McSherry et al., 2001). The challenge for many teams and organisations is in bringing about changes in culture so that evidence can be used and generated in and from practice. Similarly, healthcare professionals need to become familiar with the terms evidence-based practice and PD.

Exploring the terms evidence-based practice and practice development

To understand the systems and processes associated with getting evidence into practice, it is imperative to know what evidence-based practice and PD mean and what the similarities and differences are in making this happen.

Evidence-based practice

As identified earlier in Chapter 5 the term evidence base is a derivative of evidence-based medicine, which according to McPheeters and Lohr (1999, p. 99)

> *can be traced to a group of Anglo-American medical researchers and educators who believed medicine should be orientated more to the existing science and knowledge base than they perceived it was in the last quarter of this century.*

Muir-Gary (1997), like McPheeters and Lohr (1999), believes that this group of individuals, based at McMaster University Medical School in the 1980s, coined the phrase not because they believed that clinicians were not using science, but because they believed that they were not using evidence explicitly, carefully and in the appropriate place. Taylor (1997) expands this debate by suggesting that McMaster University regarded evidence-based medicine as a process that facilitated problem-based clinical teaching and learning involving students and clinicians, in searching for and evaluating the evidence for clinical practice. This view is regarded by McSherry and Taylor (2003) as being similar to Cochrane's early works on efficiency and effectiveness. This is because the term focuses on highlighting the outcome of a given action or intervention. Medical scholars and clinicians Rosenberg and Donaldson (1995), Sackett et al. (1997) and Muir-Gray (1997) regard Archie Cochrane, a British physician and epidemiologist, as the founder of the evidence-based movement of today. The rationale for this accolade was Cochrane's concerns that healthcare providers failed to evaluate the efficiency and effectiveness of their own practice. Wallace et al. (1997) and Thompson (2003) indicate that Cochrane considered that there was a need for wide-spread access to scientific literature, in order to improve clinical care.

Evidence-based practice embodies Cochrane's (1979) work of ensuring efficiency and effectiveness of a given intervention by placing the responsibility for engaging with and applying the best evidence with the professional and employing organisation. Furthermore, evidence-based practice provides a framework for

- using evidence in practice at an individual and organisational level (Wallin et al., 2003);
- ensuring that decisions about healthcare are based on the best available, current, valid and relevant evidence;
- recommending that decisions should be made by those receiving care, informed by the tacit and explicit knowledge of those providing care within the context of available resources (DiCenso et al., 1998);
- encouraging evidence-based practice, which requires facilitation and support at an individual and organisational level;
- pressurising organisations about the need to be able to provide the support and resources for individuals to access, critically review different forms of available evidence so that they can be implemented and evaluated (McSherry & Warr, 2006);
- offering a systematic process for getting evidence into practice.

The evidence-based process involves a series of steps:

1. Identifying a problem or posing a research question.
2. Seeking out best evidence.
3. Appraising the evidence.
4. Implementing the evidence.
5. Evaluating the effectiveness of the evidence on the patients outcome.

The evidence-based process encourages healthcare professionals to identify patients' needs or problems through information gathering skills. They then enter a critical appraisal phase, where they consider and encourage the practitioner/team to focus on devising an appropriate question along with the evidence available to answer the question. They do this by systematically reviewing and finding the best evidence from systematic reviews (where possible) to support guideline development and questioning the stages of the research process pertaining to a particular piece of evidence, that is, title and abstract, introduction/literature review, methods, results, discussions and recommendations and by asking the following:

*   Is the research of interest?
*   Why was it done?
*   How was it performed?
*   What did it show?
*   What is the possible implication for your practice?
*   What next: for information only or support practice?

For healthcare professionals to engage in evidence-based activities requires education, training and support. 'Research awareness' is about ensuring that healthcare professionals have the necessary skills, knowledge and understanding of research to base practice on best evidence or to undertake a research study (McSherry et al., 2006). Furthermore, they need to be aware of the key conditions that promote or hinder this from happening, for example by having the knowledge and skills to critique evidence. Research awareness within the context of evidence-based practice is about having an appreciation of the importance research plays in generating evidence to support individual practices and decision-making.

Practice development facilitating evidence use and generation in practice

PD as defined in Chapter 1 of this book, like evidence-based practice, has numerous definitions (Kitson, 1994; Bassett, 1996; McCormack et al., 1999; Page & Hamer, 2002; McSherry & Warr, 2006) that highlight what it is and is not. PD's primary principles are centred on promoting person centredness through the utilisation of a facilitative approach to team working, collaboration, and partnership building and by networking. By nature of design and virtue PD is not linear but a messy concept, yet amongst the mess of daily practice it does adopt a systematic and organised holistic approach to advancing and evaluating practice. Kitson (1994) and Bassett's (1996) definitions highlight the importance research as evidence plays in driving change and that the proposed change may offer an explanation of a given phenomenon. These definitions also seem to infer that PD supports the development of a more systematic and rigorous approach to Research and Development through focusing attention on the implementation and utilisation of research findings in practice. In contrast to Kitson's (1994) definition, Mallett et al. (1997) introduced the notion that PD should be based on patients' needs by arguing the case that practice and professional development although viewed synonymously at times were distinctively different. A point endorsed by McCormack and Garbett (2003), who suggest that professional development refers to developing the knowledge and skills of the individual whilst PD is about creating optimal organisational cultures and working environments to aid individuals apply such skills. Recent work by O'Neal and Manley (2007) surrounding action planning reinforces the importance of differentiating between the terms. In exploring the definitions and distinctions between practice and professional development PD offers a continuous process of quality improvement by transforming the organisational culture and working environment through targeted systematic facilitation with the real intention of providing person-centered care (McCormack et al., 1999).

By taking a critical review of Kitson's (1994) and McCormack's (1999) definitions it would appear that the role of PD is that of facilitator in supporting the creation of optimal cultures and contexts to promote innovation and changes in practice. Furthermore, the definition offered by Bassett (1996) and McSherry (2004) suggests that PD is about encouraging individuals, teams and organisations to improve practice through innovation and change. Similarly, Page and Hammer (2002) indicate that PD plays a pivotal role in fostering a culture and context that nurtures evidence-based practice because it is an approach that focuses on getting evidence into practice through innovation and change with the real intention of improving the quality of care for the patient.

PD is distinctive and unique because it happens within the professional's 'own' practice setting and is about the enhancement and growth of personal, professional and/or organisational standards and quality of services by involving and focusing on the patients' and clients' specific needs. To achieve excellence in practice McSherry (2004) argues that team working, interdisciplinary collaboration, effective communication, internal and external partnerships and a willingness to learn and share with and from each other, including users of the service, is paramount. To become excellent and effective as an individual, team and organisation, PD requires support, investment and most importantly recognition from healthcare professionals themselves. Recognition that PD is an integral part of each of our roles and everyone's responsibility is to advance and evaluate practice. Taking the above definitions and emerging debates about what PD is and means, it could be argued that PD is ideal in promoting quality improvements in care as well as one's *self* because it is pertinent to all healthcare professionals, teams and organisations. The challenges for all healthcare professionals are in using our understanding of these terms to enhance practice.

Integrating practice development and evidence-based practice to facilitate change

PD enables the development of evidence-based practice (EBP) and person-centred care. Healthcare professionals find it difficult to visualise how PD and EBP can be implemented to facilitate innovation and change in practice. Results from large projects show that the implementation of EBP depends on the ability to achieve significant and systematic behaviour change involving individuals and teams at all levels of an organisation. An analysis of 70 Dutch-funded implementation projects showed that most of the strategies used for implementation were focused on the professional and could be labelled as educational strategies such as presentations and workshops. Strategies at an organisational level were not found (Holleman & Vis, 2006). In the EBP movement emphasis has been placed on helping practitioners to find, access and critically appraise research evidence hoping that this will lead to its use in practice. This is, however, a naïve assumption; implementation is far more complex than offering the available information.

In this section, two frameworks will be presented to support this implementation process. One is a framework for facilitating change based on the works of McSherry (1999, 2004) (Figure 15.1), the second one is the PARIHS framework (Rycroft-Malone et al., 2004a).

Figure 15.1 highlights how PD, clinical governance and evidence-based practice can be integrated into one framework for professionals to use in order to bring about change or to resolve complex problems in practice. In the example provided, the integrated framework focuses on the issue of record keeping and how this may be enhanced by following the ten steps. For instance, you become aware that your organisation is concerned about the standard of record keeping and it is their intention to use an evidence-based approach to developing quality standards. You have been co-opted onto the working group. You could utilise the ten-step guide in Figure 15.1 to assist you in changing the standard of record keeping for yourself and the organisation. So how will this happen?

Figure 15.1 has been adopted from the works of McSherry and Taylor (2003) and McSherry (1999, 2004) to illustrate how PD can support healthcare professionals to use an evidence-based approach to bring about change or resolve practical problems. This provides a simple ten-step guide integrating critical appraisal within the evidence-based practice, clinical governance and best value frameworks. The ten-step guide can be modified to accommodate the diversity of practice and change across and between teams, organisations and professional groups.

Step 1: Relevance

Establish whether there is a need to review the current standards of record keeping in practice. This can only be done by informing and involving staff about why the concern has come to light, for example information from possible risk management

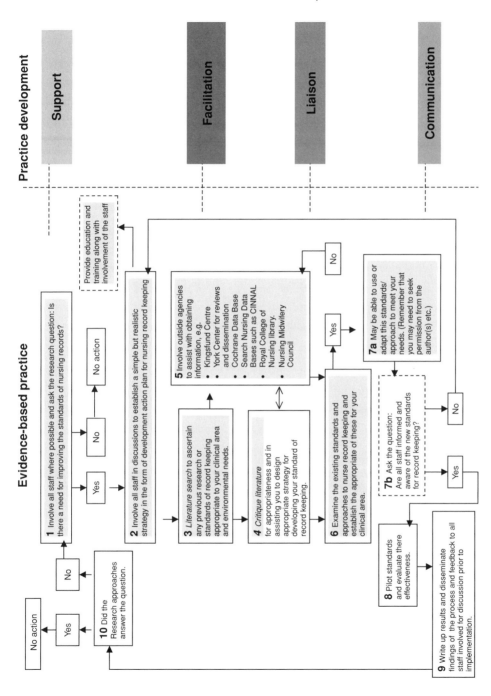

Figure 15.1 PD supporting advances and evaluations in practice.

data or complaints reporting. Time well spent at this stage in the process can lead to more effective use of time later in the process of change.

Step 2: Staff ownership

Encouraging participation can enable the development of a simple but reliable action plan that is shared, owned and most importantly agreed by all. For more information on effective action planning, see the work of O'Neal and Manley (2007). If the team or organisation are in favour and have a feeling of ownership for the proposed change or project, then the allocation of key roles and responsibilities within the process can be effectively shared.

Step 3: Literature searching

Ensure that you access all relevant literature by searching the various online databases, e.g. Cumulative Index to Nursing & Allied Health Literature (CINAHL), British Nursing Index, etc. There are several places that may be willing to offer support to aid you with improving the standards of record keeping such as your Clinical Governance Leads, Clinical Audit Department or by looking at the recommendations from your own professional bodies and departments of healthcare.

Step 4: Involve outside agencies

It is important to utilise internal and external sources of help:

> *Internally:*
> *Audit departments*
> Practice Development Centers/Departments
> Research and Development Departments
>
> *Externally:*
> *Evidence-Based Centers:*
> York Center for Reviews and Dissemination (http://www.york.ac.uk/inst/crd/crddatabases.htm; accessed 30/05/07)
> School of Health and Related Research (ScHARR) (http://www.shef.ac.uk/scharr; accessed 30/05/07)
> Joanna Briggs Institute (www.joannabriggs.edu.au; accessed 28/06/07)
>
> *Newsletters/Information:*
> Bandolier (http://www.jr2.ox.ac.uk/bandolier; accessed 30/05/07)

There are enormous sources of support, which can be easily found given the advances in information technology.

Step 5: Critiquing the literature

It is important to utilise an established approach to this part of the process such as using the frameworks offered by Crombie (1996) *The Pocket Guide to Critical Appraisal* or Greenhalgh (2006) *How to Read a Paper. The basics of Evidence-Based Medicine*. Information should be critiqued for its usefulness and effectiveness in meeting your unique set of practice needs.

Step 6: Examining existing standards

Examine the existing standards offered in the literature and associated evidence to identify which standards best meet your ward, team department or organisations needs. (Note that the emphasis should be on finding the best standards about record keeping but to remember that there may not be standards for some to use.)

Step 7: Putting the standards into practice

Having reviewed the existing standards you may be able to incorporate best practice guidelines into your practice without any or slight changes or slight modification. You must ensure that approval is obtained from author(s) and that you do not break copyright legislation by ensuring that permission is sought to use and modify work from the publishers. Following the examination of the information some practical considerations and questions need to be asked. In order to demonstrate the essence of this part of the process the example of record keeping will be utilised:

Why keep health records? Records form the basis for planning care and treatment, providing feedback on patient progress and in suggesting action for future work.

Are records a legal document? This is an essential issue and involves answering questions associated with what constitutes a legal document. Who should sign or write in the records and what should you do if you make a mistake in writing.

Types of records? It is essential to establish what constitutes a record and what will be evaluated. Records seem to be unlimited and varied making almost anything pertinent to the patients care.

How do you establish a standard of record that could be evaluated (audited)?

There are several written standards/guidelines available outlining ways of evaluating the standards of record keeping such as those advocated by professional bodies like the Nursing Midwifery Council or General Medical Council, the Health Professional Council, the National Institute of Clinical Studies (www.nhmrc.gov.au/nics/asp/index [accessed 29/06/2007]) or the Institute for Health Care Improvement (CBO).

Step 8: Pilot study

Test the effectiveness in practice via a pilot study. The pilot study will ensure that the standards are achievable and that the new initiative/innovation is practically suitable to your individuals, team, ward or department. The evaluation of set standards requires the devising of an auditing strategy and template so that the standards can be systematically audited.

Step 9: Sharing and dissemination

Communicate the information about best practice in order to ensure ongoing success. Once the audit is completed and after discussion with the team and/or organisations recommendations can be made with regard to the results and an action plan developed to implement improvements.

Step 10: Evaluation

Evaluation of the new way of working will identify how successful implementing the evidence into practice has been.

The above example highlights how evidence-based practice can be utilised within the context of a clinical governance and best value framework. Figure 15.1 shows how the research-based process provides a flexible and systematic framework directed towards improving the quality of care and services. The ten-step guide encourages an evidence-based approach by engaging professionals in the processes and, consequently, developing their skills in gathering and appraising the evidence. Furthermore, it encourages an evaluative culture by exploring the efficiency and effectiveness of interventions through audit, benchmarking or by applying evaluative approaches. PD plays a pivotal role in enabling evidence-based practice to happen because it is about facilitating, supporting, liaising and communicating with individuals, teams and/or organisations in order to maximise the best from a given situation. PD used in this way is about encouraging individuals and organisations to focus their attention on ongoing issues such as reducing risks, enhancing quality by engaging with the evidence base. This holistic approach to facilitating change is important in order to avoid misunderstandings, missed opportunities and investment in practice. PD supports the facilitation of evidence-based practice by encouraging professional to become research aware that is having the knowledge, understanding skills, confidence and support to retrieve, appraise, apply and evaluate the effectiveness of evidence (McSherry et al., 2006). However, it is important to emphasise that evidence-based practice requires time, funding and access to information technology and most importantly education and training. Furthermore, PD is about promoting a culture of evidence-based practice by involving the patients, carers and/or significant others, what we would term the 'Very Important P's': patient, public and/or people. Having identified how PD can facilitate an evidence-based practice approach within the context of clinical governance the section offers an alternative approach using the PARIHS framework.

Applying the PARIHS framework

Research exploring the reasons why practitioners might not use research in practice has focused on the individual level of the practitioner and barriers to utilisation (Coopmans, 2006). Getting research in practice requires more than focusing on the individual professionals. Practitioners cannot be isolated from the context they are working in. From analyses of several research projects, it appeared that a number of factors are key in the successful implementation of research into practice (Rycroft-Malone, 2004). The PARIHS framework acknowledges the complexity of implementation. The development of the PARIHS framework was based on experiences from PD, quality improvement and research projects (Rycroft-Malone, 2004). At the Knowledge Centre for Evidence Based Practice in the Netherlands several PD projects are using the PARIHS framework as an implementation framework. In this section, examples are used from projects in mental health and acute care settings. These include developing and implementing an evidence-based protocol on peripheral infusion in a cardiology unit and using an action research study to implement evidence-based practice in a mental healthcare organisation.

Using the PARIHS framework increases the success of implementing evidence and guides the generation of new evidence for several reasons:

– The framework is a means to consider and present the many factors influencing the uptake of evidence into practice.
– In addition, it gives an indication what factors need more attention in using evidence in practice: Are professionals sufficiently facilitated in using evidence, what kind of facilitation do they need?

The PARIHS framework consists of three elements. As far as it is known each element has equal value in successful implementation of changes in practice: evidence, context and facilitation. These three elements are placed on a continuum from low to high contributing to the success of implementation.

Evidence

Evidence refers to four sources of knowledge namely scientific evidence, professional craft knowledge or clinical expertise, patient experiences and local knowledge such as audit information.

Mental Health Care Project (MHC-project)

In a mental healthcare organisation EBP is implemented in a setting with psychotic patients. Different sources of evidence are used in this project. Clients are involved in choosing issues relevant to them. From their stories three issues were derived namely experiencing auditory hallucinations, anxiety and loneliness. Nurses confirmed that there were discrepancies between the nursing care offered and what was needed with regard to these issues. These became the focus of the project following agreement by the clients and the nurses.

The first step in involving nurses and clients in the project then was valuing evidence from clients and nurses.

The baseline for evidence-based practice was assessed by using the RICH tool (Fox & Feasy, 2001). This tool enables the research culture of the workplace to be established through a benchmarking process.

Acute Care project (AC-project)

Baseline measurement was developed, undertaken and then re-measured at 6 weeks for patients with peripheral infusion. The measurement was based on a valid instrument available in the literature, the peripheral intravascular device (Joanna

Briggs Institute for Evidence Based Nursing, 1998). The results of the baseline measurement made clear that the prevalence of phlebitis was according to the nurses, even more than expected. This unexpected high prevalence raised the awareness of nurses.

Nurses on the ward developed a new protocol based on the available evidence, professional expertise and research evidence.

From the MHC-project and AC-project it became clear that local knowledge was limited. No systematic evaluations related to the nursing care had previously taken place at either site.

Context

In the PARIHS framework, context refers to the environment or setting in which the care is delivered. An environment that is open to innovation supports the suggested changes. In the PARIHS framework, the following contextual factors are relevant: leadership, culture and evaluation.

Leadership varies on a continuum from low, meaning transactional leadership, to high, transformational leadership, which is perceived as influential in the context of evidence implementation. Transformational leaders are able to transform cultures, recognise everybody as a leader of something, inspire staff to have a shared vision Manley (2004).

MHC-project

Although the nurses were facilitated in time by their managers they still experienced insufficient time to work on the project. The managers had a different perception of the available time. This difference in perception hindered the work of the nurses for the project. The lead researcher enabled the two parties to come together to make the difference in perceptions of available time explicit.

AC-project

The manager of the ward expressed his support for the project to the ward nurses and also to others across the hospital including the hospital board.

Evidence of the project's success and a culture open to new developments resulted in the opening of a second care innovation unit in the same hospital as well as continuation of the first.

Manley (2004) after Drennan (1992) defines culture as the 'way things are done around here'. A culture at the right end of the continuum is a culture in which among other attributes, individual staff and clients are valued and learning is promoted. Towards the left end of the continuum cultures become less clear about their values and beliefs and become more task driven (Table 15.2).

Table 15.2 Key elements for implementing evidence into practice

Elements		Criteria
Evidence	Research	Well conceived, designed and executed research
		Seen as one part of a decision
		Valued as evidence
		Lack of certainty acknowledged
		Social construction acknowledged
		Judged as relevant
		Importance weighted
		Conclusions drawn
	Clinical experience	Clinical experience and expertise reflected upon, tested by individuals and groups
		Consensus within similar groups
		Valued as evidence
		Seen as one part of the decision
		Judged as relevant
		Importance weighted
		Conclusions drawn
	Patient experience	Valued as evidence
		Multiple biographies used
		Partnerships with health care professionals
		Seen as one part of a decision
		Judged as relevant
		Importance weighted
		Conclusions drawn
	Information from the local context	Valued as evidence
		Collected and analyzed systematically and rigorously
		Evaluated and reflected upon
		Conclusions drawn
Context	Receptive context	Physical, Social, Cultural, Structural, System, Professional/social networks } boundaries clearly defined and acknowledged
		Appropriate & transparent decision making processes
		Power and authority processes
		Resources – human, financial, equipment – allocated and Information and feedback
		Initiative fits with strategic goals and is a key practice/patient issue
		Receptiveness to change

(cont.)

Table 15.2 *(cont.)*

Elements		Criteria
	Culture	Able to define culture(s) in terms of prevailing values/beliefs Values individual staff and clients Promotes leaning organization Consistency of individuals role/experience to value – relationship with others – teamwork – power and authority – rewards/recognition
	Leadership	Transformational leadership Role clarity Effective teamwork Effective organizational structures Democratic inclusive decision making processes Enabling/empowering approach to teaching/ learning/managing
	Evaluation	Feedback on – individual – team } Performance – system Use of multiple sources of information on performance Use of multiple methods: – Clinical – Performance – Economic } Evaluations – Experience

Facilitation	Purpose	Task	Holistic
	Role	Doing for others – Episodic contact – Practical/technical help – Didactic, traditional approach to teaching – External agents – Low intensity – extensive coverage	Enabling others – Sustained partnership – Developmental – Adult learning approach to teaching – Internal/external agents – High intensity – limited coverage
	Skills and attributes	Task/doing for others – Project management skills – Technical skills – Marketing skills – Subject/technical/ clinical credibility	Holistic/enabling – Co-counselling – Critical reflection – Giving meaning – Flexibility of role – Realness/authenticity

Source: Rycroft-Malone et al., 2004a.

AC-project

> A protocol was developed and used within this project and there was evidence that the incidence of phlebitis decreased. Despite these positive results it appeared to be difficult to get this protocol implemented in the hospital. Several groups such as the quality assurance team had to be involved to get this new protocol implemented throughout the hospital.

Evaluation generates evidence on which to base practice. Professionals used to evaluating their work are more open to changes when these changes improve the care they provide. Evaluation within PD needs to reflect the complexity of the context and the multiple realities of the stakeholders. PD tools such as a *Claims Concerns and Issues* (CCI) exercise generates and values evidence from all stakeholders (Titchen & Manley, 2006).

MHC-project

> On a regular basis the progress and preliminary results of the mental healthcare project were presented by the researcher and the nurses to other staff members and the clients involved. Nurses were asked to reflect on the results; they supported the conclusions presented and agreed on actions to be taken.

AC-project

> The main researcher invited nurses from the ward to present the results in national journals and at international conferences. By inviting them the researcher acknowledges their work and expertise.
>
> Throughout the project evidence was gathered from the staff and the manager by using the CCI exercise. These claims, concerns and issues guided the project's focus and action plan.

Facilitation

Facilitation refers to the enablement of others to make things work. Facilitation helps practitioners and practice teams to overcome personal barriers and also barriers in the context that prevent the delivery of evidence-based and person-centred care. The continuum suggests that facilitation (Table 15.2) varies from 'doing for' to a more holistic way of facilitation, enabling others. Matching the purpose, role and skills to the needs of the situation seems to be essential for 'appropriate' facilitation (Rycroft-Malone, 2004).

MHC-project

> Nurses interested in the project were involved in searching for research evidence. They had never been to the library in their organisation. This activity took a lot of time and nurses were disappointed that they didn't find a huge amount of evidence. The researcher facilitated the nurses in appraising the discovered articles systematically and critically.

> The nurses started using an assessment instrument (Haddock, 1994) on hallucinations, which they found in the literature and checked with the other nurses whether this was a suitable instrument to use.

The PARIHS framework could be used as an assessment instrument to assess the most appropriate way to facilitate based on the available evidence and the prevailing context.

MHC-project

> The intention of the researcher was to facilitate the nurses in an emancipatory way, which means not 'doing for' them but enabling them 'to do' themselves. The researcher noticed that this did not work because of the limited opportunities for the nurses to work together with the researcher.
>
> It became increasingly clear during the research that a linear implementation model would not work because there where too many contextual factors influencing the implementation. Even when taking a less linear approach there were factors that influenced the implementation either negatively or positively.
>
> The question remains, how far can a researcher's facilitation influence an implementation study?

AC-project

> Although the second post-measurement initiative of the nurses supported the impression that there was a change in attitude towards using evidence in their own practice, there was an increase in the prevalence of phlebitis. A possible explanation for this is that facilitation was decreased in the period before the second post-measurement.

Taking the two frameworks into account, it is evident that both examples offer sound advice and guidance for advancing and evaluating practice at an individual, team and organisational level. Yet, the reality of sustained change happening is dependent on supporting practice developers themselves. So what and who are practice developers?

Practice developers

According to McCormack and Garbett (2003) and McSherry and Driscoll (2004) the characteristics and qualities of practice developers are about encouraging and motivating staff to innovate or evaluate practices regardless of size of the project in the quest for improved quality. Successful PD is dependent upon encouraging and supporting individuals to develop certain essential qualities and attributes (Table 15.3) so that they can advance and/or evaluate practice as part of the change process.

Table 15.3 Key qualities and attributes associated with practice development

Essential qualities	Individual personal attributes
Commitment	Motivate
Respect	Facilitate
Experience	Innovate
Approachable	Inform
An agent of change	Encourage
Supportive	Support
Good listener	

NB: This is not an exhaustive list and the points are not in any order of priority. For more information, see McCormack and Garbett (2003).

For some healthcare organisations PD facilitators, advisors or developers are available to support and facilitate change. However, for other organisations this is not the case, placing pressure on individuals and teams to take responsibility for advancing and evaluating their own or team's practice as part of ever-changing agenda without dedicated support. The introduction of named 'practice developers' is essential if healthcare organisations and teams are to modernise within busy, stressful and time-pressured practice areas. Several models have been reported and commented upon, which could be used as exemplars in developing these posts further within the NHS (Glover, 2002). It is also worth considering the importance of ensuring that the introduction of new PD positions is not tied in with other aspects of the governance agenda because this makes the posts too big and difficult to operationalise successfully (Garbett & McCormack, 2001).

To meet modernisation agendas it could be easy to say that all healthcare professionals have or should possess the qualities and attributes outlined in Table 15.3. Manley and Webster (2007) build on the work of McCormack et al. (2002) by offering more information about factors that enable the PD to be taken forward. However, within PD these factors become even more profound when facilitating the development and evaluation of new or existing ways of working. The individuals, team and organisation require commitment and often leadership and facilitation; a commitment to harnessing and maintaining colleague(s) enthusiasm to tackle the issues akin to advancing practice. Listening, empowering, valuing and involving the respective colleagues/users with the innovation can enhance changes in practice. This approach to PD affords respect from the facilitator to their colleagues, an essential skill that is often negated by conflicts within PD. Successful changes through initiatives depend upon the experience and approachability of the facilitator in encouraging, supporting, and where applicable, resourcing innovations in practice. The notion of the facilitator becoming a *change agent* can provide an objective, non-judgmental and open, honest approach to PD.

Successful PD from our experiences requires the utilisation and integration of the individual personal attributes with these essential skills. Thus facilitation and empowerment of individuals, teams and organisations, are based upon promoting teamwork and multi-professional collaboration via effective communication. The challenge for some professionals working in practice with or without a remit for PD is in identifying and prioritising their own individual and professional requirements and the support needed to facilitate and manage change and develop their own continued professional development and support networks.

Conclusions

Getting evidence into practice is difficult and challenging yet the potential of PD in supporting the generation of research and utilisation of evidence for individuals, teams and organisations remains untapped. PD is about facilitating individuals, teams and organisations with the development of strategies in using and generating evidence in and from practice. PD is both an efficient and effective way of supporting the use of evidence in practice because of its facilitative and systematic approach to the promotion of innovation and change. Within the context of getting evidence into practice, PD offers a coordinated approach at an individual and organisational level in both the generation and utilisation of evidence.

At an individual level, it is about improving reflexivity skills either through direct or indirect facilitation, for example by the use of action learning sets so that practice can be reviewed and evaluated. Furthermore, it is important that individuals are encouraged and supported to develop critical appraisal skills in order to regard research and evidence as an ally and not a threat. Both individuals and organisations have a duty and responsibility to develop a sound research awareness, which can be harnessed through role development or facilitation by collaborating with those in research roles in practice like the lecturer practitioner or involving students on bachelor/masters programmes for feedback.

Organisationally, it is about learning from lessons or targeting specific patient problems/needs so that practice can be reviewed and advanced. It is about acknowledging the work of the practitioner in projects/celebrating successes/showing effectiveness or change and dissemination results in order to create the 'ripple effect' for change by spreading the news both good and bad. The two frameworks provided demonstrate how PD is facilitating evidence-based practice at an international level in the United Kingdom and Netherlands, which should continue to do so in the future.

References

American Nurses Association (2002) *Code of Ethics for Nurses with Interpretive Statements*. American Nurses Publishing, Silver Spring, MD.

Australian Nursing and Midwifery Council (2003) *Code of Professional Conduct for Nurses in Australia*. ANMC, Australia.

Bassett, C. (1996) The sky's the limit. *Nursing Standard*. **10**(25), 16–19.

Clarke, C.L., Reed, J., Wainwright, D., McClelland, S., Swallow, V., Harden, J., Walton, G. & Walsh, A. (2004) The discipline of improvement: Something old, something new? *Journal of Nursing Management.* **12**(2), 85–96.

Cochrane, A. (1979) *Effectiveness and Efficiency Random Reflections on the Health Service.* Nuffield Provisional Hospital Trust, Leeds.

Coopmans, J. (2006) De betrouwbaarheid, validiteit en hanteerbaarheid van de Nederlandse versie van de Barriers scale. Master Thesis, Universiteit Maastricht.

Crombie, I. (1996) *The Pocket Guide to Critical Appraisal.* BMJ, London.

Department of Health (2005) *Creating a Patient-Led NHS: Delivering the NHS Improvement Plan.* DoH, London.

DiCenso, A., Cullum, N. & Ciliska, D. (1998) Implementation forum. Implementing evidence-based nursing: Some misconceptions. *Evidence-Based Nursing.* **1**(2), 38–40.

Drennan, D. (1992) *Transforming Company Culture.* McGraw-Hill, London.

Ferguson, L. & Day, R.A. (2005) Evidence-based nursing education: Myth or reality? *Journal of Nursing Education.* **44**(3), 107–115.

Fox, C. & Feasy, S. (2001) *Evidence based care benchmark.* The RCN Research in Child Health group, RCN, London.

French, P. (1999) The development of evidence-based nursing. *Journal of Advanced Nursing.* **29**(1), 72–78.

Funk, S.G., Champagne, M.T., Wiese, R.A. & Torquist, E.M. (1991) Barriers to using research findings in practice: The clinicians perspective. *Applied Nursing Research.* **4**(2), 90–95.

Garbett, R. & McCormack, B. (2001) The experience of practice development: An exploratory telephone interview study. *Journal of Clinical Nursing.* **10**(1), 94–2001.

General Medical Council (2001) *Good Medical Practice.* GMC, London.

Glover, D. (2002) What is practice development. In: *Practice Development in the Clinical Setting: A Guide to Implementation* (eds R. McSherry & C. Bassett). Nelson Thornes, Cheltenham.

Greenhalgh, T. (2006) *How to Read a Paper. The Basics of Evidence-Based Medicine.* Blackwell, Oxford.

Haddock, G. (1994) Auditory Hallucination Rating Scale, University of Manchester. Translated and validated by Valmaggia, L.R. (1998), Psychosencluster, APZ-Drenthe, Assen, The Netherlands.

Harvey, G., Loftus-Hill, A., Rycroft-Malone, J., Titchen, A., Kitson, A., McCormack, B. & Seers, K. (2002) Getting evidence into practice: The role and function of facilitation. *Journal of Advanced Nursing.* **37**(6), 577–588.

Health Professional Council (2003) *Standards of Conduct, Performance and Ethics. Your Duties as a Registrant 2003.* HPC, London.

Hogan, D. & Logan, J. (2004) The Ottawa model of research use: A guide to clinical innovation in the NICU. *Clinical Nurse Specialist.* **18**(5), 255–261.

Holleman, G. & Vis, J. (2006) Implementeren binnen de Verpleging & Verzorging: Feit of fictie? *Kwaliteit in Beeld.* (2), 12–13.

Ingersoll, G.L. (2000) Evidence-based nursing: What it is and what it isn't. *Nursing Outlook.* **48**(4), 151–152.

Joanna Briggs Institute for Evidence Based Nursing (1998) *Peripheral Intravascular Device Survey.* Adelaide, Australia.

Kitson, A. (1994) *Clinical Nursing Practice Development and Research Activity in the Oxford Region*. Centre for Practice Development and Research, National Institute for Nursing, Oxford.

Kitson, A.L., Ahmed, L.B., Harvey, G., Seers, K. & Thompson, D. (1996) From research to practice: One organisational model for promoting research-based practice. *Journal of Advanced Nursing*. **23**(3), 430–440.

Mallett, J., Cathmoir, D., Hughes, P. & Whitby, E. (1997) Forging new roles: professional and practice development. *Nursing Times*. **93**(18), 38–39.

Manley, K. (2004) Transformational culture; a culture of effectiveness. In: *Practice Development in Nursing* (eds B. McCormack, K. Manley & R. Garbett), pp. 51–82. Blackwell Publishing, Oxford.

Manley, K. & Webster, J. (2006) Can we keep quality alive? *Nursing Standard* Sept 27th **21**(3), 12–15.

McCormack, B., Dewar, B., Wright, J., Garbett, R., Harvey, G. & Ballantine, K. (2006) A *Realist Synthesis of Evidence Relating to Practice Development: Executive Summary*. NHS Quality Improvement Scotland and NHS Education for Scotland, Scotland.

McCormack, B. & Garbett, R. (2003) The characteristics, qualities and skills of practice developers. *Journal of Clinical Nursing*. **12**(3), 317–325.

McCormack, B., Kitson, A., Harvey, G., Rycroft-Malone, J., Titchen, A. & Seers, K. (2002) Getting evidence into practice: The meaning of 'context'. *Journal of Advanced Nursing*. **38**(1), 94–104.

McCormack, B., Manley, K., Kitson, A., Titchen, A. & Harvey, G. (1999) Towards practice development – a vision in reality or reality without vision. *Journal of Nursing Management*. **7**(5), 255–264.

McPheeters, M. & Lohr, K.N. (1999) Evidence-based practice and nursing: Commentary. *Outcomes Management for Nursing Practice*. **3**(3), 99–101.

McSherry, R. (1999) Clinical governance: Practice and professional development. *Health Care Risk Report*. **6**(1), 21–22.

McSherry, R. (2004) Practice development and. health care governance: A recipe for modernization. *Journal of Nursing Management*. **12**(2), 137–146.

McSherry, R., Artley, A. & Holloran, J. (2006) Research awareness: An important factor for evidence-based practice? *Worldviews on Evidence-Based Nursing*. **3**(3), 103–115.

McSherry, R. & Driscoll, J. (2004) Practice development: Promoting quality improvement in orthopaedic care ... as well as one's self. *Journal of Orthopaedic Nursing*. **8**(3), 171–178.

McSherry, R. & Pearce, P. (2007) *Clinical Governance. A Guide to Implementation for Health Care Professionals*, 2nd edn. Blackwell Science, Oxford.

McSherry, R., Simmons, M. & Abbott, P. (eds) (2001) *Evidence-Informed Nursing A Guide for Clinical Nurses*. Routledge, London.

McSherry, R. & Taylor, S. (2003) Developing best practice. In: *Clinical Governance and Best Value: Meeting The Modernisation Agenda* (eds S. Pickering & J. Thompson). Churchill Livingston, London.

McSherry, R. & Warr, J. (2006) Practice development: Confirming the existence of a knowledge and evidence base. *Practice Development in Health Care*. **5**(2), 55–79.

Ministerie van Volksgezondheid, Welzijn en Sport (2006) Maatschappelijke Opgaven Volksgezondheid en Gezondheidszorg. Den Haag, Ministerie van VWS.

Mohide, E.A. & King, B. (2003) Implementation forum. Building a foundation for evidence-based practice: Experiences in a tertiary hospital. *Evidence-Based Nursing.* **6**(4), 100–103.

Muir-Gray, J.A. (1997) *Evidence-Based Healthcare: How to make Health Policy and Management Decisions.* Churchill Livingston, London.

Newhouse, R., Dearholt, S.M.S., Poe, S., Pugh, L.C. & White, K.M. (2005) Evidence-based practice: A practical approach to implementation. *Journal of Nursing Administration.* **35**(1), 35–40.

Nursing and Midwifery Council (2004) *The NMC Code of Professional Conduct, Standards for Conduct, Performance and Ethics.* NMC, London.

O'Neal, H. & Manley, K. (2007) Action planning: Making your changes happen in clinical practice. *Nursing Standard.* **21**(35), 35–39.

Page, S. & Hammer, S. (2002) Practice development – time to realize the potential. *Practice Development in Health Care.* **1**(1), 2–17.

Pickering, S. & Thompson, J. (eds) (2003) *Clinical Governance and Best Value Meeting The Modernisation Agenda.* Churchill Livingstone, London.

Rosenberg, W. & Donaldson, A. (1995) Evidence-based medicine: An approach to problem solving. *British Medical Journal.* **310**, 1112–1126.

Rosswurm, A.M. & Larrabee, H.J. (1999) A model for change to evidence-based practice. *Journal of Nursing Scholarship.* **31**(4), 317–322.

Rycroft-Malone, J. (2004) PARIHS framework. In: *Practice Development in Nursing* (eds B. McCormack, K. Manley & R. Garbett). Blackwell, Oxford.

Rycroft-Malone, J., Harvey, G., Seers, K., Kitson, A. & McCormack, B. (2004a) An exploration of factors that influence the implementation of evidence into practice. *Journal of Clinical Nursing.* **13**, 913–924.

Rycroft-Malone, J., Kitson, A., Harvey, G., McCormack, B., Seers, K., Titchen, A. & Estabrooks, C. (2002) Ingredients for change: Revisiting a conceptual framework. *Quality and Safety in Health Care.* **11**, 174–180. (www.qualityhealthcare.com)

Rycroft-Malone, J., Seers, K., Titchen, A., Harvey, G.B., Kitson, A. & McCormack, B. (2004b) What counts as evidence in evidence-based practice? *Journal of Advanced Nursing.* **47**(10), 81–90.

Sackett, D.L., Rosenberg, W.M., Gray, J.A.M., Hayes, B.R. & Richardson, W.S. (1997) Evidence-based medicine: What it is and what it isn't. *British Medical Journal.* **312**, 71–72.

Snares, D. & Heliker, D. (2002) Implementation of an evidence-based nursing practice model: Disciplined clinical inquiry. *Journal for Nurses in Staff Development.* **18**(5), 233–238.

Simmons, M. (2004) Facilitation of practice development: A concept analysis. *Practice Development in Health Care.* **3**(1), 36–52.

Stetler, C.B. (1994) Stetler model of research utilisation. *Journal of Nurse Administration.* **28**(7), 45–53.

Taylor, C.M. (1997) What is evidence-based Practice. *British Journal of Occupational Therapy.* **60**(11), 470–474.

Thompson, C. (1999) A conceptual treadmill: The need for 'middle ground' in clinical decision making theory in nursing. *Journal of Advanced Nursing.* **30**(5), 1222–1229.

Thompson, C. (2003) Finding, appraising and using research evidence in practice. In: *Clinical Governance and Best Value Meeting The Modernisation Agenda* (eds S. Pickering & J. Thompson). Churchill Livingstone, London.

Titchen, A. & Manley, K. (2006) Spiralling towards transformational action research: Philosophical and practical journeys. *Educational Action Research.* **14**(3), 333–356.

Wallace, M., Shorten, A. & Russell, K. (1997) Paving the way: Stepping stones to evidence-based nursing. *International Journal of Nursing Practice.* **3**(3), 147–152.

Wallin, L., Bostrom, A.M., Wikblad, K. & Ewald, U. (2003) Sustainability in changing clinical practice promotes evidence-based nursing care. *Journal of Advanced Nursing.* **41**(5), 509–518.

Ward, M.F., Titchen, A., Morrell, C., McCormack, B. & Kitson, A. (1998) Using a supervisory framework to support and evaluate a multiproject practice development programme. *Journal of Clinical Nursing.* **7**(1), 29–36.

16. *Using Practice Development Approaches in the Development of a Managed Clinical Network*

Liz Henderson and Sandra McKillop

Introduction

A managed clinical network (MCN) is the mechanism to bring the commissioners, planners and providers of care together with service users to work collaboratively to improve the quality and effectiveness of the service. The Northern Ireland Cancer Network (NICaN) is the first regional MCN in Northern Ireland. Its aim is to continuously improve the quality of cancer care and cancer survival for the people of Northern Ireland through the provision of equitable, patient focused and clinically effective cancer services.

This chapter provides a description of how established practice development (PD) methods were used by the network's multiprofessional team to develop cancer services across the region. Given the complexity, breadth and depth of an MCN, which typically crosses geographical, organisational and professional boundaries, the PD methods discussed are in the context of leading wide-scale change at strategic, organisational and clinical levels.

As an experienced practice developer, the Lead Nurse on the team drew on PD methodology to frame and critique her own understanding with respect to the strategic development of the network. Through this lens, she then contributed to the team debate and, when relevant, made explicit the links between actions proposed and the theory underpinning her proposal. In this chapter, the team critically reflect on some of the processes used in developing the network and explicitly link these to a PD conceptual framework. The key learning is identified, illustrating the team's growing awareness of PD as a methodology with relevance to achieving sustainable cultural change, and the development of person-centred services.

The final section compares and contrasts PD and service improvement (SI), the latter being the approach typically associated with the development of MCNs. The discussion presents an analysis of the two approaches and the applicability, and added value they provide when working to effect large-scale complex changes. It presents the argument that both SI and PD approaches are needed to achieve sustainable improvement across an MCN.

Given that networks as an organisational concept are to become a main form of health service organisation, this chapter may be of interest to those involved in policy development, MCN development, or to those interested in SI and PD approaches.

Background

What is a managed clinical network?

There is growing interest worldwide, within and outside the healthcare environment, in networks as an organisational concept. This is based on the recognition, amongst other things, that the problems we face are interconnected and, increasingly, beyond the capacity of single organisations to address.

The concept of network in health service was first aired in Scotland in *The Acute Services Review* (SE, 1999) and was defined as '[l]inked groups of healthcare professionals and organisations from primary, secondary and tertiary care, working in a coordinated manner, unconstrained by existing professional and organisational boundaries, to ensure equitable provision of high quality, clinically effective services'. At present, care is perceived broadly within separate professions and organisations. It is over and through this obstacle course that patients make their 'cancer journey'. The main aim of a managed clinical network is the provision of seamless, managed care that is founded upon standards and evidence-based 'best practice' care pathways (Figure 16.1).

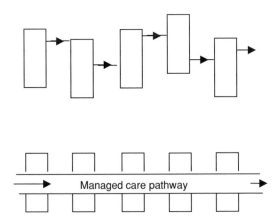

Figure 16.1   Fragmented to managed care pathways.

The concept of a network is not new to the health service. Both managers and clinicians would see themselves as part of various informal networks. The development, however, of MCNs as a way of planning and delivering services in the health service is growing. A statement that a network is proposed is insufficient to guarantee its effectiveness. As in Scotland (SE, 1999), and more recently in Northern Ireland (NICaN, 2005a), MCNs need to be underpinned by sound principles such as clarity about the management arrangements; multidisciplinary and multiprofessional approach, service user representation, evidence-based practice, clinical audit, training and effective clinical and social care governance.

In considering the impact and positive benefits of MCNs to date, there are indications that they improve the patient's journey, engage clinicians and reduce inequalities in care (NHS Confederation, 2002; Edwards & Fraser, 2001; NAO, 2005).

What is the Northern Ireland Cancer Network?

The development of a MCN for cancer services in Northern Ireland emanated from the considerable work progressed under the Campbell Commissioning Project. Established by the four Health and Social Service Boards in 1998, the project was tasked with taking forward the recommendations of the report *Cancer Services: Investing in the Future* (DHSS, 1996), commonly referred to as *The Campbell Report*.

Amongst others the recommendations included the following: creating five cancer units, building a new cancer centre on an acute hospital site; developing multiprofessional specialist cancer teams at the centre and units; and progressing clinical trials. Having largely fulfilled its remit in 2002, the project board considered the most appropriate arrangements to take forward this work. There was a genuine desire to ensure that the highest quality of cancer care was available to the people of Northern Ireland and to further encourage multidisciplinary working and a regional approach to service planning. Having explored a number of available options, it was recommended that an MCN be established for cancer services.

In addition to the above ambition, other drivers for establishing the Cancer Network include the prevalence of the disease, increased incidence, complexity of treatment, increased expectation from the public and the scale of resources required to deliver the service.

The establishment of the Cancer Network in Northern Ireland has been generally received with support and enthusiasm. There is a great spirit of determination to provide a regional improvement in cancer services.

How the Cancer Network gets its work done

NICaN board

The NICaN board oversees the development of the Cancer Network. The inaugural meeting was held in February 2004. The purpose of the board is to provide strategic direction for the network and support continuous improvement in the quality and coordination of cancer services. Board members consist of Chief Executives or their representatives of the commissioners and providers, primary care and patient perspectives, the Department of Health and Social Services and Public

Safety (DHSSPS), Macmillan Cancer Support (as funder) and the lead members of the network team.

Network team

A small core team facilitates the development of the Cancer Network. Appointments were made from end 2003 and initially included three clinical leads each seconded 2 days to the network, namely Network Lead GP (Dermott, a practicing General Practitioner), Network Lead Clinician (Gerard, a practicing Consultant Respiratory Physician), Network Lead Nurse (Liz, also Lead Cancer Nurse at the Northern Ireland Cancer Centre), a full time Network Manager (Sandra), Network Administrator (Lisa) and Administrative Assistant. In response to identified priorities, additional funding was sought and appointments made, which included a part-time Supportive and Palliative Care Regional Coordinator (Lorna), and a Patient and Public Involvement Coordinator (Janis). The team explicitly links and includes relevant regional post holders, for example Regional Coordinator Cancer Services Pharmacist (Fionnuala and Maire).

Tumour and theme clinical networks

The work of the Cancer Network is being progressed by supporting 'groups' of health professionals, patients and voluntary sector representatives to work together in a coordinated way across geographical, organisational and professional boundaries.

These 'groups' or 'clinical networks' are responsible for the development of regional standards, audit, patient pathways, service redesign, quality assurance and the identification of funding priorities. They are the principal source of advice to planners, commissioners and providers of services to indicate the service reconfiguration and resource implications required to achieve the highest quality care. There are both 'tumour-specific groups' and 'theme groups' (Figure 16.2).

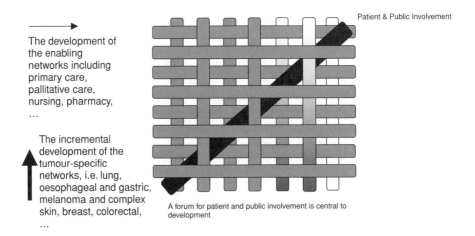

The development of the enabling networks including primary care, pallitative care, nursing, pharmacy, ...

The incremental development of the tumour-specific networks, i.e. lung, oesophageal and gastric, melanoma and complex skin, breast, colorectal, ...

Patient & Public Involvement

A forum for patient and public involvement is central to development

Figure 16.2 The matrix of tumour and theme clinical networks.

Working collaboratively, they are taking forward a programme to ensure a high-quality, equitable cancer service across the region for patients, carers and their families.

Across the Cancer Network there are a number of *local lead cancer teams* with responsibility for the coordination, planning, management and development of services in line with regionally agreed standards and guidelines.

Practice development approaches in an MCN

PD is a well-established movement in UK healthcare and increasingly is becoming an international movement (McCormack & Titchen, 2006). It is concerned with creating transformational cultures of effectiveness in order to deliver person-centred, evidence-based healthcare.

As Lead Nurse for Cancer Services, both at a local and at regional level, I (Liz) have a particular interest in improving the quality of care for people affected by cancer, by enabling practitioners to realise their potential and to develop a person-centred approach to practice. So although not in a named PD role, I view PD as being integral to how I work.

The worldview of PD that informs my practice is emancipatory PD (EPD) underpinned by critical social science, as outlined by Manley and McCormack (2003). A concept analysis of PD undertaken by Garbett and McCormack (2002) forms the basis for what is now a widely accepted definition of PD:

- PD is a continuous process of improvement towards increased effectiveness in patient-centred care.
- This is brought about by helping healthcare teams to develop their knowledge and skills and to transform the culture and context of care.
- It is enabled and supported by facilitators committed to systematic, rigorous processes of emancipatory change that reflect the perspectives of service users (Garbett & McCormack, 2002, p. 88).

My interest in EPD as a methodology for individual growth and sustainable practice change has developed over these past few years, beginning with the International PD Collaborative (IPDC) Practice Development School, and further strengthened as a participant on a 2-year PD programme. Subsequent to this I undertook a facilitation e-learning course (http://campusone.ulster.ac.uk), completed the RCN facilitation accreditation scheme (http://www.rcn.org.uk/resources/practicedeveloment/about-pd/processes/facilitation/) and gained further experience by facilitating a number of PD programmes.

However, each of these experiences was uni-disciplinary in nature with participants from a nursing background who worked at clinical or organisational levels. The complexities of developing a regional MCN, with a wide range of disciplines working at all levels and across various settings, each with its unique culture, therefore posed a significant challenge. I decided that I would continue to use my knowledge and experience of PD and of the underpinning critical social science (Fay, 1987) in the following ways:

- Given my responsibility to contribute to network development I would use PD to frame and critique my own understanding and to determine actions or responses needed.
- Given the team's responsibility to develop the network I would contribute to team discussions from this perspective and be deliberate in my intent of raising the team's awareness of PD as a methodology with relevance to the development of the Cancer Network.

The team reflection

For the purpose of this chapter, we engaged in a team reflection around the question 'what processes have we used that have enabled the development of the network?' The initial question considered was 'how have we used PD in developing the network?' But given that the team were not overly familiar with PD methodology or always aware of an explicit PD link in relation to some of the methods, the broader question was more appropriate. I noted down the responses gleaned, subsequently read and re-read the notes to identify the processes used, which are established PD methods. In doing so, clusters emerged around five key areas (Figure 16.3).

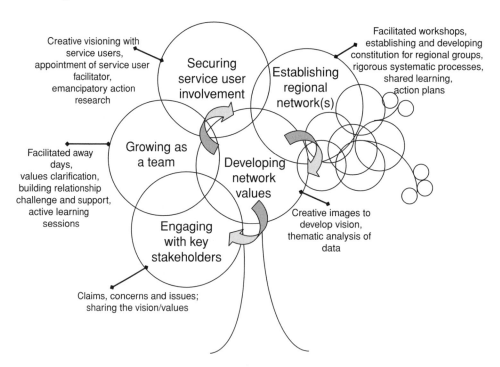

Figure 16.3 Using PD approaches in the growth of an MCN.

The clusters are depicted as a series of cycles forming a growing tree, with the identified PD processes located beside each cycle. The arrows indicate a flowing movement between the development cycles, since each cycle overlaps with and blends into the other cycles to indicate the integrated nature of the work. The metaphor of a tree is apt in describing the network, since although starting small, it continues to grow, for example, with increasing numbers of tumour-specific and enabling network groups being established (as depicted by the increasing number of smaller cycles).

In the following section, for each of the five circles we

1. briefly describe the PD processes used,
2. undertake a team reflection and
3. identify the team's key learning.

Developing network values
Practice development processes

The inaugural residential board meeting was held in February 2004. The purpose of the meeting was to prompt discussion around the principles for MCNs, invite members to engage in an exercise to outline the vision and values of the Cancer Network and outline a work programme for the first year.

The team had agreed at our planning day to try a creative approach to developing a vision for the network. Board members were invited to select two or three images from a pack of professional photographs, which helped to encapsulate their vision for cancer services in Northern Ireland. It was evident from the metaphors used, and how members expressed themselves, that core values were being tapped into. The rich dialogue generated at each table was recorded in note form by the team members and subsequently subjected to thematic analysis. Notes of the meeting, the themes identified and audit trail were collated in a report and returned to board members for verification.

Team reflection

This was our first exposure to the board, and as such, this creative approach represented quite a risk to our credibility as a newly formed team, so we felt relieved and very pleased that the whole process worked well. Had we gone along with a more straightforward form-filling exercise or straight discussion, we would have missed the emotional nuances, which emerged and contributed significantly to shaping the vision. Yet, when planning the meeting we almost rejected a creative approach and had to challenge our own thinking around 'we could not ask Chief Executives to be creative with images!' The very real cultural norms and social constraints almost stifled our innovation. In many ways, this epitomises daily practice in the health service, where it is safer to do things the way they have always been done.

Team key learning

A key learning point is that indeed the use of creative expression can enable individuals, or groups, to articulate values that otherwise may be submerged under taken-for-granted assumptions and healthcare complexities.

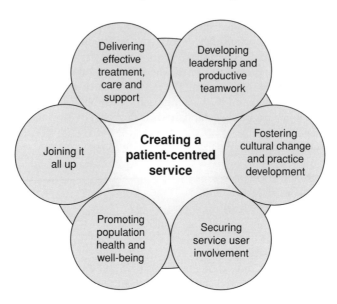

Figure 16.4 The seven values of the NICaN.

At the time, we did not really appreciate the significance of this exercise, or how it would support the continued development of the network. On reflection, we can now see that the vision, articulated as underpinning values (Figure 16.4), has been pivotal in helping plot the course for NICaN. Unsurprisingly, the values map to the five major themes that govern the future HPSS in Northern Ireland and to the quality standards for health and social care. By making explicit this mapping, the values are now perceived at having greater legitimacy. According to Schon (1991), raising ideas such as this over the threshold of public consciousness, rouses interested people around them. They then begin to 'sloganise' the ideas, and in so doing, create emotional meaning and energy, which moves the ideas onto the conceptual structure of the social system, making them appear obvious in retrospect. We have reflected on this alignment, and whilst it could be argued that this is being coercive, we consider it a pragmatic synthesis between healthcare policy and practitioner values, with the intent of developing greater person-centred services.

There is no doubt that the Cancer Network values have helped to guide us in a healthcare context that is turbulent, perpetually fluctuating and changing. We now draw upon the values, not only to share with, support or challenge key stakeholders, but also to enable us reach decisions with regard to appropriateness of intent or action.

Stakeholder engagement
Practice development processes

Networks are relationship based. One of the early objectives therefore of the NICaN team was to develop relationships with key personnel across the region and to engender a shared sense of ownership of the network values/vision. The exercise also helped to establish effective channels of communication, determine a baseline of activity, collate information to facilitate the development of common standards and audit processes, and gather information and evidence to help inform the evaluation framework for the network.

We used a modified fourth-generation evaluation approach (Guba & Lincoln, 1989) and distributed a questionnaire at each meeting, which asked stakeholders to identify their 'claims, concerns and issues' with regard to the developing Cancer Network and gave them time to complete. The 'claims' we phrased as 'expectations'. Over the course of year 1, claims/expectations and concerns from over 230 stakeholders, including those of the NICaN board and the team, were collated, read and subsequently analysed. Through a process of thematic analysis, 11 overarching issues emerged. These were presented to the NICaN board and used to inform the 3-year Cancer Network Development Plan.

Team reflection

On evaluating the meetings we agreed that the objectives had been met. As this was one of the first coordinated activities undertaken by the NICaN team, it was also felt that the exercise had proven to be a constructive team development activity, clarifying the team's understanding of, as well as helping to develop, a shared vision for the network.

The reception by clinicians was generally very positive, and the emerging Cancer Network was greeted with much enthusiasm. There was an acknowledgement of the effort made by the team to engage with key personnel and to ensure that their perspective (and voice) was heard at this formative stage of development of the network.

While meeting with and actively listening to stakeholders was invaluable in terms of building relationships, we felt we could have made more effective use of the claims, concerns and issues process. Initially, there was confusion amongst us as to the purpose, with some of us thinking that it was about assessing stakeholder knowledge of the proposed network, as opposed to its being a means of taking into account their particular 'constructions' or realities, and working with these multiple perspectives in order to strengthen stakeholder empowerment. Had we had a shared understanding, as well as the conviction and confidence to structure the meetings more around identified issues, we could have engaged in a much more mutually educative and empowering activity, rather than rendering this aspect a mere form-filling exercise. That said, the value of ultimately identifying the core issues from numerous stakeholder perspectives should not be minimised as it provided unique insights and helped us to determine network direction.

Team key learning

As an MCN is relationship based, the value of engaging with stakeholders should not be underestimated. In analysing the data, we adopted a systematic and rigorous approach by working in pairs to theme the data, before member cross-checking and leaving a clear audit trail. This was a learning experience for us all.

According to Guba and Lincoln (1989), fourth-generation evaluations are never complete; they simply pause until a further need and opportunity arise. Therefore, to make full use of this process, we need to periodically invite each of the network groups and constituent components of the network to evaluate their current claims, concerns and issues, thus eliciting their constructions about network progress. This will not only be of benefit to their network groups but also cross-fertilise with the constructions of the other network groups, making self-evaluation through reflection, planning and action of an ongoing, and owned activity.

Understanding and using an empowerment methodology to identify stakeholder perspectives acknowledges those potentially 'at risk' from the change process. It values their input, not only in identifying issues for further action, but also in evaluating if, from their point of view, progress has been made. This process thus enables stakeholders to have more of a sense of ownership and control and helps to develop a more open culture. Undertaking this process in a rigorous, truly participatory fashion requires those facilitating it to have an understanding of the underpinning methodology and the skills and confidence to commit to such a systematic process, despite the prevailing workplace culture of just getting on with the 'real business'.

From a practice developer's perspective, I (Liz) have learned that sometimes I too readily accommodate to the safer option and hide within the team. I need to have the courage of my convictions, and take responsibility to risk role-modelling processes that I believe to be appropriate.

Growing as a team

The network team is central to the development and operation of the Cancer Network. Transformational leadership (Bass, 1993) is required, which recognises that each of us can take the lead depending on the situation, as we seek to inspire others towards the vision for person-centred cancer services. Within the team, expertise, credibility and relationships with key stakeholders are pivotal to enable improvements in the quality of cancer care. As with guidance on network team composition, the Cancer Network team is multiprofessional and multidisciplinary. There are varying arrangements regarding hosting and contracts, secondments, and human resource management. Although there is an office base, members have bases that are geographically dispersed across Northern Ireland rendering diary alignment quite a challenge. Given this complexity, and the recognition that transformational leadership and effective team working enables network development, it is critical that the team take time to continually review and develop their role. In addition to the value of building a team, it also helps to ensure that team members are equipped and supported to enable them to effectively fulfil their responsibilities.

Practice development processes
Setting core objectives
The identification of core objectives for year 1, which focused on establishing the foundations for the network, provided a systematic framework. It not only helped to keep the team on track and provide a means to monitor progress, but also helped

clarify others' expectations regarding the realistic achievements of a fledgling network.

Team-building events

Developing as an effective team was one of the initial core objectives. Hence a team-building residential programme was arranged at which we engaged in a creative process to agree ground rules. This was followed by a group disclosure exercise, which, according to Luft (1987) and Benson (2001), is important if relationships based on trust are to develop. An analysis of our team roles using Belbin (1998) was also included.

Values clarification

As an exercise, values clarification has helped us to reach understanding and consensus at times when our diverse professional backgrounds and worldviews hindered effective communication or conceptual clarity. For example, despite using the language of 'service user involvement' we had very different understandings of what this involved. The values clarification process and negotiations involved, which included the input from a service user, achieved common understanding and proffered significant learning for all.

Reflective dialogue

Frequent engagement in reflective team dialogue on our performance, various activities and evaluation of the network, has further enabled our learning and identified areas for action.

Presentations

A formal presentation on 'methodological approaches' by a leading PD expert was aimed at helping us to make some sense of our paradigmatic differences. Ongoing internal discussion around PD together with a formal presentation has helped us achieve some further understanding of this methodology.

Team reflection

Drawing on the managerial knowledge and expertise within the team, a process to establish *clear objectives* was undertaken. Clearly, in developing and growing as a team, relevant management techniques as well as PD approaches have been used.

Resoundingly, there is agreement that weaving the two together is helpful in many ways, and our reflections are framed using Adair's (1986) model, Figure 16.5.

In relation to the initial *team-building* event, we concur that this was not a particularly enjoyable experience, with some of us well out of our comfort zones, both with the creative approach and the level of disclosure. Both processes felt awkward, strained and uncomfortable. Equally, the subsequent 'Belbin Team Role' exercise aimed at providing insight into our different styles gave some of us the sense of being monitored. A subtle group coerciveness to participate seemed to permeate the session.

On reflection, there were assumptions made as to all of us agreeing on the usefulness of undertaking such activities (when there were important business items

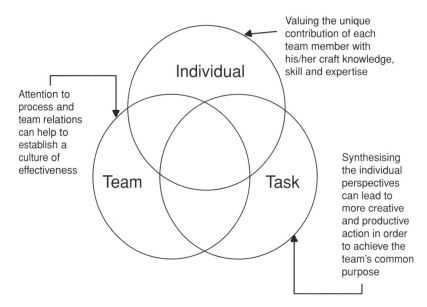

Figure 16.5 Management and practice development approaches for team effectiveness.

to address), as well as assumptions made about the readiness of team members to risk being so open. This had the potential to damage, rather than develop team relations. Despite the strain of the event, there was deepening of our understanding of each other as very different individuals and an obvious commitment to work synergistically for the benefit of the common goal. Subsequent team meetings, residential network workshops and just generally working together have helped us to develop effective team relationships even as new team members have joined.

On evaluating a recent team development workshop, team members felt that it had achieved its objectives in reviewing the current format and effectiveness of the team, and sharing perceptions and assumptions about aims and performance criteria. We also used this opportunity to challenge each other in a supportive way and acknowledged that more work is required to clarify individual roles and responsibilities, and those roles that are interdependent.

Within the team, trust and respect for each other is evident, and we now operate with high levels of challenge and support. We have learned how to make the most of each other's strengths and permit our 'allowable weaknesses' (Belbin, 1998). With regard to functioning and interacting with others, explicit team values of process transparency, integrity and professionalism are held high.

Key learning

Given the complexities of the team, as noted in the introductory paragraph of this section, the team's continual growth and the complexity of the Cancer Network agenda, the team clearly recognise the value of stopping the 'doing' and taking time to engage in active learning, either as part of team meetings, informally and formally at dedicated times.

In looking at some aspects in more detail, a number of other key learning points have emerged. With respect to the first *team-building* session, possibly more attention should have been given to planning and structuring the event. Although nominally agreed by us all, it was unrealistic to cover both team development and core business in one day. Furthermore, when setting the ground rules and subsequent disclosure exercise, not enough attention was paid to individuals or to making the 'hidden' visible. We doggedly persisted with the 'creative' process. In this case, creativity itself became the task, and the professional artistry required when facilitating (Titchen & Higgs, 2001), such as attunement, synchronicity and improvisation, was sadly lacking. On reflection, we should have paused and examined what was happening in the group. If attention had been drawn to the dynamics within the group it may have enabled the concerns of members to be expressed, and either productive dissent, shared understanding or a negotiated group consensus regarding the purpose of the session achieved.

Through engaging in the process of *reflection* for this chapter, we are beginning to see that our team reflections are inclined to be of a superficial nature. We describe the situation, outline the positives and negative aspects, share how we feel about it, and what we could do better in future, which in itself is helpful. However, we tend not to examine our underlying thought processes, assumptions or value judgements that have led us to arrive at our conclusions. For deeper learning to occur we need to actively engage in critical reflection. Critical awareness according to Mezirow (1981) is 'becoming aware of our awareness' and critiquing it. Thus this type of critical debate, either individually or collectively, may develop one's ability to look at things as other than that they appear. Personal and professional issues and meanings in the situation are exposed, and the influence of historical, cultural, social and political constraints explored (Titchen, 2004). Reflecting at this deeper conceptual and theoretical level engenders fresh insights about 'self', which, according to Mezirow (1981), is essential for transformative learning, as it relates to knowledge generation.

With this in mind a few of us have recently established a team *action learning set*, as a means of engaging in shared critical reflection, and to enable us to more effectively facilitate network activities. Although there is a tendency for us to let more pressing 'legitimate' network matters take precedence, we acknowledge the necessity of such critical space to enable individual and team development amidst the turbulent and demanding healthcare culture.

The difference between the *culture* 'out there' and that within the team was highlighted by one of the new team members in terms of the later being 'person centred' and open to learning.

We realise that role-modelling person centredness and *transformational leadership* within our 'home team' are vitally important, as we seek, in various ways, to facilitate the ongoing development of positive relationships and effective multi-professional specialist cancer teams across the network.

Involving service users

One of the seven guiding principles of the Cancer Network is to secure user involvement. From the outset we engaged with a number of local cancer support groups and facilitated two creative workshops during which group members painted and themed their vision for cancer services in Northern Ireland (NICaN, 2005b). Part of their vision was active service user involvement in the planning and monitoring of cancer services.

Practice development processes

In line with MCNs elsewhere two service users were appointed to the network board. Within the network team, we worked in partnership with a person who had her own experience of cancer, to develop a draft strategy. Her contribution clarified team understanding of the concept and significantly influenced the tone of the report, *Cancer Service and Service User Involvement: Not Why, but How?* (NICaN, 2005c). Pivotal among its recommendations was the requirement to appoint a Service User Facilitator to take the lead in securing meaningful service user involvement, and Janis was subsequently appointed.

Service users – definition (NICaN, 2005c):

> Service users include patients, carers, family, friends, advocates, members of organisations representing service users' interests, community and minority groups as well as members of the public affected by, or interested in, cancer services.

To establish the infrastructure for active and ongoing service user involvement, five workshops for those 'interested in the development of cancer services' were hosted in various localities around Northern Ireland. Approximately 30 people attended each session, and comprised those with their own experience of cancer as well as carers. From these meetings it was agreed to establish an NICaN Cancer Experience Forum, as a way to connect the various cancer support groups and interested individuals in order to maximise their contribution to cancer service development. Although in the formative stage, members of this forum are now shaping their work plan and exploring multiple methods for meaningful and active network involvement. In discussion with the team, Janis was encouraged to consider an emancipatory action research approach to service user involvement for her doctoral studies, and subsequently linked with a supervisor who is an international expert in PD.

Team reflection

As a team we have made quite a journey in appreciating the value and importance of involving service users in the development of services. Whilst believing the concept laudable, and publicly endorsing it as a network value, initially a few of us quietly questioned such strong emphasis, given the practical difficulties of overcoming tokenism and securing meaningful engagement. Coming from cultures that historically have adopted paternalistic attitudes in knowing what is best

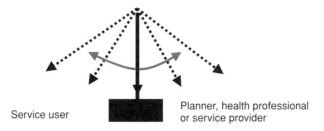

Figure 16.6   Negotiation pendulum for consensus decision-making.

for patients, the political and policy context have clearly changed with service user involvement, which is now one of the dominant ideologies.

In practice, however, we have observed how health professionals often feel uncomfortable with service user inputs, yet their response tends to privilege such contributions, even when their comments appear to be misinformed or out of context. Whilst it seems that the will is there to involve users in service development, professionals are not quite sure how best to go about it, which produces at times a sense of dissonance. We can see that this in itself could be an inverted form of paternalism manifest through a 'tyranny of niceness' (Sommers, 2005) as opposed to disagreement.

It is clear that securing true partnership working based on respect, mutuality and reciprocity will be a major challenge. This will require new mechanisms or processes to enable consensus decision-making, based on meaningful negotiation between service users and healthcare professionals. We have thought of this as a pendulum with the debate moving between parties until consensus is reached (Figure 16.6) (NICaN, 2005c).

However, over the months through regular contact, working with and listening to service users, we have collectively started to see the real potential of partnership working, with better understanding of the others agenda. We also believe that working collaboratively on these agendas increases the potential to effect cultural change, make an impact on population health and well-being and achieve improvements right along the 'patient pathway'. Our aim within the network therefore is to enable a power balance where true partnership working is achieved. We now feel excited about the prospect of leading on this within the Northern Ireland Health Service and, through evaluating the processes used and the impact of these on service development, make a contribution also to the research agenda.

Team key learning

In reflecting critically on this, we have challenged ourselves if we too are being paternalistic in pursuing a research study around the impact of service users, when, for example, to date other professional network groups are not researching their impact. However, we have concluded that there is a clear case for knowledge generation around the factors that enable disenfranchised groups such as 'service users' to become empowered for collective action towards social and cultural change. An empowerment methodology therefore such as emancipatory action research befits that intent.

Establishing network groups

The work of the Cancer Network is progressed by 'groups' or 'clinical networks' that are responsible for the development of regional standards, audit, patient pathways, service redesign, quality assurance and the identification of funding priorities. There are both 'tumour-specific groups' and 'theme groups'; see Figure 16.2. In the rest of the United Kingdom, these networks, working with their respective network/executive board and network team, have the mandate from their government to implement national policy and are the recognised model for cancer services planning and delivery.

In Northern Ireland, the Cancer Network had very different 'roots' in being set up under the auspices of the commissioners. In the formative development of the network, there was also an absence of regional policy on cancer services and MCNs. Working in a 'policy vacuum' clearly there was a need to focus on helping the groups to identify a shared sense of purpose and reaching consensus on a regionally agreed work plan.

Practice development processes

In preparation for the initial meetings of the groups, much time and effort was spent on being clear on the objectives of the meetings, identifying 'best practice' elsewhere, securing senior executive buy-in and using transparent and appropriate processes to actively engage all interested parties. During the meetings, a systematic approach was utilised to achieve a group remit and identify the core constituency required to take forward the remit. Having sought agreement on these two aspects, membership for the group was sought, again using a transparent and inclusive approach. Having achieved clarity on the purpose and added value of the 'group', members were encouraged to consider their draft work plan.

Through the process of working towards the establishment of these groups the constitution for network regional groups was developed and refined. This included group purpose (which was refined by each of the groups), core membership requirements, details on meeting frequency and core work strands. It also included the accountability arrangements, made explicit the underpinning network values and highlighted the need for a clear and managed communication strategy across the network.

Team reflection

Although the objective of working towards the establishment of four groups within the first year was achieved, there may have been disquiet over the time and effort expended on 'forming' the network groups without enough attention to task or 'product delivery'. On reflection by the team, it is evident that the process of slowly establishing and building the groups was crucial to secure the buy-in and ownership. Although the same attention to the process is still applied when establishing new groups, the constitution provides the framework for swifter group development and ensures a commonality of approach. This is essential within an MCN as it supports the management of communication, information sharing and inter-relationships between various groups.

In establishing regional network groups, reflexivity featured strongly as each group setup required a flexibility of process, a willingness to move with the emerging dynamic, and an 'openness' to learn and amend our processes accordingly. Each of the regional network groups has its own unique climate, culture and focus. With some groups, creative sessions were used to enable members to articulate the direction of travel; with others this would have been inappropriate at this particular place and time.

Using creative approaches in establishing network regional groups

A creative workshop was facilitated with the network pharmacy group, to explore how they could move to a more person-centred pharmacy service. Group members at this event undertook a creative concept analysis and identified key points for action. The nursing group used images as metaphors to describe how they were experiencing their roles, and subsequently identified the enabling and inhibiting factors for effectiveness. The strategic work programme of the nursing group explicitly embraces PD as the means to achieve transformational cultures of effectiveness.

As we now reflect on establishing regional network groups, we can see that a lot of our energies in year 1 went into establishing 'enabling' or 'cross-cutting' network groups such as Nursing, Supportive and Palliative Care, Primary Care, Pharmacy, and Service User groups. With tumour groups such as NICaN, lung, haematology and gastrointestinal groups were also established. Although some have critiqued this early balance as not being focused enough on tumour network groups, there is a clear benefit to having created an enabling infrastructure from which to draw appropriate membership for those groups still to be formed. The network gives voice to all key stakeholders, not only voice, but through the managed links and strategic alliances provides a mechanism to hear multiple perspectives, and in harnessing these rich intelligence sources offers a means to enable organisations, individuals and teams to make sense of and work with cancer service complexity.

Key learning

Clearly, the use of participatory, inclusive and collaborative approaches has enabled participation and shared ownership across the constituent members of the network. As identified earlier in the discussion on stakeholder engagement, the MCN is relationship based and therefore the value of engaging with stakeholders and securing their buy-in should not be underestimated.

By using rigorous and systematic processes to establish these groups, and continually reviewing and refining the group constitution, the network is now in a strong position to move forward its development. Focus will now be on the development and implementation of evidence and standards based care pathways, service audit and monitoring via the tumour-specific networks.

The external evaluation of the setup (Hamilton, 2005) and initial operation of the Cancer Network indicated a 'relatively stable foundation phase' and in the

Table 16.1 Summary of key learning from team reflection on PD processes used

- Use of creative process enables articulation of values
- Making values explicit provides a solid foundation and shapes the future
- Proactive engagement with key stakeholders develops shared ownership
- Using systematic rigorous approaches increases reliability of data
- Working with an empowerment methodology requires skilled facilitation
- Valuing each person's unique experience and craft knowledge maximises the team's potential
- Attention to process and group dynamics provides a climate conducive for working
- Prioritising time and space for critical reflection is an investment not a luxury
- Transformational leadership enables the development of an effective workplace culture

absence of regional guidance, the report suggested that there was a dependence of the 'enthusiasm and commitment of the NICaN team, closely monitored by the network board'. It concluded though that the efforts may not sustain the progress and proposed that the *'shape and operating principles* be derived from the Department of Health and Social Services in Northern Ireland'.

In the new climate of healthcare reform, access targets and performance management, the network will need to embrace the opportunities afforded by a clearer mandate. Crucially though, the same rigour and attention to process need to be applied in establishing and continuing to build the network.

Summary of learning from shared team reflection

A summary of the team's key learning points is outlined with respect to using PD methods to progress the work of the MCN (Table 16.1).

To take this a step further in terms of learning, we have mapped the developmental processes used onto the PD conceptual framework developed by Garbett and McCormack (2002); see Figure 16.7.

The process of having critically reflected on the methods used to enable network development has given us more of an insight into PD methodology. We now understand PD to be an ongoing process, which has a twofold purpose:

- To achieve improvements in patient-centred care.
- To enable healthcare teams develop cultures of effectiveness.

Achieving this requires facilitators who adopt 'systematic and rigorous processes' and who understand and work with 'emancipatory' change principles. The latter include working with individuals' and teams' values and beliefs, and surfacing assumptions as a means of raising awareness between the values they espouse, and the values enacted in the 'swampy lowlands' of everyday practice (Schon, 1991). Bringing to consciousness the tension between the professed values, and those lived out, is what helps to increase dissatisfaction with the status quo and generate a desire for change (Manley, 2004).

Adopting active learning processes that foster critical reflection underpins this 'emancipatory' approach to PD. In so doing, practitioners learn to view things

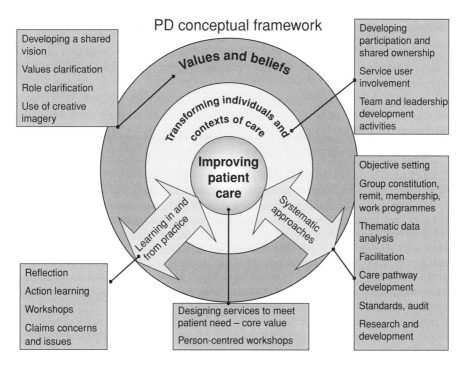

Figure 16.7 PD approaches mapped to conceptual framework.

as other than they appear, thus gaining fresh insights into and new knowledge about their culture and their practice. All knowledge is valued in PD as it provides 'evidence' to inform practice change (McCormack, 2003). Experience is seen as a valuable source of knowledge (Benner, 1984) as is feedback from service users and empirical research (Sackett et al., 1997), and includes evaluation of the practice context and culture (McCormack & Manley, 2004).

Workplace culture is often defined as 'the way things are done around here' (Drennan, 1992), and is heavily influenced by a set of unwritten rules. These 'rules' are often carried over from practices, attitudes or behaviours that have worked well in the past, which are absorbed by individuals unquestioningly, and then perpetuated. In practice, this can manifest itself in many ways, from outmoded routines and rituals to learned helplessness, to strained relationships and dysfunctional teamwork. Active learning processes, which include critical reflection and action with high challenge and high support, are aimed at enabling practitioners to become more aware of self and how our inherited dispositions and social influences place limits on how we view ourselves in the world, influence our attitude to practice, and how we relate to others (McCormack & Titchen, 2006). The whole thrust therefore of EPD is to enable practitioners not only to be 'enlightened' as to the nature of their situation, but also to be 'empowered' to take action, to overcome obstacles and bring about identified changes in self, in practice or the practice context. In so doing, they become freed or 'emancipated' from the forces or assumptions that previously constrained them. Respect for individuals under-pins this way of working, where each is valued as a unique person and not as a role. This person-centred ethos help to provide a milieu much more conducive to effective patient care.

As we reflect it is clear that we have *not* been engaged in a systematic PD pro-gramme, but simply have used a number of methods associated with PD, whilst not fully appreciating that connection. It is also evident that many of the devel-opment processes employed are not exclusive to PD. For example, whilst 'setting clear objectives' is in line with PD's 'systematic rigorous approach', it is known by team members as a general change management principle. Likewise, the im-portance of 'team-building events', which are in line with PD's 'enablement of effective teamwork', are understood by team members as group development and management theories. By contrast, methods used such as working with values and beliefs, developing a shared vision, action learning and stakeholder claims concerns and issues are directly attributable to a PD source. Therefore as each member of the team contributes to network planning and development we draw on our individual craft knowledge (Titchen, 2001), skill and expertise, and through debate harness this rich diversity of knowledge to arrive at decisions. Often we are in accord with the actions required, albeit informed from different knowledge sources.

However, the exercise of mapping the PD processes to a conceptual framework is extremely useful, as it starts to connect methods to a methodology. In view of the ease at which the methods link, can it be assumed that PD has a role to play in helping an MCN achieve effective patient centredness?

Discussion

Patient-centred services and effectiveness are at the heart of the UK government's programme of reform for the health service, with cancer services given high pri-ority (DH, 2000). In response to this, Cancer Networks elsewhere in the United Kingdom have proactively embraced Service Improvement (SI), not PD, as a means of delivering on reform. For example, in Scotland the Cancer Services Improve-ment Programme began with a broad aim of 'improving the patient experience' (SE, 2006). In England, national funded programmes such as the Cancer Services Collaborative Improvement Partnership are established, which likewise describe their goal as, 'improving the experience and outcome of care for people with sus-pected or diagnosed cancer, by improving the way in which care is delivered' (CSC, 2003, 2006). These collaborative programmes have historically been time limited and focus on specific projects, although they emphasise that improvement needs to continue beyond the life of the project. Since both SI and PD are concerned with improving patient care, the question arises: Are they one and the same thing?

A closer look at how they are operationalised may shed some light. In terms of similarities, it is clear that both PD and SI take a 'systematic rigorous ap-proach' to change. Both advocate the need for facilitators to enable healthcare teams to effect the improvements. Both approaches champion service user involvement, patient-centred care, valuing evidence generated from practice and sharing the learning from this. A review of SI (http://www.institute.nhs.uk; formerly www.modern.nhs.uk/cancer) and toolkits reveals, amongst others, a concern for 'managing the human dimensions of change' (NHS, 2004a), 'building and nurturing an improvement culture (NHS, 2004b)' and 'working with groups (NHS, 2004c)'. Collectively, they aim to 'empower' front-line staff to work together to provide high-quality care that is safe, effective, patient centred, timely and efficient. More recently, the NHS-integrated SI programme claims to be leading a 'fresh approach to transformational change' (NHS ISIP, 2006). It provides tools and techniques that encourage joined-up working across local health and social care communities for maximum benefits for patients and staff.

It is evident from this review that a significant number of ideas and approaches are shared between SI and PD. In a systematic review of the evidence base supporting PD, McCormack et al. (2006) summarised the concepts found in definitions of PD. When compared with SI, the only concept identified as unique to PD is the concept of 'emancipation'.

Yet, in practice, there are obvious differences in the methods and tools that each use. To help elucidate this further, a table comparing SI and PD is presented (Table 16.2). In order to aid clarity, the table has distilled each approach with the purpose of accentuating their difference.

It is clear that both SI and PD are aimed at improving healthcare outcomes, which include the experience of patients, but the means of achieving this differs significantly. In simplistic terms, the former focuses primarily, but not exclusively, on systems and processes, the latter on people and their practice. What is the relevance of this, and what do each have to contribute to MCNs?

What can service improvement contribute?

Evidence from elsewhere in the United Kingdom demonstrates that engaging in SI can make a significant difference to outcomes of care and improve patient satisfaction with services. With the accumulated evidence from thousands of projects, 'high impact changes' to develop services have been clearly identified, along with key change principles, which place the patient firmly at the centre of the process (NHS, 2005). Joining up the patient journey by improving access, reducing delays, improving information and support, developing the team around the patient are some of the foci for change. By involving managers as well as clinicians and securing executive sponsorship, key stakeholders are included from the outset, and an accountability structure established. Given this portfolio, it is clear that SI is of direct relevance, and indeed is essential to deliver on MCN's work programmes.

What can practice development contribute?

PD on the other hand focuses on individual empowerment and developing workplace cultures of effectiveness, both of which, it is argued, are necessary for *sustainable* change (Manley, 2004). Located in an empowerment methodology, PD largely involves reflective learning strategies, which focus on the active engagement of participants in learning, consistent with adult learning theories. A number of PD

Table 16.2 SI and PD compared and contrasted

Components	Service improvement	Practice development
Stated purpose(s)	Improve experience and outcome of care	Increased effectiveness in patient-centred care Transforming culture and context of care
Main focus	Improving processes/systems and services Integrated SI	Developing clinical practice
Patient aspect	Optimises care delivery systems across the whole pathway of care: • Connect up the patient journey • Develop the team around the patient journey • Make the patient experience central	Person-centred practice, concerned with the following: • Rights and social justice • Sharing of power relationship between practitioner and patient • Autonomy of individual to determine own destiny • Centrality of values between patient and practitioner Respect for personhood Organisation of care to facilitate person-centred practice Enabling relationships
Concepts specific to each	Human resource management Process management Benefits realisation Added value	Enlightenment Empowerment Emancipation Human-flourishing
Theoretical underpinning	Systems theory Improvement science	Critical social science
Underpinning knowledge	Practical and technical knowledge to effect change	Increased critical awareness: • Enlightened as to the 'oppressive forces' and barriers to change • Empowered to take action • Freed from taken-for-granted aspects of practice that previously constrained Self-knowledge, Individual growth and development

Methods specific to each	Improvement toolkits Plan, Do, Study, Act model of change Process Mapping Redesigning clinical pathways Capacity planning Service redesign Benchmarking	Systematic methods to facilitate: Using and generating knowledge: • Facilitating evidence into practice • Critical inquiry • Critical reflection • Critical dialogue • Active learning • Critical companionship Practice changes Process and outcome evaluation
Facilitation style	Technical facilitation: Helping practitioners to effect change supported by above tools, techniques and processes	Holistic facilitation: Helping practitioners to effect change through person-centred facilitation (relationship based), critical reflection and enabling processes
Focus of learning	Learning about improvement processes and sharing learning	Learning to learn Active reflective learning
Product	Focused on benefits and outcomes	Focused on process outcomes as well as outcomes
Evaluation	Measurement – numerical variables Cost savings	Personal/collective development Evaluation of culture Measurement – numerical variables
Outcomes	Systems change Process redesign, right person, right training, right place	Care processes change Empowered practitioners Learned processes of sustainability Workplace culture change
Key references for above	DH (2005) Clarke et al. (2004) Habermas (1972) http://www.institute.nhs.uk http://www.wise.nhs.uk/cmsWISE/Cross+Cutting+Themes/Imp/Imp.htm www.cancerimprovement.nhs.uk	Fay (1987) Habermas (1972) Manley and McCormack (2003) McCormack and Manley (2004) McCormack (2004), McCormack et al. (2006)

programmes illustrate the type of systematic approach adopted (e.g. McCormack & Henderson, 2006; Dewing, 2003; Wilson et al., 2005). Programmes differ from the approach of the network team previously described in this chapter, in that the same participants are involved throughout the duration of the programme, which runs for an agreed period of time (e.g. 6–18 months). Typically these programmes include the following:

- Developing a collective sense of ownership and purpose for the programme.
- Establishing active learning sets (through reflection and action).
- Developing transformational leadership skills (runs throughout the programme).
- Identifying personal work-based learning objectives.
- Creating a shared vision for the service.
- Evaluating the context of care and analysing workplace culture.
- Eliciting service user feedback.
- Theming and learning from the data.
- Developing and implementing action plans.
- Reevaluating the service.
- Identification of ongoing development work.

Patient centredness is at the heart of PD, with the focus being on helping practitioners identify ways they can engage more effectively with patients in order to better identify and meet their care needs. Viewed as a person first and a patient second, there is a sharing of power relationship between practitioner and patient, with the autonomy and right of the patient respected. Practice is organised in such a way as to facilitate such engagement, and the focus is on 'working with' the person rather than achieving tasks or 'doing to' them. More recently, the concept of 'person centredness' is identified in PD literature (e.g. McCormack, 2004). Person centredness includes patient centredness but involves a way of 'being' with others, including members of the healthcare team. Inherent in both concepts is the notion of respect for personhood, which is equally applicable to team members as it is to patients. It is argued that positive relationship between multiprofessional team members is essential for an effective workplace culture, and that this enables each person to grow and flourish (McCormack & Titchen, 2006). In this type of culture everyone is a leader of something, innovation is evident, scholarship and competency are valued, quality is everyone's concern, and practice is developed (Manley, 2004).

From experience, many workplace cultures are not effective. In reality, relationships in many uni-disciplinary and multidisciplinary teams are often time fraught with difficulty. Hierarchical ways of working exist, and there is a preoccupation with achieving the task at the expense of developing team relations and open communications. Yet West (2005) has demonstrated that the quality of multidisciplinary team working can impact on clinical outcomes. This is of particular relevance to cancer services, since MDTs are core to clinical effectiveness. It is therefore clear that PD with its interest in empowerment, sustainable development and effective workplace cultures can also contribute significantly to networks' agendas.

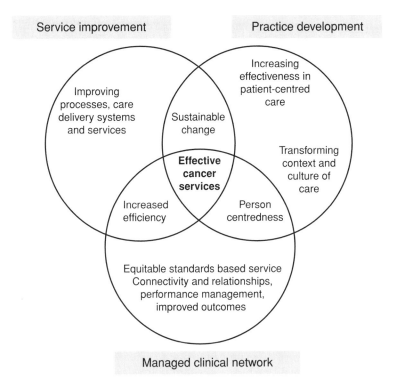

Figure 16.8   Synergistic model for development of effective services across an MCN.

Service improvement and practice development in a managed clinical network

This chapter presents the argument that both SI and PD approaches are needed to achieve sustainable improvement across an MCN. Figure 16.8 represents the proposed synergistic relationship between SI, PD and an MCN, all of which, we suggest, are necessary to enable more efficient and effective person-centred services across a region with the potential for sustainable improvement. We have attempted to identify a particular contribution of each and the particular property emerging when blended with another field.

MCNs, as we have seen, are concerned with continuous improvement in clinical outcomes as well as improving the quality of cancer care and services. To achieve this, evidence-based, clinical and organisational standards are required, with monitoring processes in place and practitioners held to account. Organisational standards involve connecting up the various components of the 'patient journey' and connecting the various statutory and non-statutory providers to work collaboratively to improve the quality of service offered. However, collaboration depends on establishing trust and positive relationships so that there can be partnership working between healthcare professionals, commissioners and planners, and between healthcare professionals and service users.

This is a huge change agenda and describes changes in the patterns of interactions between the various parties, which, according to Bate (1994) is *cultural change*. The values of NICaN explicitly state the need for such cultural change. However, Davies and Nutley (2000) argue that this cannot be easily wrought from the top-down by simple mandates but successful strategies need to actively involve staff in the process. This is a significant challenge, given the scale and complexity of the network, with numerous teams, organisations and myriad workplace cultures involved.

SI recognises cultural change as a key element of a whole systems approach for sustainable improvement (CSCIP, 2006), yet in reality there appears to be little attention paid to this aspect. Rather the translation of the holistic change principles into practice has, in many instances, been reduced to a driven, task-orientated, time-specified project. Indeed the Scottish Cancer SI Programme (SE, 2006) explicitly acknowledges its narrowing of focus from improving the patient experience to achieving cancer access targets. From a network perspective, increasing efficiency by meeting targets and streamlining services on its own is inadequate, offering purely a quick-fix solution that fails to take into account developments in inter- and intra-team relationships, so essential for effectiveness. It is focusing on the task at the expense of engaging with people. This type of 'driven' change, supported by short-term projects is difficult to sustain once the facilitation support is withdrawn (CSCIP, 2006).

Whilst all improvements are to be welcomed, for *sustainable change* there is a clear need to enable local teams to become innovators, where they accept responsibility for developing their own practice, and continually strive to improve the quality of care and improve their service. This involves moving from closed, controlling, negative workplace cultures to those that become and remain patient centred, with open communication and participative safety, where feedback is welcomed, innovation is fostered, and positive team relationships exist.

PD's focus is on enabling healthcare teams to develop such cultures of effectiveness where practice is evidence based and person centred. But it would be naïve and frankly misleading to suggest that PD approaches or whole-scale PD programmes would automatically achieve such transformation, since it is well recognised that changing cultures is a long, slow, inherently difficult process. What PD offers is help to foster the conditions that make such change possible. Yet, even if MCNs adopted PD as a means to achieve greater person centredness and evidence-informed practice, unless, Manley (2004) points out, the focus of practitioners development work is strategically appropriate, they could not be termed effective. In other words, there needs to be a fit between PD and the organisational goals. Given the reality of a policy-driven heath service, where standards, targets and performance management are a facet of daily life, a pragmatic PD approach is needed across networks, where practitioners are enabled to develop critical insights into their practice in relation to the drivers for change, and an informed understanding of appropriate actions to take, which will enable person centredness even within the current climate.

What this chapter argues is that both SI and PD approaches are needed to foster sustainable change across MCNs, since both approaches contribute to improvements in practice. Given the overlaps in the areas of interest, we would suggest that they are located at two ends of a continuum, with SI towards a technical end, and PD towards the other more 'holistic' end. Both SI and PD depend on facilitators to support the change process. We suggest that there is a need for MCNs to be supported by holistic facilitators who have the skill and knowledge not only to use SI methods and tools, but who also understand and are skilled in PD approaches, to enable them to move appropriately in either direction along the continuum, according to the particular circumstances.

In summary therefore, SI's major contribution is systems related, with excellent resources and models for analysis and redesign to achieve streamlined patient journeys. PD's major contribution is on the 'human dimensions of change' with methods and approaches to enable practitioner empowerment and person-centred practice. In today's healthcare environment, strategically appropriate organisations must be efficient and effective, able to deliver on targets, whilst at the same time endeavouring to improve the patient experience through joined-up services, increased choice, timely information and effective person-centred care. But irrespective of whether the impetus for change is external or internal, whether it is 'driven' or 'enabled', those involved in the process need to value the person for their intrinsic worth, as opposed to seeing people only of value if they contribute in some way to achieving the organisational goal.

For a more effective service across a region, we submit that what is required is not an 'either–or' situation, but a synthesis of both approaches applied to an MCN as the organisational model, to deal with the complexity of whole systems change.

Conclusion

In true PD style, learning from reflection should lead to action. Hence, as a result of reflecting and writing this chapter there are a number of actions emerging for the team to take. Both as individuals and as a team we need to apply the new learning as summarised in Table 16.1 to ourselves and to our practice. As we engage with regional network groups, lead cancer teams and local multidisciplinary teams, we need to draw more explicitly on PD knowledge, to find new ways of engaging in a manner that is 'appropriate' to the group', which respects where different stakeholders are, but which at the same time starts to challenge some of the social and cultural norms.

However, our most significant action will be to raise awareness at organisational and strategic level of the need for a much more holistic approach to the complex and challenging change agenda than the 'driven' ethos that currently exist. Taking an MCN view, we propose a combination of SI and PD approaches as a way to keep the balance needed, and working with the inherent tensions in that suggestion. We fully recognise the importance of achieving the task but recommend that it is done in a manner that truly values the team. In this way, the person for whom the service exists has an increased chance of an efficient, effective and person-centred experience.

Acknowledgements

We thank Gerard Daly, Dermott Davison, Fionnuala Green, Janis McCulla, Maire McGrady, Lisa McWilliams, Lorna Nevin for their critical dialogue that has helped to inform the structures and processes described in this chapter.

References

Adair, J. (1986)*Effective Teambuilding – How to Make a Winning Team*. Pan Books, London.

Bass, B. (1993) Transformational leadership: A response to critiques. In: *Leadership Theory and Research: Perspective and Direction* (eds M.M. Chemers & R. Ayman). Academic, San Diego, CA.

Bate, P. (1994) *Strategies for Cultural Change*. Butterworth-Heinemann, Oxford.

Belbin, R.M. (1998) *Team Roles at Work*. Butterworth-Heinemann, Oxford.

Benner, P. (1984) *From Novice to Expert: Excellence and Power in Clinical Nursing Practice*. Addison-Wesley, Menlo Park, CA.

Benson, J.F. (2001) *Working More Creatively with Groups*. Routledge, London.

Clarke, C.L., Reed, J., Wainwright, D., McClelland, S., Swallow, V., Harden, J., Walton, G. & Walsh, A. (2004) The discipline of improvement: Something old, something new? *Journal of Nursing Management*. **12**(2), 85–96.

CSC (2003) *Cancer Services Collaborative: Improvement Partnership – A Quick Guide*. NHS Modernisation Agency, Leicester.

CSC (2006) Cancer Services Collaborative. (www.cancerimprovement.nhs.uk)

CSCIP (2006) The Challenge of Implementing Sustainable Changes in Cancer Services. NHS Cancer Services Collaborative Improvement Partnership. (www.cancerim-provement.nhs.uk)

Davies, H.T.O. & Nutley, S.M. (2000) Organisational culture and quality of health care. *Quality in Health Care*. **9**, 111–119.

Dewing, J. (2003) A practice development project for nurses working with older people. *Practice Development in Health Care*. **2**(1), 13–28.

DH (2000) The NHS Cancer Plan: A Plan for Investment. A Plan for Reform. (www.doh.gov.uk/cancerplan)

DH (2005) NHS modernisation agency. *Improvement Leaders' Guide: Improvement Knowledge and Skills*. DOH Publications, London.

DHSS (1996) *Cancer Services: Investing in the Future*. Department of Health and Social Services, Belfast.

Drennan, D. (1992) *Transforming Company Culture*. McGraw-Hill, London.

Edwards, M. & Fraser, S.W. (2001) *Clinical Networks – A Discussion Paper*. NHS Confederation, London. (www.nhsconfed.net)

Fay, B. (1987) *Critical Social Science*. Blackwell, Oxford.

Garbett, R. & McCormack, B. (2002) A concept analysis of practice development. *Nursing Times Research*. **7**(2), 87–100.

Guba, E.G. & Lincoln, Y.S. (1989) *Fourth Generation Evaluation*. Sage, Thousand Oaks, CA.

Habermas, J. (1972) *Knowledge and Human Interests* (Trans. J.J. Shapiro). Heinemann, London.

Hamilton, K. (2005) The Foundation Phase: An Independent Review of First Year Activities of the Northern Ireland Cancer Network. (www.nican.n-i.nhs.uk)

Luft, J. (1987) *Group Processes: An Introduction to Group Dynamics*, 2nd edn. Mayfield Publishing, Palo Alto, CA.

Manley, K. (2004) Transformational culture: A culture of effectiveness. In: *Practice Development in Nursing* (eds B. McCormack, K. Manley & R. Garbett). Blackwell, Oxford.

Manley, K. & McCormack, B. (2003) Practice development: Purpose, methodology, facilitation and evaluation. *Nursing in Critical Care.* **8**(1), 22–29.

McCormack, B. (2003) Focus. Knowing and acting: A strategic practitioner focused approach to nursing research and practice development. *NT Research.* **8**(2), 86–100.

McCormack, B. (2004) Person-centredness in gerontological nursing: An overview of the literature. Practice development – person-centred practice. *International Journal of Older People Nursing.* **13**(3a), 31–38.

McCormack, B., Dewar, B., Wright, J., Garbett, R., Harvey, J. & Ballantine, K. (2006) *A Realist Synthesis of Evidence Relating to Practice Development: Final Report to NHS Education for Scotland and NHS Quality Improvement Scotland.* NHS Quality Improvement Scotland, Edinburgh. (www.nhshealthquality.org)

McCormack, B. & Henderson, L. (2006) Critical reflection and clinical supervision: Facilitating transformation. In: *Clinical Supervision in Practice, 2nd Edition, Some Questions, Answers and Guidelines for Professionals in Health and Social Care* (ed V. Bishop), pp. 108–140. Palgrave Macmillan, New York.

McCormack, B. & Manley, K. (2004) Evaluating practice developments. In: *Practice Development in Nursing* (eds B. McCormack, K. Manley & R. Garbett). Blackwell, Oxford.

McCormack, B. & Titchen, A. (2006) Critical creativity: Melding, exploding, blending. *Educational Action Research.* **14**(2), 239–266.

Mezirow, J. (1981) A critical theory of adult learning and education. *Adult Education.* **32**(1), 3–24.

NAO (2005) The NHS Cancer Plan: A Progress Report. National Audit Office.

NHS (2004a) *Modernisation Agency Series 3: Improvement Leaders' Guide to Managing the Human Dimensions of Change.* NSH Modernisation Agency, London.

NHS (2004b) *Modernisation Agency Series 3: Improvement Leaders' Guide to Building and nurturing an improvement culture.* NSH Modernisation Agency, London.

NHS (2004c) *Modernisation Agency Series 3: Improvement Leaders' Guide to Working with Groups.* NSH Modernisation Agency, London.

NHS (2005) *Improvement Leaders Guide: Improvement Knowledge and Skills.* NSH Modernisation Agency, London.

NHS Confederation (2002) Clinical Networks, Nexus. Background Briefings, NHS Confederation. Managerial, London.

NHS ISIP (2006) NHS Integrated Service Improvement Programme. London. (www.isip.nhs.uk)

NICaN (2005a) Northern Ireland Cancer Network. (www.nican.n-i.nhs.uk)

NICaN (2005b) Developing the vision for the Northern Ireland Cancer Network: Cancer Choices, Dungannon. (www.nican.n-i.nhs.uk)

NICaN (2005c) Cancer Services and Service User Involvement in Cancer Services: Not Why, But How? (www.nican.n-i.nhs.uk)

Sackett, L.D., Scott-Richardson, W., Rosenburg, W. & Haynes, B.R. (1997) Evidence-based medicine: How to practice and teach. *Evidence Based Medicine*. Churchill Livingstone, London.

Schon, D.A. (1991) *The Reflective Practitioner: How Professionals Think in Action*. Avebury, Aldershot.

SE (1999) *The Introduction of Managed Clinical Networks within the NHS in Scotland*. Management Executive Letter Circular MEL 10. (http://www.show.scot.nhs.uk/sehd/mels/1999_10.htm)

SE (2006) *Cancer Service Improvement Programme*. Scottish Executive, Edinburgh. (www.cci.scot.uk)

Sommers, E.K. (2005) *Tyranny of Niceness: Unmasking the Need for Approval*. Gazelle Book Services, Lancaster.

Titchen, A. (2001) Critical companionship: A conceptual framework for developing expertise. In: *Practice Knowledge and Expertise in the Health Professions* (eds J. Higgs & A.Titchen), pp. 80–90. Butterworth-Heinemann, Oxford.

Titchen, A. (2004) Helping relationships for practice development: Critical companionship. In: *Practice Development in Nursing* (eds B. McCormack, K. Manley & R. Garbett). Blackwell, Oxford.

Titchen, A. & Higgs, J. (2001) Towards professional artistry and creativity in practice. In: *Professional Practice in Health, Education and the Creative Arts* (eds J. Higgs & A. Titchen). Blackwell, Oxford.

West, M. (2005) *The Aston Team Facilitation Programme*. Power Point presentation. Aston Business School. (Lynnm@astonod.com)

Wilson, V., McCormack, B. & Ives, G. (2005) Understanding the workplace culture of a special care nursery. *Journal of Advanced Nursing*. **50**(1), 27–38.

17. *Accrediting Practice Development Activity: An Approach for Achieving Person-Centred and Evidence-Based Care*

Kim Manley, Jane Canny, Jill Down, Jane-Marie Hamill, Elaine Manderson, Natalie Moroney, Jenny Newton, Alyce A. Schultz and Helen Young

Introduction

This chapter focuses on accreditation and credentialing activity as a means for developing the practice of teams and organisations towards providing care that is person centred, evidence based and continually modernising (Manley, 2004), and a culture where all can flourish (McCormack & Titchen, 2006). Different accreditation/credentialing experiences and purposes are drawn on. All have relevance to achieving the purposes of practice development (PD), whether that is through developing and using standards in the workplace or enabling others to develop their practice through clinical or educational programmes that aim to develop PD expertise.

The chapter first draws on three different experiences that outline how standards describing an effective workplace culture are developed and used in practice, how evidence is collected and corroborated to demonstrate achievement of the standards, and the impact this approach has on patients, facilitators and practice teams.

The second focus is on developing evidence-based practice through a Clinical Scholars programme that supports practitioners to develop expertise in evidence-based practice within the context of Magnet organisations in the United States (Schultz, 2005a, 2005b). The Magnet Recognition Program® accentuates and

Box 17.1   Accreditation and credentialing terms

> **Accreditation**: recognition by a non-governmental, external agency of a school, pro-
> gramme or service that has met certain standards beyond those that are minimally
> acceptable. Participation in the process is voluntary (International Council of Nurses,
> 1997).
>
> **Credentialing** is a term applied to the processes used to designate that an individ-
> ual, programme, institution or product have met established standards set by an
> agent (governmental or non-governmental) recognised as qualified to carry out this
> task. The standards may be minimal and mandatory or above the minimum and
> voluntary (Styles & Affara, 1998).

supports nursing within the interdisciplinary team and recognises a hospital-wide
culture of development through achievement of standards. Finally, the accreditation of a joint Master's programme in Australia with the University of Ulster (Northern Ireland) is described, one that aims to build a foundation of PD
expertise.

Accreditation and credentialing (Box 17.1), amongst other terms, are global approaches increasingly used to kite-mark various healthcare and education-related
services and providers. Both involve external assessment of internally generated
evidence against predetermined standards with regard to the endpoints desired
at the organisation, team, programme or individual level. This chapter focuses
on using standards, a component of all credentialing/accreditation approaches,
as a tool for PD at the *team* and *organisational* level in healthcare and educational
settings rather than focusing on the achievement of that final quality mark. Chapter 12 focuses on the *individual* and the development of facilitation knowledge
and expertise through formalised processes of learning and development– the
key skill-set for helping others to develop their practice (PD) (Manley & Webster,
2006).

Three different sets of standards are referred to in this chapter:

- RCN *Standards for an effective workplace culture*. A set of standards framed around
  the purposes of PD, namely
  - developing person centredness;
  - developing individual, team and service effectiveness;
  - developing evidence-based care, including knowledge utilisation and evi-
    dence development;
  - developing effective workplace culture.
- Standards developed by the Magnet Programme – an international credentialing
  approach used with healthcare organisations.
- Meeting education standards to accredit a new Master's programme in PD.

Part of the chapter is dedicated to practitioners' experiences with developing and
using the RCN *Standards for an effective workplace culture* (RCN, 2007) in a number
of different specialisms first at unit level, and then at organisational level, as a tool

for developing practice and capturing impact. The journey starts with the story of two practitioners, Elaine Manderson and Jane-Marie Hamill, who work within a nursing development unit based within a critical care setting. They describe the process used to develop the standards and the impact of this involvement on their unit.

This is followed by experiences of practitioners and PD facilitators across two acute hospital organisations and one primary care organisation who were involved in piloting the standards at unit level.

Jill Down, with organisation-wide responsibility for PD within a large acute hospital, and Helen Young, a senior practitioner, share their experience of using the standards as a PD tool and identify both insights and outcomes. First at unit level in a centre caring for people who have experienced stroke and then transferring this learning to a community team.

Piloting the standards also provides the impetus for achieving organisational learning and development, when Jane Canny, who is responsible for improving the patients' experience across another large acute hospital, and Natalie Moloney, a specialist nurse, worked with the standards within a colorectal specialist unit and then across the organisation.

In the second part of the chapter, Alyce Schultz identifies how the standards developed by the Magnet Recognition Program are relevant to PD, specifically with regard to achieving evidence-based practice through a programme of support. Finally, the role of educational accreditation in the development of an innovative Master's programme in PD is shared by Jenny Newton, a key initiative for developing future expertise in PD.

Developing and using standards for an effective workplace culture at the unit level

Chelsea and Westminster Intensive Care Unit (ICU) became accredited through the Kings Fund as a Nursing Development Unit in 1991. Ten years later, although the unit was constantly developing nurses and nursing, there was no longer a formal process for accrediting the work undertaken. For this reason, the ICU team met with the Royal College of Nursing (RCN) Accreditation Unit to explore the potential for accrediting workplaces. A project group was established and consisted of representatives from Chelsea and Westminster and Addenbrookes's Hospitals, the RCN Accreditation Unit and practice developers from Bournemouth University.

Purpose of the project
The purpose of the project was to develop standards that enabled specific workplaces to be recognised for being person centred, evidence based and effective. The resulting standards reflected local, national and international agendas for healthcare. The evidence base was derived from research and transcended all boundaries (systems, people and process boundaries).

Box 17.2 Attributes associated with working effectively and providing quality in Magnet Hospitals

---

Attributes
- Support for education
- Working with nurses who are clinically competent
- Positive nurse/physician relationships
- Autonomous nursing practice
- A culture that values nursing
- Control of and over nursing practice
- Perceived adequacy of staffing
- Nurse-manager support.

Background to workplace culture

Studying the workplace and identifying what makes a good place to work is not new. Kramer and Schmalenberg (2004) in their study revisiting Magnet Hospitals identified eight attributes that staff nurses considered as essential in order to work effectively and produce quality care (Box 17.2)

The role of culture is also mentioned in terms of shared values and norms, as a 'culture of excellence' has always been associated with the concepts of the magnetic work. The specific cultural processes necessary to enable these values to be integrated in the practice environment are evaluated in the Magnet Recognition Program as processes for producing a culture of excellence, along with its structures and outcomes.

Some of these processes are also reflected in the Promoting Action on Research Implementation in Health Services (PARIHS) framework (Kitson et al., 1998; Rycroft-Malone et al., 2002, 2004). The PARIHS framework identified a number of factors influential on evidence use including a context with an effective workplace culture, linked to leaders with ability to transform cultures to one that is more conducive to evidence use in practice and a focus on. A finding endorsed by Manley (1997) whilst researching workplace culture in the context of developing the consultant nurse role. She identified three attributes of quality patient services: practitioner empowerment, practice development and a number of other workplace characteristics, all encompassed by the term 'transformational culture'.

Transformational culture is synonymous with the characteristics of an effective workplace culture, composed of a number of interrelated factors that have an effect on the way individuals and teams work. A transformational culture is one where adapting to change has become a way of life for all members, and continuing to develop a quality service is everyone's business (Manley, 1997, 2004).

The workplace standards and the process of becoming accredited enable a key purpose of PD to be achieved, that is, to transform the culture of care so that it becomes and remains person centred, evidence based and continually effective within a changing healthcare context.

The standards sought to address a number of key UK government recommendations reflecting the policy context (Table 17.1). So their development was timely as they also set out to achieve the quality outcomes of clinical governance.

Table 17.1   Key U.K policy initiatives that the standards sought to address

Focus of government policy	Publication

• Linking quality improvement with
  ○ clear national standards,
  ○ effective care and treatment,
  ○ team effort, collaboration and partnership extending to patients, families and carers.
	Making a Difference (DH, 1999)

• The culture of the workplace is emphasised through the introduction of Improving Working Lives Standard. Here organisations must demonstrate that they are investing in more flexible, supportive work arrangements, tackling discrimination and harassment and developing skills of all staff to improve patient services.	NHS Plan (DH, 2000)
• The focus of NHS reform was shifting more towards improving the quality of care patients receive.	Standards for Better Health (DH, 2004a)

Developing the standards

The first phase of the project was to identify a shared vision and an action plan for how to achieve the vision. In order to develop this vision and to ensure that it was representative of all the members of the steering group a values clarification exercise was used (Warfield & Manley, 1990) as outlined in Table 17.2. This exercise is used to identify common ground and collective values by drawing individual thoughts together through buzz groups and a nominal group technique.

The steering group believed that it was important to evaluate the progress of the project and selected fourth-generation evaluation (Guba & Lincoln, 1989) for this purpose. This form of evaluation is based on a series of interactive processes involving the engagement and empowerment of stakeholders (Guba & Lincoln, 1989; Clendon, 2003; Koch, 2000). In practice, this means identifying the stakeholders involved in the project, including those who may gain or lose from the project (McCormack & Manley, 2004). The steering group then asked stakeholders to identify their claims, concerns and issues (Titchen & Manley, 2006) to guide the project's implementation and the development of the standards.

As part of the vision implementation, a sub-group was identified to work on the standards development comprising a

- PD senior fellow from the RCN
- PD nurse in medicine
- PD nurse from ICU
- Clinical leader from ICU
- Deputy director of nursing.

Table 17.2   Values clarification exercise and resulting vision

Questions asked
I/we believe the purpose of the 'accreditation of workplaces project' is . . . .
I/we believe that this purpose can be achieved by . . . .
I believe that my role in this project is . . . .
 	
Vision resulting
The ultimate vision of the project is to enable sustainable person-centred and effective cultures to develop through the process of workplace accreditation. This involves
• sharing good practice and dissemination,
• recognising and celebrating individual achievement and identifying good places to work.
 	
Achieving the vision
To achieve this vision we need the following:
• A project group committed to the vision and project management, but one that also
  ○ involves and uses the skills of others enabling critique and mutual development;
  ○ identifies benefits, beneficiaries, promotes and creates a business case;
  ○ communicates with key stakeholders internally and externally.
• A sub-group to develop specific, measurable, achievable, realistic and time-bounded (SMART) standards that build on existing standards and evidence.

The group then met to develop the framework for the standards and to identify what needed to be included. The outcome of this sub-group was to be the basis of a developmental tool that could be used to identify effectiveness through the development of a portfolio of evidence. A number of key themes emerged and these informed the four standards (see Table 17.3 – right-hand column).

The next stage was the creation of sub-elements for each standard, for example, Standard 1 – *developing person centredness* – included the sub-element of participation. The workplace was required to demonstrate how it achieved genuine involvement in order to achieve a person-centred approach to care. Specific questions were identified that could enable a team to consider how it met a particular standard, for example, under the participation sub-element:

• How are service users encouraged to participate in their care?
• How do they work in partnership with service users to enable them to plan, monitor and evaluate the service provided?

Once the standards were drafted they were disseminated for critique to a wide number of stakeholders across the United Kingdom. This critique was essential as part of the *fourth-generation evaluation* and provided the sub-group with valuable feedback allowing further refinement.

The final aspect of work was to cross-reference the standards against the 'Standards for Better Health' – organisational standards that apply to all health and social organisations across the United Kingdom (Department of Health, 2004a). There were a number of areas that linked well with our unit/team level standards

Table 17.3 Standards for effective healthcare in overview

	Standard title	What it means	Main themes
1	Developing person centredness	Focusing every aspect of 'care' around the person who is receiving care in relation to how they see their healthcare needs in the context of their life plan. It involves valuing all individuals, teams, organisations, communities and other members and their contributions.	• Participation • Information • Diversity • Values • Fundamental aspects of care
2	Developing individual, team and service effectiveness	Developing effectiveness in self and others to enable and sustain person-centred, evidence-based care. Lifelong learning is integral to the standard and is linked with formal systems enabling continuous critique and reflection.	• Facilitation • Teamwork • Knowing and involving stakeholders • Personal and professional development • Continued competence, skill development and utilisation
3	Developing evidence-based healthcare including knowledge utilisation, transfer and evidence development	Actual knowledge and evidence used in a practice rather than what is known and may not be used. How knowledge is used and articulated as practical know-how continues to be refined through structured reflection and critique, thus promoting effective care (Titchen, 2000). Evaluation and indicators of effectiveness.	• Knowledge development • Evidence utilisation • Transfer of knowledge • Evaluation • Evaluating indicators of effectiveness at individual, team and service level
4	Developing effective workplace culture	An effective culture (termed a transformational culture; Manley, 2004) is recognised by the presence of three components: practice development with its focus on person-centred and evidence-based care; staff empowerment; and, other workplace characteristics, namely the following: • Shared values and practices. A common mission, consistency and involvement. • Adaptability internally and externally reflected by a learning culture. • Services match needs. • Stakeholders are valued. • Leadership is valued and its potential developed at all levels.	• Living and experiencing espoused values • Effective communication • A culture of innovation • Participation and shared decision-making by stakeholders • Learning culture • Leadership development • Empowerment

and it was felt that the PD strategies we used would work for organisations trying to provide effective person-centred care.

Standards for effective healthcare

The final standards (see Table 17.3) reflect the elements that make up the vision of what makes a healthcare setting beneficial to users and a good place to work for staff. They have been developed using the concept of PD (Garbett & McCormack, 2002) and through understanding and valuing the concept of transformational culture (Manley, 2004). They have been developed not only as a method of assessment but also as a tool to assist with the development of a transformational culture through the use of PD activities at the unit level.

The workplace standards are different from any other standards for the following reasons:

- They focus specifically on workplace culture.
- They encompass the importance and presence of facilitators.
- They have an explicit evidence base derived from research rather than expert opinion.
- They can be used in all healthcare settings across the NHS, independent and voluntary sector.
- They have international application potential.

Integrating the standards with practice

The standards have been used in practice at Chelsea and Westminster Hospital ICU in two ways:

1. To develop evidence to demonstrate that we achieve them in practice.
2. To guide the further development of practice.

Many of the PD initiatives used at Chelsea and Westminster Hospital ICU demonstrate the standards in action. Evidence of this action is presented through examples of a range of documents and activity outlined in Table 17.4.

The workplace standards have enabled the unit to consider a number of different ways in which to improve practice. For example, in relation to the patient's experience, we have used focus groups where ex-patients were invited to share their experiences. As a result of this feedback, we have developed a patient information folder for particular conditions that nursing staff can use to help patients understand their disease process. The standards have also been used successfully to guide the implementation of action learning sets for senior staff. In addition, they helped with developing a PD strategy that links the workplace standards to the business plan. The workplace standards have placed the unit in a unique position through the ability to articulate the role that PD plays within a modern healthcare setting.

Table 17.4 Examples of evidence from Chelsea and Westminster ICU that can be used to demonstrate the workplace standards

Activity on the ICU	Links to workplace standards			
	1	2	3	4
Development of a philosophy of care	✓	✓	✓	✓
Practicing primary nursing	✓	✓	✓	✓
Shared values and beliefs – values clarification for inter-team project groups – a mechanism for achieving shared governance within the unit	✓	✓	✓	✓
Action learning sets and clinical supervision for staff (group and individual)		✓	✓	✓
Inter-team project groups deliver on standards	✓			✓
Action plans on essence of care benchmarks (fundamental aspects of care important to users)	✓		✓	✓
Reflective reviews – Patients – Project groups	✓	✓	✓	✓
Patient and relative involvement – patient and relative advocate, surveys, focus groups	✓	✓		✓
Patient representatives on steering group	✓	✓		✓
Information books for admission to and discharge from ICU (available in various languages)	✓			
Staff satisfaction surveys	✓			✓
Development plans for staff		✓		✓
Evidence-based guidelines in use			✓	
Observations of care			✓	

The RCN *Standards for an effective workplace culture* once developed were then piloted by practitioners in other areas; their experiences and outcomes are described next.

Using the workplace standards in acute and primary care settings at the unit level
Context and purpose

The Lewin Unit is a 30-bed stroke and rehabilitation unit that provides both acute and rehabilitation care for patients suffering a stroke and also those requiring rehabilitation following neurological events. The service has required reconfiguring in order to provide effective and timely care to improve patient outcomes and quality of life, ensuring timely thrombolysis in the early hours followed by rehabilitation provided by an effective multi-disciplinary team (Department of Health, 2001b).

Staff on the unit seized the opportunity to become involved in a project to develop the service, the culture of their workplace, and to develop evidence from their clinical area mapped against workplace standards, whilst contributing to the refinement of four pilot workplace standards (RCN, 2007). The project was facilitated by an RCN PD facilitator and an internal facilitator using action learning (McGill & Beaty, 1997) with a group of five staff from the Lewin Unit and four staff from another unit who also participated in the project. Action learning underpinned by a critical theory approach is concerned with identifying the barriers to action and dismantling them. The barriers may be within individuals or within the systems in which they work or a combination of both (Fay, 1987). Helping the team to develop, review and use the evidence from their workplace (Kitson et al., 1998), I (Jill) experienced challenges, developed insights and can identify outcomes from the journey with the team. Neither unit knew the other and had limited experience of action learning. We had ten, two and a half sessions to begin the journey of exploration, so a clear purpose of the project and action learning was developed with the set using a values clarification exercise (RCN, 2006) (Box 17.3). This was an important process to develop a common vision, as sometimes there may be a contradiction between what we say our values and beliefs are and what we actually do in practice.

Box 17.3 Values clarification questions for identifying project and action learning purposes

---

What are our values and beliefs in relation to the workplace standards project?
1. I/we believe the ultimate purpose of this project is . . . .
2. I/we believe this purpose will be/can be achieved by . . . .
3. I/we believe my/our personal responsibility to the project is . . . .
4. Other beliefs we have about the project . . . .

The purpose of the workplace standards project is:
Through the process of engagement and participation, we will create an effective culture that will improve the quality of patient care.

– Requires facilitators, enablement

The purpose of action learning in the workplace standards project is:
- To keep the action going
- To learn by reflection but also be future orientated
- Looking at different solutions and overcoming barriers
- Challenge boundaries and make us think outside the box
- To achieve actions and change practice through learning
- To help people be more effective in their work
- To help us to help others to achieve the workplace standards
- Demonstrate that our workplace meets WP standards for an effective workplace culture

---

Challenges

Exploring, challenging and reviewing the work of a team requires a culture where giving and receiving feedback is valued and acted upon (Manley, 1997). Most of the staff were unfamiliar with the process of action learning and it provided a new way of working for them, helping them to critique their work, develop insights and identify actions.

The team initially identified multiple sources of evidence from the unit to support the achievement of the workplace standards and these are illustrated in Table 17.5.

They realised that if the evidence to support the standards was to impact on the development of a transformational culture (Manley, 1997), rather than become a paper exercise, they needed to explore it further and develop the processes for collecting and using it. In essence it highlighted the need to ask the 'so what?' questions of the evidence, identifying further questions regarding the evidence (Box 17.4).

The process of working with the team in an environment that enabled them to grow and learn, helped them to develop and explore insights about their workplace culture through the pilot period (Table 17.6). It was not always a comfortable journey but strengthened the team who became more challenging of each other in a supportive way.

Impact of using the workplace standards

Once the pilot period was completed, the journey continued using the standards as a developmental tool to guide the progress of the unit. The most significant impact was not in the technical development of the service but the enlightenment and enablement of staff so that they could make changes in their service as a team. These changes were related to helping staff develop their skills in helping others to learn in the workplace and become more effective in their practice (see also Chapter 12). As a result of the project, patient focus groups have been introduced, action learning is used for staff development, there is focused development of leadership skills in the team, and there is the development of team projects with patient and staff involvement that address the questions in Box 17.4.

A strengthened multi-disciplinary team has resulted and an environment where staff are driving changes and responding to organisational influences in a positive way that are sustainable and where evaluation is evident. The standards have also

Box 17.4 Questions raised by the evidence

- What difference does this make to patients and staff?
- How do we know what difference it makes?
- How can we be sure that our espoused values and beliefs are experienced by staff and patients?
- How can we ensure that all our work is multi-disciplinary?
- How can we involve all the team in this work?

Table 17.5 Evidence identified to support the achievement of the workplace standards

Standards 1–4	1	2	3	4
Types of evidence used to demonstrate achievement of the standards	Developing person centredness	Developing individual, team and service effectiveness	Developing evidence-based healthcare	Developing effective workplace culture
	Patient stories and surveys	Leadership development for team leaders	Development of guidelines, policies and procedures	Student and staff survey feedback
	Shared patient goal planning with MDT	Team meeting notes and action plans	Hospital acquired infection data	Use of compliments and complaints and risk data to change practice
	Essence of care audit results	Personal reflective reviews	Clinical research projects	Observations of practice
	Patient forum and focus groups	Staff training and development records	Integrated care pathway development	Leadership development
		Patient environment action team reviews		Ward philosophy

Table 17.6 Insights developed about the workplace culture

Person centredness
- We need to develop a philosophy that is based on the values and beliefs of all our staff and patients
- Working with staff to develop processes to develop the culture is part of a journey, not an end point

Developing individual, team and service effectiveness
- We could prioritise our projects and be incremental rather than trying to do everything at once

Developing evidence-based healthcare including knowledge utilisation, transfer and evidence development
- To involve all staff and the multi-disciplinary team in using feedback and developing action plans from audits and other evidence

Developing an effective workplace culture
- We need to be careful not to develop a culture that is a 'tyranny of niceness' (Street, 1995)
- Need to focus more on developing leadership potential in all staff
- Need to balance technical skills development with developing other quality processes with staff and patients

helped to direct and support work driven by national policy initiatives (Department of Health, 2001a, 2001b, 2004a).

One of the team leaders during the pilot project, Helen, was then provided with an opportunity to use the standards in a primary care setting.

The journey in primary care

My (Helen's) promotion to a position within a primary healthcare organisation as a Neurological Rehabilitation Manager for two teams afforded me the opportunity to take the work forward in a different setting. My previous experience of working with the workplace standards had highlighted the need for complete team involvement from the start. One multi-disciplinary team was made up of 11 staff:

- 3 physiotherapists
- 2 occupational therapists
- 1 nurse
- 4 rehabilitation technical instructors
- 1 administrative assistant

With careful preparation I worked with the team. They decided to focus upon one standard at a time. They selected Standard 1, *developing person centredness*, and began by identifying evidence to show how they could demonstrate that they achieved the different aspects of the standard. From the evidence collected, a narrative was written (Box 17.5) – this was a synthesis that described and captured

Box 17.5 Narrative describing evidence to support Standard One

---

**Workplace accreditation
standards for effective healthcare
Standard 1**

The staff of the Neuro Rehab Team North (NRTN) believe that the ethos of the team reflect a person-centred approach. This can be identified in the way that all members of the multi-disciplinary team (MDT) work together towards common goals. The staff of the NRTN feel that this ability of the whole team to work together in this manner is central to effective person-centred care and fosters mutual respect and friendship amongst the different professionals and the patients. This can be demonstrated by feedback received from both staff and patients (Individual Performance Development Review [IPDR] documents, Thank you letters). The MDT endeavour to create an atmosphere of positive encouragement and reinforcement of progress made. It is believed that the NRTN can only be effective if care is focused around the patient, and every patient, relative and member of staff are treated as individuals in their own right.

The NRTN facilitates patient-centred goal planning. Evidence has shown that patient's goals should be central to the care delivery. The goals are set by collaboration between MDT members and individual patients. These goals form the basis of treatment, and are regularly reviewed to determine progress (sample goal planning documentation; Functional Independence Measure & Functional Assessment Measure [FIM/FAM] [Turner-Stokes et al., 1999]). The NRTN work closely with other specialised therapy groups and charitable organisations, such as the Multiple Sclerosis (MS) Therapy Centre, Headway and the Green Gym, enabling the patient to achieve their optimum potential during their rehabilitation period.

As a team, the NRTN is responsive to the needs and comments of all disciplines. Feedback is encouraged from staff members at their individual development performance review (IPDR) (sample IPDR document), regular meetings and away days (minutes). Patients are invited to give feedback via individual goal setting meetings (sample care plans; evaluation sheets). Relatives and friends are also encouraged to provide feedback (thank you letters; complaints). One new initiative currently being considered by the team is to demonstrate to the patients the progress they have made during their rehabilitation by involving them in reviewing their FIM/FAM results.

The ability of the MDT and the patient and their family to work together in a coordinated and well organised way, ensuring that everyone is kept informed and updated, is central to the success of our care. We believe that the person-centred approach adopted by the NRTN enables us to do this in a way that is meaningful and beneficial to all concerned.

---

how the team felt they met the standard. This narrative was then underpinned and cross-referenced to a range of other supporting evidence.

At this time the team also needed to address a number of UK policy initiatives to do with job evaluation and job profiles (Department of Health, 2004c), competency (Department of Health, 2004a) and new government standards for healthcare organisations (Department of Health, 2004a). The evidence emerging from working with the workplace standards was used to demonstrate the achievement of these latter standards.

I then chose to use the RCN *Standards for an effective workplace culture* as a guidance tool to help the development of the second team. This team was smaller:

- 1 physiotherapist
- 2 occupational therapists
- 3 rehabilitation technical instructors

Using the standards with this team enabled me to explore with the team members where the gaps in the service and team were and what needed to be done. The team members were very keen to develop and change and wanted to know how they could be more effective and improve patient satisfaction. One of the aspects that the team recognised quickly was the necessity to involve the patient when planning goals for their rehabilitation. This was something that had been in place very informally in the past and needed to be strengthened with greater patient involvement, and the use of a tool that would enable some standardisation and evaluation. The team began setting formal goals with their patients and started using a functional assessment tool – the Functional Independence Measure & Functional Assessment Measure (FIM/FAM) (Turner-Stokes et al., 1999) – as an outcome measure to demonstrate whether goals had been achieved. This measure is now shared with the patients, their families and their General Practitioner (GP) and also with the person who refers the patient to the service.

Workplace standards as a catalyst for change

Picking up on the work that the NRTN had been doing, the second of my teams, the Neuro Rehab Team South (NRTS) quickly recognised that their high caseload was preventing them from providing quality of care, meaning that the care was not always person centred. The team felt that they were 'scratching the surface' and knew that they could do better. They had not previously been able to identify a catalyst to effect this change. I carried out some calculations to identify individual capacity within each person's caseload. This enabled me to find ways of enabling the team to provide the quality care they were anxious to give. The team then became more effective with their discharge planning in relation to their existing caseload. It became clear through this work that the standards could be used as a way of helping staff to develop their service for patients.

As a follow-up to all the change and development that the team had been involved in, a patient satisfaction survey was used. This seeks patients' opinions about how they rate the team, how useful the team's input was, how goal orientated the team is, and whether the patient was involved in the planning of their rehabilitation. The feedback portrayed the team very favourably, which was a testament to their hard work and dedication. Furthermore, the activities by the team members provided evidence for their individual appraisal, career and personal development plans.

As a result of 'Commissioning a Patient Led NHS' (Department of Health, 2005), GPs will commission services. This policy position provides another opportunity to use the evidence and insights generated from using the workplace standards to inform the commissioning process. In order to be commissioned, the team needs to demonstrate what it is they do, and how effective they are, in line with Standards for Better Health (Department of Health, 2004b). Because of our experience with using the RCN standards, much of what will be required to fulfil this new agenda is already in place. For example, the FIM/FAM functional assessment provides a means of demonstrating progress made by patients. This evidence can therefore be used to help commissioners recognise both the quality and value for money service provided by the team to patients.

Start small think big: using the RCN workplace standards from unit to organisational level

How we began

A colorectal surgical ward took up the opportunity to pilot the standards, in January 2005. Piloting the standards was considered to be mutually beneficial and the RCN offered to work with the internal facilitator, for the duration of the pilot (6–9 months).

Piloting the standards would benefit the following:

- *The clinical area*, by facilitating and supporting the team to realise improvements in quality care and gain recognition for the team's work.
- *The hospital*, by further embedding PD processes across the organisation; increasing the number of people with PD expertise who can help others; developing expertise in the use of evidence from practice; achieve kudos from being associated with this UK-wide initiative.
- *The participants*, by providing the opportunity to further develop skills in facilitation, action learning, leadership and inter-professional team working.
- *The RCN*, by helping them to gain further information to build on, develop and refine the effective workplace standards and accreditation processes.

The resource implications were 3 hours a month for 6–9 months for all the project team members plus administration time and the energy and effort needed to implement and support the changes that came as a result of the pilot.

Reflection on the process

The aim of facilitation is to make things easier for others (Harvey et al., 2002). However, it does not always seem like that to the people and groups involved. A preliminary meeting was held with the ward team to discuss the work plan for the facilitated sessions. It was evident from this meeting that a senior nurse and doctor in the team were determined to undertake a PD initiative and were driving the process.

The aim of the first session was to clarify hopes, fears and expectations of the group members. Ground rules for working together were set and the group undertook their first experience of action learning – the approach selected to support them.

Observations made at this point included the impact of the leadership style, relationships between individual group members and the level of engagement with the process. There was willingness for team members to work together and help each other find solutions to problems. However, participation in the discussions was not equal, and there was some impatience with the pace of the process. At the end of the session group members could identify learning in three areas:

1. Learning from the scenario that was presented.
2. Learning from the action learning process.
3. Learning to connect this to the workplace standards.

Learning from the scenario included the following:

- What it means to put espoused values into practice and the need for consistency in values at different levels of the organisation.
- Recognising the needs of other groups of staff and managing conflict.

Learning from the action learning process included the following:

- How to reflect and help someone in a non-confrontation way.
- Not to make assumptions and to seek solutions.

Connections with the workplace standards included the following:

- Identifying elements of a learning culture (a learning culture includes having a non-blame culture [Wilson et al., 2005]).
- Demonstrating person centredness by giving an individual time to focus on issues important to them and focusing on values and beliefs.

At the next session, the group reported that they had found it difficult to make a connection between the action learning they had experienced, and achieving the outcomes they wanted. Action learning was considered to be time consuming when time was of a premium. This issue had been discussed and a way forward decided, in between meetings, by the team leaders.

In retrospect, it became clear that the purpose of the initial action learning experience was unclear to the participants and that instead of viewing it as an example of the process in action, they struggled to make a connection between the content of the discussion and the aims of the project.

It is possible that having a clear idea of what was to be achieved impacted on the group's preparedness to take part in action learning; a process where the outcome measures are allowed to develop over time. Tolerance for unexpected developments was low and this was characterised by the response to disagreements with or questions as to the value of the proposed changes, from the wider ward team. These were sometimes talked about in our sessions as examples of others either failing to understand the project or dismissed as troublesome behaviour. Utilisation of critical feedback, communication and relationships with team members who were not in the project group became themes for the group discussion.

In subsequent sessions the 'concerns, claims and issues' evaluation tool (Guba & Lincoln, 1989) was used to summarise information about the achievements, identify barriers to the work and plan the next steps. Some group members highlighted that they had never worked like this before and enjoyed it a great deal.

The opportunity to engage in genuine teamwork, discussion and planning was new and welcome. Group members felt involved, their views listened to and their input valued. In subsequent meetings the team was supported to plan next steps, organise evaluation and learn from the ongoing experiences of group members. A significant change was evidenced by the way the team handled difficulties with their processes. When the team experienced difficulties in making links between the different forms of evidence and how they related to the standards, this was experienced as a team issue and the solutions sought collectively, with the intention of achieving collective understanding. Facilitation in using the workplace standards enabled and supported a clinical team to identify and articulate goals, learn from their experience and use their experience to implement improvements in practice.

The major practice change resulting was the way that the patient ward rounds were conducted. An inter-professional and patient-centred ward round was introduced to improve communication and information between patients and all the members of the healthcare team involved in their care. This change facilitated other improvements such as an increased accuracy in predicted discharge dates and better information for patients, reducing length of stay and more favourable feedback from patients. These matched directorate and organisational priorities at the time.

Clinical leadership within the team provided the motivation and direction for improving practice, and inter-professional working established the environment where different roles and expertise were valued and team members learn from each other.

What goes up must come down

Sharing best practice is a key ingredient of the NHS Institute for Innovation and Improvement's strategy for promoting quality and effectiveness within the National Health Service (NHS) (NHS Institute for Innovation and Improvement, 2005). In the early stages, the sharing and promotion of our work were undertaken at a local level through presentations to team members at inter-professional meetings and informal discussions with colleagues and managers. The response received was optimistic and encouraging, and this increased confidence and motivation to build on the work. The work was judged to be a success owing to the improvements in the outcome measures identified above. We were asked by senior managers to assist them in promoting the work throughout the trust with a view to making it trust's policy. We had access to larger groups of people, medical councils, senior nurses and PD events. Having the opportunity to speak to influential people who would be crucial to the success of further implementation was inspiring. However, the positive and enthusiastic response that we had come to expect from colleagues started to waver. Resistance from medical and nursing professionals became apparent and we realised that what started as a 'bottom-up' drive for improvement was now perceived as a top-down dictation. This manifested itself through very different responses to the work, often characterised by defiance and conflict.

Lewin (1946), a leading theorist in change management and the force-field analysis model, has often been criticised for having a top-down approach. Perhaps misinterpreted, Lewin did acknowledge that effective change could only take place if there was a 'felt need' by everyone concerned and he later recognised that what mattered was not whether the initiative came from top, middle or bottom but that the change had the support and active equal participation of all involved.

To gain this participation, Schein (1992) emphasises the importance of understanding the culture within which the change is being implemented and warns that overriding the development of this understanding is a short-term fix with no staying power. Studies carried out using the Myers-Briggs evaluation tool (Myers et al., 1998) demonstrate that different types of people enter the healthcare professions so it should be no surprise that different outlooks will be evident (Frith-Cozens & Mowbray, 2001). Bujak (2003) identifies that, while physicians profess to want to create efficient services, they are unwilling to engage in organisational initiatives. This may in some part be a manifestation of sometimes turbulent and untrusting relationships between healthcare professionals and health service managers. With this in mind we set about to understand the priorities of the different services and discuss with them the potential benefits to staff and patients that could arise from implementing a different style of ward round. This strategy enabled discussions about the change initiative to be focused on the context in which it was being implemented rather than on the organisation as a whole.

Changing the organisation and format of the ward rounds was a change in a system that resulted in learning and change in other aspects of the 'way things were done'. The workplace standards provided the framework to identify, articulate and further develop practice. For example, when patients' views about the new ward round were sought, maintaining privacy was identified as an area for further development work.

The chapter now moves from a focus on practitioners' personal experiences of developing and using standards as a mechanism for achieving a culture of effectiveness that is person centred at unit level to organisations deemed centres of excellence, through magnet credentialing. An initiative is described that supports practitioners to lead on achieving evidence-based practice in relation to clinically relevant issues within their organisations.

Evidence-based practice in Magnet facilities

The Magnet Recognition Program for Excellence in Nursing Services® through the American Nurses Credentialing Centre (ANCC) identifies healthcare facilities and systems that epitomise excellence in patient outcomes through nursing leadership, shared governance, and the translation of available evidence and knowledge into practice. In 1990, the ANCC was designated by the American Nurses Association (ANA) Board of Directors to develop and maintain an application programme based on the essential components of magnetism identified in 41 hospitals in the 1980s that were able to retain professional nurses and provide exemplar nursing care during a time of severe nursing shortage. The Magnet Recognition Program has been extended internationally with facilities in the United Kingdom and Australia being designated Magnet facilities. The Forces of Magnetism (McClure & Hinshaw, 2002) provide an organisational conceptual framework for demonstrating the highest quality of nursing leadership and patient care.

In a large tertiary care hospital recently designated as a Magnet facility, the Clinical Scholar Mentorship Model (CS Model) received commendation as an exemplar of a sustainable programme of research and evidence-based practice at the point of care. The model is based on the premise that 'knowledge users produce better patient outcomes' and is advanced through a decentralised mentorship programme of bedside Clinical Scholars. The CS Model (Schultz, 2005a) for promoting and sustaining evidence-based practice (EBP) within nursing evolved inductively through the mentorship of a clinically based nurse researcher and motivated point of care nurses.

Early initiatives included pressure ulcer prevalence and incidence studies, falls prevention and pain management. From this early work, several funded and unfunded studies developed. The studies were disseminated at local, regional, national and international conferences, and manuscripts were written collaboratively and published in respective specialty journals (Conley et al., 1999; Schultz et al., 2002, 2003). Nurses who served as coordinators of the early projects became the first Clinical Scholars (Box 17.6).

Clinical Scholars exude a 'Spirit of Inquiry', a key element for moving evidence into practice. With the first Clinical Scholars serving as facilitators of smaller practice-based groups, a series of workshops based on the CS Model was conducted (Schultz, 2005b). The CS Model encompasses five basic concepts for promoting and sustaining the use of evidence in practice:

- Observation
- Analysis
- Synthesis
- Application/evaluation
- Dissemination

Box 17.6 Clinical Scholars

Clinical Scholars are defined as nurses who exhibit a high level of curiosity, critical thinking, continuously search for new knowledge, reflect on their experiences, seek and utilise a wide variety of resources, and use evidence to improve the effectiveness of interventions (Clinical Scholar Task Force, 1999).

The workshops were designed with these concepts as the overarching themes. The purposes of the workshops were to

1. promote an organisational culture of EBP and clinical scholarship, and
2. prepare direct care providers to initiate and evaluate EBP.

Administrative support

Administrative support was provided through paid time to attend the workshops and paid time for preparation and implementation of the projects. All clinical managers attended a full-day workshop prior to the start of the series so they would understand the expectations of the nurses involved in the Clinical Scholar programme and the expectations of themselves as support persons. Medical librarians assisted in the programme and provided access to library resources, with at least 30 nursing journals available on-site. Travel and registration expenses were paid when nursing abstracts were accepted at clinical conferences.

The Clinical Scholar model

Observation

Clinical scholarship begins in the creative and curious mind. The first workshop in the series furthered the powers of observation by centring on how to ask a researchable question based on observation of patient, family and provider issues (Honess, 2005). Once questions were clear in regard to patient population, the new intervention or treatment, the current practice and desired outcomes, the participants were taught how to conduct an electronic library search by the medical librarian. All staff nurses had access to the internet and the capability of conducting a literature search from computers on their respective units. Project teams were formed based on similar clinical issues and began thoughtful deliberation on the potential risk, harm, benefit and cost to changing practice and which stakeholders were needed on their teams.

Analysis

Selection of appropriate research manuscripts and analysis of the research evidence that is appropriate and meaningful in changing practice are often cited as barriers to EBP (Funk et al., 1995); however, when the educational format is guided by adult learning principles, with content meaningful to the participant, this step of the CS Model is more fully comprehended. Articles for group review were selected based on their clinical relevance, not on their study design or statistical outcomes. Basic concepts of research design and statistics, related to the clinical questions, were included in didactic presentations to facilitate understanding. Practice-specific group meetings focused on critiquing research studies that had clinical meaning. Clinical teams completed evaluation forms for individual studies that answered their clinical questions (Gallant, 2005). Published clinical guidelines were searched and evaluated for use in the projects (Lancaster, 2005).

Synthesis

Synthesis of the research evidence is critical in determining whether or not a practice change is ready for implementation without further generation of supporting evidence. The individual evaluation forms were used to develop synthesis tables of relevant evidence (Kent, 2005). Table 17.7 provides an example.

Once the synthesis tables were completed, the level and quality of the evidence were determined and decisions were made on whether the proposed practice change was ready for implementation (Stetler et al., 1998).

Application and evaluation

In this phase, additional stakeholders were informed of the projects or added to the project teams. If the teams were not interdisciplinary prior to this phase, members of all disciplines who would be affected by the practice change were now involved in some way. New practice guidelines or clinical protocols were developed based on the strength of the evidence. Plans were made for the practice change to be piloted on a single unit. If the evidence did not support a practice change, a clinical research study was proposed with the staff nurse serving as the principal investigator. An ethical review proposal was completed.

This phase of the CS Model requires interdisciplinary, administrative and collegial support (Keane, 2005). If the organisational structures are not in place for implementation of the project and the staff nurses involved in the project are not highly committed and supported during implementation and data collection, the project may fail. In organisations where innovation and autonomy are supported as evident in Magnet facilities, money and time are available for staff nurses to incorporate clinical inquiry into their daily practice. Unit-based managers support staff nurse involvement and staff nurses are rewarded for their innovative thinking.

Dissemination

The process and the results of EBP changes must be shared with interdisciplinary colleagues. Nurses were taught how to write abstracts and develop slide presentations. The climax of the first workshop series was a full day of 'Evidence in Motion' presentations by the 45 new Clinical Scholars for all administrators and staff. The participants described how their participation in the Clinical Scholar programme changed the way they thought about their work, resulting in a shift in attitude and a return to the values and commitment that first motivated them to become professional nurses (Strout, 2005).

Outcomes of the Clinical Scholar model

Fourteen clinical projects were planned during the first series; nine of the projects have been presented at local, regional, national or international conferences. One project received the research abstract award from the American Nephrology Nursing Association in 2005. Several more clinical projects evolved from the clinical inquiry of the Clinical Scholars. Five of the six original facilitators are currently in academic graduate programmes. As a group, they have conducted two additional

Table 17.7 Synthesis table (bed rest following cardiac procedure)

Author (date) funding	Sample research design	I independent variable/ intervention	Dependent variable outcome	Significant results	Limitations/ gaps	Generalisability level of evidence (AHRQ)
Vlasic et al. (2001) University of Western Ontario, Canada	Randomised, controlled, single centre trial Blinded until hemostasis $N = 101$; 6 hrs • Bed rest $N = 99$; 4 hrs • Bed rest $N = 99$; 2 hrs • Bed rest Total = 299	Bed rest: 2, 4 or 6 hrs	Vascular complications Major: requiring blood transfusion, surgical repair, ultrasound guided compression prolonged hospital stay Minor: only requiring site compression, hematoma $< 5 \times 5$ cm^2, bleeding – soaking two 4×4 gauzes	6 hrs bed rest • 5% hematoma • 2% rebleeding 4 hrs bed rest • 6% hematoma • 3% rebleeding 2 hrs bed rest • 3% hematoma • 4% rebleeding • 1% pseudo-aneurysm & surgical repair*	Trial became unblinded after hemostasis	Yes ------------ B
Bogart et al. (1999) Kansas City, MO	Randomised experimental design 100 control group 100 experimental group • 6 hrs bed rest • 4 hrs bed rest	Control group: 6 hrs of bed rest Experimental group: 4 hrs of bed rest	Vascular complications Rebleeding, hematoma, AV fistula, pseudoaneurysm, limb ischemia, thrombosis of femoral artery Hematoma: • Small < 5 cm • Medium 6–10 cm • Large >10 cm	Experimental group 6 hrs bed rest 1% sm hematoma Control group 4 hrs bed rest 2% rebleeding 1% pseudoaneurysm	Post– cardiac catheterisation patients 79% of experimental group; 71% of control group received heparin during the procedure Patients were not on plavix or ticlid	Yes ------------ B

Source: Agency for Healthcare Research and Quality.
* One patient.

series of workshops based on the Clinical Scholar model. Even though the nurse researcher who was originator and facilitator of the programme has left the hospital, the CS mentors have continued to educate more bedside Clinical Scholars, a measure of sustainability supported by the model. Members of other disciplines, particularly physicians, are now asking the Clinical Scholars to be members of their research teams and to help develop studies that will answer clinically meaningful questions.

The 'individual capacity to change the system is directly dependent on the organisational infrastructure, culture, and capacity to change' (Stetler, 2003). The individual capacity to change is directly dependent on possessing the characteristics of a Clinical Scholar.

Developing Clinical Scholars in practice is also the focus of a university programme that values work-based learning and PD through facilitation. This next section discusses the genesis of a Master's programme in PD that arose from the idea to harness the expertise of colleagues across two countries – Australia and Northern Ireland – into a collective and collaborative strategy to generate substantial knowledge for and about PD. It highlights the processes through which a PD programme needs to pass to meet rigorous academic standards.

Demystifying practice development through an academic pathway

PD as an academic outcome

Developing an academic programme in PD has many parallels with establishing a PD project in clinical practice. The seeds for the Master of Practice Development programme between Monash University (Victoria, Australia) and the University of Ulster (Northern Ireland) were germinated in 2003. As with any change in practice it did not occur overnight. Three years of development and negotiation preceded university approval.

In line with the inherent philosophy of PD, the first step in developing the programme was to ensure that the key stakeholders shared the same vision with regard to the purpose and intent of the course. This required considerable discussion and debate, particularly as within the academic environment there is also a requirement that the learning outcomes of any course be consistent with the establishment's strategic directions and graduate attributes. The learning outcomes for the Master of Practice Development are stated in Box 17.7.

Having agreed on the purpose, the next step was to consider the structure of the programme and its fit within the course profile offered by the university. The underlying philosophical tenets of PD, empowerment, enlightenment and emancipation informed the programme development. This was consistent with the programme's aim of developing understanding of the philosophical frameworks and theoretical underpinnings of PD so as to develop facilitative and critical reflectivity skills and enhance and develop knowledge and skills for improving effectiveness of client outcomes.

Box 17.7   Learning outcomes for a Master's in Practice Development

- Broaden critical understanding of PD knowledge, its influence on work-based practices, encourage and enable continuing professional and personal development.
- Develop practitioners' written and oral communication skills; their capacity to work in a team through facilitated action learning and enhance their ability to use technology effectively through the Web-based learning.
- Foster development of intellectual curiosity in relation to PD and awareness of cultural diversity through international partnerships with academics and students.

Placing the programme in context

The proposal to develop a new Master's degree was presented to a Faculty committee, comprising academics, from diverse medical and health science backgrounds, who were unfamiliar with the concept of PD. Therefore having a clear vision of the course's intent was critical in articulating the what, where and why of the PD programme. Undertaking a values clarification exercise proved an invaluable tool for presenting the intent of the programme to a wider audience.

Three learning outcomes (see Box 17.7) guided the programme's development and the establishment of partnerships with clinical health agencies interested in and or utilising PD within their organisations was critical. These partnerships provided access to experienced PD facilitators, clinicians, nurse managers, clinical educators and directors of PD, who provided expertise to inform course development and design.

Recognising students' progression through a post-graduate course requires careful planning. The use of an entry equivalence matrix provided a useful tool to recognise the professional development and clinical experience practitioners were bringing to their academic post-graduate studies. For example, the Post-Graduate Certificate in Life Long Learning/Facilitation offered by the University of Ulster (http://campusone.ulster.ac.uk/potential/postgraduate.php?cid=G732PJ [accessed 30/06/2007]) was identified as one avenue for access into the Master's programme developed by Monash University with the University of Ulster.

To ensure that the first learning outcome could be achieved the course development team specified working in a practice environment as an essential criterion for entering the programme so that the knowledge and skills gained through the course could be utilised. Practice in this context referred to any healthcare, education, learning or management/leadership activity.

The pedagogical approaches used within the Master of PD were primarily e-learning activities incorporating asynchronous learning groups, reflective activities and assessment strategies that would complement and develop the practitioners' knowledge, critical understanding and skills in the implementation and evaluation of PD.

Box 17.8   Interaction attributes

Interaction attributes (Northrup, 2001) necessary for facilitators to help clinicians in the use of Web-based learning materials: • Interaction with content • Collaboration • Conversation • Intrapersonal interaction • Performance support

Interaction attributes

As the programme drew predominantly on e-learning, it was important that educators developing the teaching and learning material have the necessary skills to be confident and competent facilitators of clinicians using this mode (Wilson & Stacey, 2004). Five interaction attributes necessary to facilitate interaction through Web-based learning have been identified by Northrup (2001, p. 31) (see Box 17.8). Development of these attributes necessitates professional development support through workshops, short courses and action learning projects (Wilson & Stacey, 2004).

Development of these attributes in academic staff enables them to support clinicians with activities such as critical reflectivity and reflective conversations required to engage in PD activities within their workplaces.

In summary, establishing a new academic course is a systematic process in common with PD activities. The success of the course from an academic perspective will be determined at school, faculty and university levels (Table 17.8).

From a PD perspective the course success will be determined by its impact on practice. This may require the establishment of a longitudinal study! As this section has indicated, developing an academic programme for PD is not too dissimilar to the journey required to develop a project in practice – developing a common vision, working with stakeholders, systematically implementing the vision and evaluating its impact.

Concluding comments

Whilst only aspects of the accreditation/credentialing process has been drawn on in this chapter, it is clear that the processes of working with specific standards can in itself help practitioners and practice teams develop their practice, improve patient care, articulate their impact and flourish in the process. Whilst such tools are a resource for those who help others to develop their practice, the underlying factors influential on success do not change. There has to be genuine organisational support and sign-up reflected in appropriate structures and processes that enable skilled support to be provided to those who work most closely with patients and users. This chapter has shared some of the PD processes that can contribute to achieving such a culture.

Table 17.8 Evaluation and quality assurance mechanisms for PD programme

---

School level

Course Advisory Committee, comprising faculty staff from both universities, external members from associated health service industries with receive.

- Informal and formal feedback from and about
  - ○ students,
  - ○ research outcomes generated through the student project work.

Faculty level

New courses are given a 3-year lead in time to demonstrate their viability by

- attracting sufficient enrolments to justify the cost of programme provision;
- evaluation of units annually through quality cycles;
- presentation of evaluation data to academic board; underperforming units are required to demonstrate how they will improve.

University level

- Linked to the enhancement and development of practitioners' in-depth understanding of practice development processes and the generation of discourse on practice development.
- Monitoring of impact on learners' learning in the workplace.
- Above linked to increased research, teaching and learning grants.

References

Bogart, M.A., Bogart, D.B., Ryder, L.B., et al. (1999) A Prospective randomised trial of early ambulation following 8F diagnostic cardiac catheterisation. *Catheterisation and Cardiovascular Intervention.* **47**, 175–178.

Bujak, M.D. (2003) How to improve hospital–physician relationships. *Frontiers of Health Services Management, Winter.* **20**(2), 3–21.

Clendon, J.M. (2003) Nurse-managed clinics: Issues in evaluation. *Journal of Advanced Nursing.* **44**(6), 558–565.

Clinical Scholar Task Force (1999) Sigma Theta Tau International Clinical Scholarship white paper. Available from www.nursingsociety.org/new/CSwhite paper.pdf [accessed 05/01/2005].

Conley, D., Schultz, A.A. & Selvin, R. (1999) The challenges of predicting patients at risk for falling: Development of the Conley scale. *MEDSURG Nursing.* **8**, 348–354.

Department of Health (1999) *Making a Difference.* Department of Health, London.

Department of Health (2000) *The NHS Plan. A Plan for Investment. A Plan for Reform.* Department of Health, London.

Department of Health (2001a) *National Service Framework for Older People.* Department of Health, London.

Department of Health (2001b) *Essence of Care. Patient – Focused Benchmarks for Clinical Governance.* Department of Health, London.

Department of Health (2004a). *Standards for Better Health.* Department of Health, London.

Department of Health (2004b) *The NHS Knowledge and Skills Framework (NHS KSF) and the Development Review Process.* Department of Health, London.

Department of Health (2004c) *Agenda for Change Final Agreement.* Department of Health, London.

Department of Health (2005) *Commissioning a Patient Led NHS.* Department of Health, London.

Fay, B. (1987) *Critical Social Science: Liberations and its Limits.* Polity, Cambridge.

Frith-Cozens, J. & Mowbray, D. (2001) Leadership and the quality of care. *Quality in Health Care.* **10**, ii3–ii7.

Funk, S., Tornquist, E. & Champagne, M. (1995) Barriers and facilitators of research utilization: An integrative review. *Nursing Clinics North America.* **30**, 395–407.

Gallant, P. (February 2005) Analysis: What's all the speak about critique? *Excellence in Nursing Knowledge.* 5.

Garbett, R. & McCormack, B. (2002) A concept analysis of practice development. *NT Research.* **2**(7), 87–99.

Guba, E. & Lincoln, Y. (1989) *Fourth Generation Evaluation.* Sage, Newbury Park, CA.

Harvey, G., Loftus-Hills, A., Rycroft-Malone, J., Titchen, A., Kitson, A., McCormack, B. & Seers, K. (2002) Getting evidence into practice: The role and function of facilitation. *Journal of Advanced Nursing.* **37**(6), 577–588.

Honess, C. (2005) Observation: Conceptualizing a researchable clinical issue. *Excellence in Nursing Knowledge.* 3.

International Council of Nurses (1997) *Registry of Credentialing Research Definitions/ Glossary (2001 ICN Credentialing framework).* International Council of Nurses, Geneva.

Keane, K. (2005) Dear diary: Rewards and challenges of applying the evidence. *Excellence in Nursing Knowledge.* 7.

Kent, G. (2005) Synthesis and evaluation: The clinical scholar model in practice. *Excellence in Nursing Knowledge.* 4.

Kitson, A., Harvey, G. & McCormack, B. (1998) Enabling the implementation of evidence based practice: A conceptual framework. *Quality in Healthcare.* **7**, 149–151.

Kramer, M. & Schmalenberg, C. (2004) Essentials of a magnetic work environment. *Nursing.* **34**(6, pt 1), 50–54.

Koch, T. (2000) 'Having a say'; negotiation in fourth-generation evaluation. *Journal of Advanced Nursing.* **31**(1), 117–125.

Lancaster, K. (2005) Critiquing clinical guidelines. *Excellence in Nursing Knowledge.* 5.

Lewin, K. (1946) Action research and minority problems. *Journal of Social Issues.* **2**, 34–46.

Manley, K. (1997) A conceptual framework for advanced practice: An action research project operationalising: An advanced practitioner/consultant nurse role. *Journal of Clinical Nursing.* **6**(3), 179–190.

Manley, K. (2004) Transformational culture: A culture of effectiveness. In: *Practice Development in Nursing* (eds B. McCormack, K. Manley & R. Garbett), pp. 51–82. Blackwell, Oxford.

Manley, K. & Webster, J. (2006) Can we keep quality care alive? *Nursing Standard.* **21**(3), 12–15.

McClure, M.L. & Hinshaw, A.D. (2002) *Magnet Hospitals Revisited: Attraction and Retention of Professional Nurses.* American Nurses Association, Silver Spring, MD.

McCormack, B. & Manley, K. (2004) Evaluating practice developments. In: *Practice Development in Nursing* (eds B. McCormack, K. Manley & R. Garbett), pp. 83–117. Blackwell, Oxford.

McCormack, B. & Titchen, A. (2006) Critical creativity: Melding, exploding, blending. *Educational Action Research.* **14**(2), 239–266.

McGill, I. & Beaty, L. (1997) *Action Learning.* Kogan Page, London.

Myers, I.B., McCaulley, M., Querk, N. & Hammer, A. (1998) *MBTI A Guide to the Development and Use of the Myers Briggs Type Indicator*, 3rd edn. Consulting Psychologists Press, Washington, DC.

NHS Institute for Innovation and Improvement (2005) *Improvement Leaders' Guides.* NHS, Nottingham.

Northrup, P. (2001) A framework for designing interactivity in web-based instruction. *Educational Technology.* **41**(2), 31–39.

RCN (2007) *Workplace Resources for Practice Development.* Practice Development Team, RCN, London.

RCN Practice Development Team. (2006) Available from http://www.rcn.org.uk/resources/practicedevelopment/about-pd/tools/values-clarification.php [accessed 20/08/2006].

Rycroft-Malone, J., Harvey, G., Seers, K., Kitson, A.L., McCormack, B. & Titchen, A. (2004) An exploration of the factors that influence the implementation of evidence into practice. *Journal of Clinical Nursing.* **13**(8), 913–924.

Rycroft-Malone, J., Kitson, A., Harvey, G., McCormack, B., Seers, K., Titchen, A. & Estabrooks, C. (2002) Ingredients for change: Revisiting a conceptual framework. *Quality and Safety in Health Care.* **11**, 174–180. (www.qualityhealthcare.com)

Schein, E.H. (1992) *The Corporate Culture Survival Guide. Sense and Nonsense about Culture Change.* Jossey-Bass, New York.

Schultz, A.A. (2005a) Origins and aspirations: Conceiving the clinical scholar model. *Excellence in Nursing Knowledge.* 4.

Schultz, A.A. (2005b) Clinical scholars at the bedside: An EBP mentorship model for today. *Excellence in Nursing Knowledge.* 8.

Stetler, C.B. (2003) Role of the organization in translating research into evidence-based practice. *Outcomes Management.* **7**(3), 97–105.

Stetler, C.B., Morsi, D., Rucki, S., et al. (1998) Utilization-focused integrative reviews in a nursing service. *Applied Nursing Research.* **11**, 195–206.

Street, A. (1995) *Nursing Replay: Researching Nursing Culture Together.* Churchill Livingstone, Melbourne.

Strout, T.D. (2005) Curiosity and reflective thinking: Renewal of the spirit. *Excellence in Nursing Knowledge.* 3.

Styles, M. & Affara, F.A. (1998) *ICN on Regulation: Towards 21st Century Models.* ICN, Geneva.

Titchen, A. & Manley, K. (2006) Spiralling towards transformational action research: Philosophical and practical journeys. *Educational Action Research.* **14**(3), 333–356.

Turner-Stokes, L., Nyein, K., Turner-Stokes, T. & Gatehouse, C. (1999) The UK FIM+FAM: Development and evaluation. *Clinical Rehabilitation.* **13**, 277–288.

Vlasic, W., Almound, D. & Massel, D. (2001) Reducing bed rest following arterial puncture for coronary interventional procedures (BAC trial). *Journal of Invasive Cardiology.* **13**(12), 788–792.

Warfield, C. & Manley, K. (1990) Developing a new philosophy in the NDU. *Nursing Standard.* **4** (4), 27–30.

Wilson, G. & Stacey, E. (2004) Online interactions impacts on learning. Teaching the teachers to teach online. *Australasian Journal of Educational Technology.* **20**(1), 33–48. Available from http://www.ascilite.org.au/ajet/ajet20/wilson.html [accessed 11/08/06].

Wilson, V., McCormack, B. & Ives, G. (2005) Understanding the workplace culture of a special care nursery. *Journal of Advanced Nursing.* **50**(1), 27–38.

18. *The Future Contribution of Practice Development in a Changing Healthcare Context*

Kim Manley, Brendan McCormack, Val Wilson and Debra Thoms

Introduction

Practice development (PD) has grown and evolved since its early beginnings in the 1980s in the United Kingdom. Originally associated with nursing, it is now an international development spanning both northern and southern hemispheres, one that includes and enables all the personnel that comprise healthcare teams, in partnership with users, to provide person-centred and clinically effective healthcare services – a focus that is articulated by authors in this book.

PD today is associated with a explicit methodology and a broad set of methods underpinned by specific principles, values and beliefs for developing and redesigning systems that can sustain person-centred and clinically effective care (Chapters 1 and 2) integrated with learning in the workplace (Chapters 6 and 14). The workplace cultures that result from implementing these methods and principles are associated with increased individual, team and organisational effectiveness (Manley et al. (2007) and Chapter 11) and subsequently services that are efficient and effective in their use of human and economic resources provided through a culture experienced as flourishing for all – patients, users and staff (McCormack & Titchen, 2006).

However, the full contribution of PD to contemporary healthcare agendas globally has yet to be realised. Policy leaders and commissioners have been slow to recognise the potential of PD methodology as an approach for simultaneously improving and redesigning services to ensure that they are fit for purpose. In this book, McCormack, Manley and Walsh (Chapter 2) uncovered some of the reasons for this situation and primarily highlighted the contribution that PD makes to understanding 'patterns' in systems redesign – something that is often given least priority in modernisation strategies. McCormack et al. (2006) identified a number of factors that contributed to the alienation of PD from service development, innovation and improvement strategies. These include the containment of PD in a nursing context, challenges associated with the language of PD and the complexity of the integrated methods used. We suggest that the findings of McCormack et al. (2006) are reinforced by many of the perspectives articulated in this book and provide a key strategic agenda for the future enhancement of PD at a policy level.

The aim of this chapter is to therefore explore two questions:

- What does PD have to offer to a changing healthcare context reflected in the healthcare trends that will influence the next generation?
- What are the influencing strategies that will enable PD to become more widely adopted in clinical redesign?

Both questions are informed by an inquiry undertaken with the members of the International Practice Development Colloquium (IPDC) comprising practice developers who integrate improvement work using PD methodology and methods with roles as practitioner–researchers and enablers of learning in the workplace, working alongside practitioners and practice teams. The inquiry undertaken to inform both questions involved identifying healthcare trends for the next generation. These trends, it was anticipated, would drive healthcare policy and would therefore be significant in arguing PD's ongoing contribution to healthcare as well as expressing the mechanisms through which PD could address them.

A political influencing framework developed to improve influencing skills (Antrobus, 2003) is used to frame the discussion and is informed by the findings from the inquiry, evidence from previous chapters in this book and the findings of the systematic review of the PD evidence undertaken by McCormack et al. (2006). This framework will help identify the influencing strategies to be used to enable the potential of PD to be both recognised and adopted more widely by healthcare leaders and commissioners. The chapter will conclude with a commentary by Debra Thoms, the Chief Nurse for New South Wales, Australia, who will provide further comments and insights about the influencing process.

What does practice development have to offer to a changing healthcare context?

When considering the value of any theory or specific methodology and associated methods, such as those that characterise PD (Chapter 1), theory analysis frameworks enable systematic identification and analysis of core concepts, their internal relationships and structure. External analysis explores the relevance of theories to everyday practice – termed social utility.

Theory from PD is arrived at from researching practice in a way that is always inclusive, participative and collaborative (McCormack et al., 2006) that is, it is underpinned by a set of values and principles. Investigation of practice draws on these values and principles to simultaneously integrate cycles of development and growth that encompass planning, designing, reflection, implementation and evaluation. The ongoing systematic analysis of this work and engagement in scholarly inquiry have resulted in greater clarification of fundamental PD principles as well as making explicit the theoretical and philosophical foundations of PD. The theoretical, methodological and principles development have been described in detail in Chapter 1. Whilst PD, through its very nature, is a practical endeavour undertaken with practitioners and practice teams, its social utility in relation to its methods has not been made sufficiently explicit This has been in part due to the lack of formal recognition of PD methods in clinical redesign. In a systematic review of the evidence relating to PD, including evidence from key stakeholders involved in PD, McCormack et al. (2006) propose for the first time a number of methods that are deemed 'essential' in emancipatory PD work, and these have been outlined in Chapter 1 of this book.

One approach to identifying social utility involves a retrospective analysis of PD projects that meet the criteria of including specific methods, something that was the focus of the first systematic review conducted by McCormack et al. (2006). The inquiry informing this chapter has built on this systematic review and utilised a critical dialogue approach to uncovering challenges and opportunities associated with embedding PD in healthcare policy, strategy and practice innovation. This analysis further informs the influencing strategies that will position PD with policy leaders and commissioners in healthcare more notably in the future.

Future healthcare trends: a collaborative inquiry

There are analyses of current healthcare trends in the literature (WHO, 2006); however, to identify those that have significance for PD an inquiry into future healthcare trends as perceived by members of the IPDC was undertaken. Two assumptions underpinned the inquiry, firstly that future healthcare trends will be drivers for future healthcare policy, and secondly, practice developers are well positioned to identify the full potential of PD than those without such understanding.

The purpose of the inquiry was to identify the

- key healthcare trends for the next 25 years;
- contributions that PD can make to these trends;
- influencing strategies and priorities that those involved in PD need to address if PD is to become more mainstream and influential internationally.

The inquiry was undertaken in two stages. The first phase involved surveying 18 (of which 12 responded) members of the IPDC using a short semi-structured questionnaire. This was analysed and themed to inform the second stage, which was a more detailed analysis with a number of IPDC members using two focus groups (Box 18.1). One focus group was held through a teleconference involving members from the United Kingdom and the Netherlands, and the other was held

Box 18.1 Focus group discussion schedule included:

---

1. Verifying the themes that emerged from the first phase analysis in relation to
   - heathcare themes for next 25 years;
   - how practice development can contribute to future healthcare trends.
2. Exploring the following questions:
   - Briefly consider whether PD has a role within *developing* as well as *developed* countries and what that role would be.
   - Identify priority areas/new directions for PD activity with regard to the global trends identified.
   - Explore in more depth the *arguments* and *language* that PD needs to use to make what it has to offer more attractive to commissioners and policy makers.
   - Identify priority actions required to gain global recognition for what it has to offer.
   - Identify other influencing strategies that will position PD more strongly within the policy arena.

---

in Australia and involving members participating in person from Australia, New Zealand and the United Kingdom. The findings of the inquiry have informed the themes emerging with regard to healthcare trends and what PD has to offer as well as strategies for ensuring that commissioners and policy developers know of PD's contribution. Quotations are drawn from the focus groups to illustrate the findings.

The key healthcare themes for next 25 years identified are explained under the broad headings of Society, Health Issues, Changes in Health Systems and Workforce and Technology (Table 18.1).

There was recognition within the focus groups that a number of healthcare trends were associated more with either the developed or developing countries; for example increased mental and physical health chronicity, increasing demand, increased aging population in the context of reduced resources were characteristics of the developed world. Developing countries were associated with high levels of sexually transmitted diseases such as HIV and infectious diseases, often associated with poverty and lack of education; similar trends in the developed world resulted from increased mobility of people and complacency. Whilst technology was clearly something that was not readily available in developing countries the potential of technology to be influential in both the developed and developing world was clearly recognised through, for example, the use of mobile phones, telemedicine and technological development.

The contribution of PD to healthcare trends

The ways that PD can contribute to addressing future healthcare trends are presented in Table 18.2. The resulting themes are derived from a thematic analysis of the questionnaire data, followed by verification and further refinement in the two focus groups. The themes not surprisingly echo the content of the chapters of this book and the threads that weave them together.

Table 18.1   Health trends: key themes

SOCIETY in relation to health will experience: • *Changing population profiles that impact on health need and health provision,* e.g. an increasing population and aging profile with shortfall in care providers (in the Western world). • *Continuing economic drivers at all levels of health organisation,* e.g. health continuing to develop as a market economy with increased consumer knowledge, control, choice and expectations; public resourcing and private funding issues as costs of healthcare increase; funding/incentives for changing lifestyle increased. • *Closer inter-relationships between healthcare and social care,* e.g. long-term conditions relocated under social services. • *Greater personal responsibility for health.* Citizen's responsibility to make decisions and accept the consequences. • *Continuing inequality between developing and developed countries linked to the fundamentals of health.* • *Effects of global warming as it impacts on economics and health,* particularly in developed countries because of the economic consequences of diminishing fossil fuels. There will subsequently be greater valuing of innovation and sharing to address global warming. • *Continuing multi-culturalism* and the recognition that people have different needs.	**CHANGES in health systems and workforce SYSTEMS** will increasingly focus on: • *Community care,* e.g. informal care, prevention, low tech care, less hospital beds, risk associated with hospitals, local cooperatives supported by virtual electronic resources. • *Development of specialist centres* further away from people's homes. • *Performance, targets, outcomes* continuing focus on clinical and economic outcomes and accreditation systems. • *Greater availability and need for evidence to support practice.* • *Larger, more complex and more costly healthcare systems.* • *Political directives for organisational restructure* to provide more effective service planning and delivery models. **WORKFORCE** issues will emphasise: • *Increased team, interdisciplinary, inter-agency, cross-boundary working.* • *Recruiting, retaining healthcare staff* linked to developing effective workplaces cultures. • *Reducing professional boundaries, specialism vs generalism.*
HEALTH ISSUES, an increased: • *Focus on prevention rather than cure* with financial incentives for former. • *Chronicity, palliative care and co-morbidity* linked to ageing population. • *Physical and mental ill-health,* e.g. heart disease, diabetes, obesity, depression, alcohol and drug abuse. • *Infectious diseases,* e.g. HIV, TB, pandemic flu.	**TECHNOLOGICAL development will lead to:** **BENEFITS:** • *Increased accessibility to healthcare and expertise.* • *Biomedical advances.* • *Gene technology tracking those who are vulnerable.* • *Local and virtual networks.* **CONSEQUENCES:** • *Ways of working,* e.g. electronic records and telemedicine consultations; knowledge management issues. • *Ethical issues* as a result of technological advances. • *Increasing specialisation* with potential devaluing of generalist skills.

Table 18.2 Key themes emerging from the question: How do you see practice development contributing to future healthcare trends?

Theme	Sub-theme
1. Keeping persons at the centre of care	• Keeping the person at the centre of care and involving patients and clients in decision-making • Enabling others to value consumers and be advocates for them, and enabling patients and users to be their own advocates
2. Involving patients and clients in decision-making	• Active and meaningful involvement of key stakeholders
3. Developing systems and cultures for quality services	• Enabling team building and interdisciplinary care • Changing cultures of care driven by needs of users • Restructuring and modernising systems • Strategic development of services
4. Investing in staff towards new ways of working	• Fostering creativity, innovation and development • Helping staff to work more smartly
5. Enabling evidence-based practice	• Enabling practice expertise to influence policy • Enabling practice-based research, learning and evidence-based practice
6. Systematic change and evaluation	• Working with change/changes in an intentional, systematic and rigorous way towards a clear purpose

Whilst the majority of trends identified in Table 18.1 and the approaches in Table 18.2 may be challenged for being aligned with the experiences of developed countries, there was a strong consensus within the focus groups that PD had a lot to offer both developing and developed countries.

The contribution of PD is not linked with any one specific healthcare trend but to all areas of healthcare. This is because of the specific way in which PD works with people regardless of the healthcare issue and also the way the patient/ person in healthcare is viewed.

For example, working with the healthcare trend of increasing multi-culturalism and its ensuing complexity was linked to using a multi-stakeholder approach – a core principle of PD. In response to diminishing resources within any context, the PD principle of creativity was seen to be of value as it offers possibilities to be more creative with limited resources. Working with limited resources was a key issue for many people involved in PD interviewed in the systematic review by McCormack et al. (2006). Having to find creative ways to maximise the impact of limited resources and needing to work creatively to do so was a key issue.

Regardless of the location of PD work, 'Westernised or Eurocentric ideas' were considered to be easily taken for granted. The need for PD to have an understanding of, and appreciation for, any culture and context in which it worked was strongly endorsed and this meant working with its associated reality, cultural nuances and goals. This is an issue discussed in some depth by Moss and Chittenden (Chapter 9) and one that clearly needs careful consideration in the future evolution of PD methodologies.

Working in different cultural contexts requires keeping in mind the 'raw principles' of PD. An example was given in one focus group of how in one PD school it was uncovered that the notions of providing high challenge and high support (a key strategy in the workplace for helping others to become more effective) were antithetical to the cultural notions common in some Asian cultures where to challenge a 'superior' would be unthinkable. 'Seeing PD as a collection of tools and methods rather than as the core principles of participation, collaboration, inclusion, and equity, endangered the pitfall of getting caught in the concrete operational stage (after Piaget (1955) – rather than being comfortable with what PD is about (principles and values) and using tools in a fluid, flexible way'.

Whilst endorsing the approaches that PD offers (Table 18.2) there was an initial sense by focus group participants that the healthcare trends identified (Table 18.1) seemed bewildering if trying to articulate how PD may specifically contribute to each – they seemed so big!. This was accounted for by the fact that PD tends to work at the more micro-level than the mega-macro-level of these global trends. However, if we examine the focus of many of the chapters of this book (e.g. Chapters 10, 11, 16, 17) where authors grapple with methods of engaging with practitioners and patients, then it could be argued that these methods could be explored further to embrace broader healthcare agendas. Global trends are about the ways that things are changing and PD helps people cope with and work with change regardless of where the trend comes from. Global trends do not shift the fundamental centre of what PD is about. PD activities help local trends and changes to be integrated as a matter of course through the way it works. This point can be illustrated through the example of the shift away from acute care and large hospitals to community and primary healthcare provision. PD strategies can contribute to this redesign of service and service transition through the methods/themes' outlined in Table 18.2 and the engagement with the developmental principles articulated in Chapter 1. Further, PD would be expected to involve working with people who are more geographically disparate and subsequently would need to be more diversified in the way it works. This point has been reiterated in Chapter 3 where the authors argue for a language in PD that is inclusive and which is translatable in different contexts.

Changing workforce trends are highly relevant to future work in PD. A key issue is the lack of multidisciplinary engagement with PD; an issue that was raised by some participants in the focus groups, and identified as having negative impact on the progress of PD if not actively addressed. This perspective reinforces the findings of McCormack et al. (2006) who found a diverse range of PD literature with a nursing focus but a limited range of material from a multidisciplinary perspective. In addition, the literature available failed to provide any conclusive evidence of the value of multidisciplinary over unidisciplinary approaches to PD. The authors concluded that it is the focus of the PD work that should determine whether it is uni- or multidisciplinary orientated. However, it is clear that further work is needed to determine strategies for multidisciplinary engagement in PD work. Existing strategies have largely been ineffective in engaging with multidisciplinary teams and new and innovative strategies are required. The nursing workface in particular is also changing and moving into areas that require a reconsideration of what it is that nurses do in relation to other professional groups and new and emerging groups. PD needs to grapple with the reality of change in the workforce and how this challenges its core principles. For example, this might mean that recruitment and retention issues challenge our notion of continuity of care and perhaps we need to grapple with the notion that continuity of care does not mean continuity of carer. There is also a key future role in working with non-registered practitioners as well as whoever is involved in healthcare provision whether they be caregivers or lay practitioners.

In summary, there is an overwhelming view that PD needs to shift its gaze in terms of how to contribute and position itself in relation to the big picture associated with the global health themes identified. The positioning of PD in this broader context would enable greater understanding of the effectiveness of the methods used and the impact of PD on major healthcare agendas. As a participant in the focus groups warned: 'not to do so is to run the risk of missing (or failing to influence) some key priorities or trends or issues that may impact upon us'.

Whilst acknowledging that there is a need to understand the big picture it is also recognised that this should not detract from the core PD business of making the interface between staff and users of services more effective. The notion of a skilled practice developer working at all levels as a political operator and translator therefore comes through in the available evidence (McCormack et al., 2006) and in the focus group data. PD processes need to work across all levels of staff not just the practitioners at the 'coal face' thereby integrating and translating trends across levels from individual charge nurses, to area directors of nursing, to people in policy. For these people, their world is not just local but is 'further out'. Focus group participants suggested that it is not possible to be an effective practice developer and not take into account the area beyond the grassroots registered nurse. The policy and strategy areas and the work of the registered nurse should not be isolated from each other:

There needs to be some sort of 'interface' or 'filter' that can translate the global trends and what those trends may mean at a micro-level of the individual clinician in a clinical area.

Helping policy makers and commissioners understand the value of PD

In recognising the need to influence policy makers and commissioners if the potential for PD is to be achieved, two themes need consideration: the first is to do with the language and the second with the arguments that could be used to make PD more attractive. Both are inextricably interwoven with PD's purpose and underlying principles.

Language and PD

Two issues about language merit discussion when promoting PD as a strategy for addressing present and future healthcare issues:

- Differentiating PD from other terms and approaches.
- Making the language more attractive to policy makers and commissioners.

A whole gambit of different terms across the quality agenda are recognised as having differences and similarities with PD causing widespread confusion and therefore lack of recognition about what PD has to offer. It is felt that some of these terms are better understood than PD by key stakeholders, for example *quality improvement, organisational development, professional development*. Some approaches have much in common with PD, for example *community development approaches* such as community action research (Senge & Scharmer, 2000) as an approach for achieving improvement and increased effectiveness, although it is recognised that little serious debate has been given to this in the PD community and its literature. Then there are the new and in-vogue ideas that are often a repackaging of previous approaches or developed externally to healthcare, for example the *LEAN methodology* (Institute for Innovation and Improvement, 2007). There are also similar terms such as *practice improvement* and *developing practice* that cloud the concept of PD.

Discussions with the focus groups explored labels that may be more appropriate to use and that captured the intents and processes of PD for policy makers. Person-centred care and the patient's experience with its focus on the outcomes of PD were considered to be terms that were not strange to policy makers. However, policy makers have multiple agendas:

> *Policy makers are not just interested in the one stakeholder; they will be making policies that will drive all institutions that are providing healthcare – we need to talk a bit wider in terms of multi-stakeholders and not just limit it to patients and clients. We need to look at terminology like developing working practices developing efficiency and effectiveness – the sort of jargon that will appeal to policy makers. The problem is that it is very difficult to incorporate it in a short snappy title.*

Quality improvement and professional development are linked by policy makers to increasing efficiency and effectiveness, although the concepts themselves may not capture the humanistic approaches that underpin emancipatory PD and are articulated through many of the chapters of this book. The use of the term 'improvement' can be used glibly and is currently seen as an in-vogue term, but often without the substance about how improvements are achieved. However, PD itself is not immune from being used as a glib term. Whilst being aware of other movements that move in and out of vogue, PD too needs to be aware of the impact of 'hype' on its own reputation and for it not to be just a flavour of the month: 'if it is not delivered in a way that is meaningful and useful it will be a "Bit like Britney Spears" – really popular a few years ago and now not so much – with some huge shocking things happening along the way'. Against the recognition that terms change over time, different things become topical in policy and it is important to go with the policy direction and to speak the same language. However, these developments and strategic directions need to be considered carefully as there can also be a danger of subsuming PD under the managerial mantle with a consequential loss of both its focus and direction. The terms can become meaningless and without substance if the words are so malleable that they can mean anything we want them to mean. PD can thus become more about style than substance. This line of argument leads to two conclusions about the language used in PD. The first relates to ensuring that people understand what PD means and the fact that we need to be more vigilant in making sure that we explain ourselves and make sure people understand what PD means. If people are confused by the language we use we need to take the time to help them understand and work harder at being more understandable ourselves.

The second relates to being more assertive about the outcomes of PD. McCormack et al. (2006) have provided some insights into this. Their study highlighted the need to be assertive about the outcomes arising from PD work and showing that these outcomes have synergies with the key influences and policy trends. Thus the agenda shifts from one of 'language' to that of outcomes. Being assertive, showing our evidence and being systematic about the way we collect the evidence are key agendas for the future development of evaluation strategies in PD – an issue discussed by Wilson, Brown and Hardy in Chapter 7. These authors reinforce the message of McCormack et al. (2006) regarding the importance of being clear about the evaluation methods used and the desired outcomes and they go some way to advancing methodologies for designing such studies.

What are the arguments for PD and how do we get the message across?

This section is framed by two key themes:

- Articulating the contribution of PD.
- Getting the message across.

The following quote expresses the challenges underpinning the two themes:

> *How do we get the message across around the value of the processes as that is the thing that I would argue enables PD to stand aside from many of the other activities that might be going on. Albeit there might be areas of common ground and opportunities for integrating common methods. But it would seem that the hardest thing is getting across the value of the processes, . . . 'we talk to the converted' we maybe don't make our arguments strong enough so when faced with those who are more sceptical it is very easy*

for PD to be brushed aside and something else that seems to be a quicker fix to be put in place and taken on board. So the challenge is how do we share examples and experiences of the value of the process and that it is worth investment, that it can make a difference and doesn't always have to take for ever, rather than people turning to what appear to be much quicker strategies but don't appear to have the longer term benefits of developing and enabling people, which is where I think we make a difference – its looking at the balance between the quick fix and the sustainability. The argument that is often given about PD is that its all very well talking to people and exploring what they think but the reality is that we have to get the job done when there is a strong patient imperative.

Key messages that needed to be emphasised in relation to PD contribution are as follows:

PD is about

- working with the needs and wants of all stakeholders and through this approach achieving efficiency and effectiveness;
- listening to and working with front-line workers who know if the service is effective and whether the needs of clients are being met;
- achieving sustainable change by working with PD processes within an explicit workplace context;
- investing in staff towards new ways of working that involves developing individuals and teams to do much more than just address a specific issue – they go on to develop and change practice all the time;
- learning in the workplace that makes a difference;
- achieving the implementation of evidence-based practice and the integration of multiples sources of evidence in the workplace.

These themes are captured in the latest definition of PD presented in Chapter 1:

Practice development is a continuous process of improvement towards increased effectiveness in patient centred care. This is brought about by helping healthcare teams to develop their knowledge and skills and to transform the culture and context of care. It is enabled and supported by facilitators committed to systematic, rigorous continuous processes of emancipatory change that reflect the perspectives of service users.

This definition reflects the key themes of person centredness, holistic engagement, facilitation, learning and the sustainability of change through embedding them in corporate strategies and many of these themes have been addressed in previous chapters and explored in Chapter 1. This definition of PD demonstrates that it is not just a set of tools and that it is a particular worldview with underpinning philosophical principles (McCormack & Titchen, 2006). It does not fit easily with other worldviews and thus finds itself in a 'methodological battleground' for space in a healthcare context that requires 'quick fixes' to address intransigent problems. Whilst PD clearly has to be seen to contribute to addressing many of these problems, the danger of it becoming 'mainstream' is that PD becomes just another set of tools and its essence 'lost in translation', rather than a set of principles underpinned by inclusivity, participation and collaboration. Thus the need for those engaged in PD to influence policy and strategy agendas is paramount.

What are the influencing strategies that will enable practice development to become more widely adopted in policy design?

PD needs to become more political in enabling others to draw on and use what it has to offer. Linked to this is the challenge of articulating its social utility more persuasively. The framework for political influencing developed by Antrobus (2003; RCN, 2006) is useful for adopting a systematic and focused approach to achieving policy change by ensuring that

- PD is presented as a proposal for policy change;
- supporters are identified and worked with to develop a collective voice;
- the policy outcomes desired are articulated;
- stakeholders are identified and key messages developed for each group that reflect what PD can deliver on;
- common goals are aligned with other groups' agendas.

A 'benefits realisation exercise' (RCN, 2006) inclusive of a stakeholder analysis and the recommendations put forward by McCormack et al. (2006) would provide the robust development of an action plan/PD proposal, which would influence policy makers to support the achievement of strategic policy goals. Getting a head start by articulating a proposal as a policy solution, which is aligned to national directives, will bridge the language of policy and practice resulting in a creative and effective partnership that will have positive benefits for performance, quality/safety and the enhanced patient experience.

The principles of developing a shared vision, identifying stakeholders and working collaboratively are central principles to PD when working with practitioners and clinical teams in practice, as evidenced throughout this book. Within the context of influencing policy-making this activity takes place with stakeholders at a more strategic level. Therefore when thinking about both supporters and stakeholders, three strategies are necessary:

- Making links with the agendas of other disciplines, e.g. social workers, medicine.
- Making links with the agendas of international healthcare organisations, e.g. World Health Organization, Council of Europe, International Council of Nurses by using existing international connections.
- Shifting the gaze to Chief Nurse and Chief Executive level, in order to understand how strategic leaders understand key concepts used in PD, e.g. person centredness.

PD needs to develop strategic relationships to enhance the sphere of understanding of what it can achieve as policy makers are usually eager to support effective robust systems and tools that are timely responsive and provide solutions. The concept of social engineering (Schneier, 2000) as a concept in political science influences attitudes and social behaviour on a large scale, whether by governments or smaller groups in the political arena. Within PD we need to extend the explanation of reliable information in a language that may be common to all stakeholders.

Influencing strategies that will position PD more strongly within the policy arena

Throughout the chapters of this book and in focus group discussions, a number of strategies can be proposed to advance PD at a policy level:

- Tapping into commissioners of healthcare, finding out who they are, how to access them and their criteria for quality.
- Aligning PD with the vision of the organisation showing how PD can be one of the things that can enable the vision to be achieved.
- Showing PD's role in the translation of evidence into practice.
- Demonstrating local outcomes.
- Contextualising PD at a number of different levels, with a number of different foci.
- Lobbying and networking with important political stakeholders, e.g. politicians and political parties.
- Using 'joined-up writing' opportunities so that good works going on in different areas and at different levels are brought together.
- Drawing on accreditation processes as a means and an end to promote the role of PD.

Members of the IPDC in this enquiry strongly articulated a single most important key priority. This was to both provide and strengthen the evidence base underpinning PD in relation to its outcomes, improved efficiency and effectiveness and to present this evidence to groups other than 'those already in the know'. Strategies advocated for this purpose are outlined in Box 18.2.

Box 18.2 Strategies for providing and strengthening the evidence base of the impact of PD

- Obtaining matched funding and subsidies from European and international sources.
- Improving how we handle different kinds of data.
- Pooling data internationally to demonstrate outcomes.
- More follow-up studies of PD projects after external facilitators have withdrawn to illustrate impact and sustainability.
- Drawing on evidence from other disciplines that use similar processes, e.g. participatory management, community development approaches, health promotion.
- Link evidence to team motivation, increased productivity increased efficiency and effectiveness.
- Draw on more community-based and cross-boundary opportunities for PD.

A view from above – a Chief Nurse's perspective: Debra Thoms Chief Nurse, New South Wales, Australia

Health systems across the developed world are being faced by similar pressures in meeting service demands amid the ongoing challenge of ensuring the provision of an adequately educated and available workforce. The contribution that PD can make to healthcare delivery has been set out in this book and recognition of the key healthcare trends that are evident today discussed in this chapter. So how can policy makers be influenced to embrace PD?

Many of the strategies applied to modern heath systems have numeric indicators or targets. The strategies implemented to achieve these targets are sometimes seen as a 'quick fix' but if the achievements are to be sustained there will need to be broader cultural change within the organisation. These goals often have a stated focus on the patient journey or patient flow or similar terms and the person-centred focus of PD can assist in enabling the improvements to move beyond the short term. PD provides an added dimension to approaches such as clinical redesign, lean thinking or similar strategies. This will contribute to the desired changes becoming embedded into the functioning of the system as PD assists in changing the culture of the organisation.

It has been highlighted in this chapter (and Chapters 1 and 2) that PD is seen to work at the micro-level in the face of large system-wide changes. The long-term sustainability of some of large system-wide changes is potentially fragile and approaches such as PD enable these to become more clearly embedded in the overall operation of the organisation. Proponents of large change at times do not recognise the impact on the 'micro' level and it is later questioned why the change has not been sustained. Ultimately, if there is no change at the micro-level the macro-change will not last.

For some staff and particularly younger staff joining health services, the culture of organisations can at times be challenging – changes utilising PD will assist in the retention of staff and thereby the recruitment of staff. This assists in meeting the challenge of a sustainable workforce. At the same time a contribution will be made to improved patient outcomes and consumer satisfaction with the service.

The authors correctly highlight the importance of both the language and the arguments proffered to support a PD approach when attempting to influence policy makers. There are many in policy positions in organisations that come from a clinical background. One of the inherent strengths of PD is the resonance it has with practitioners. This connects with a language that potentially has some commonality for those who are proponents of PD and those in policy positions from a clinical background. Identifying key people in such positions and developing their understanding of what PD has to offer in line with their goals can assist in raising the profile of PD within health systems. These clinician policy makers may then be able to assist in further translating the contribution of PD for other senior policy makers who may not be from a clinical background or who initially find the concepts more difficult to understand.

PD also provides skill development for those who take on facilitator roles. These skills are transferable into other settings and can be used as a means to demonstrate the positive impact of a PD approach. Taking advantage of opportunities for roles that may not specifically be identified as PD but which allow practitioners to influence the understanding of others of the contribution that PD has to make should be utilised. Demonstrating through these avenues and through other organisational activities such as forums and seminars enables a broader audience to gain an understanding and perhaps seek further knowledge so that they can achieve similar outcomes in their own areas of work.

The involvement of consumers in health and the recognition of the positive impact their involvement can have provide an opportunity for practice developers to demonstrate the impact and contribution that a person-centred approach to care can provide. Again, skills particularly in facilitation that practice developers have gained can assist in engaging a broader community and enable the contribution that PD can make to be demonstrated.

Identifying key stakeholders who potentially will understand the concepts of PD and can then become a 'champion' is another way of influencing. There may be an opportunity to employ practice developers within key areas of departments where they can use their skills and gradually develop the shared understanding of the broader work group. At the same time the improved output from that workgroup will demonstrate to the larger organisation that there is something different about the way this group works. In addition, as the evidence base demonstrating the positive impact of PD builds, support is provided to those in key positions in influencing broader systems.

Perhaps what is needed is to recognise a capacity for 'upward leadership'. Useem (2001) provides some thoughts and guidance on how to 'lead up'. It is necessary to have clarity and a good understanding of the organisation's goals and purpose so that PD can be placed well within that context and so that it can demonstrate how it will help these be achieved. Building a relationship with senior leaders and managers will provide opportunities to influence the organisation in the way that it functions and in the adoption of the underpinning principles of PD. There is a need to build the confidence of those above in the capacity to achieve outcomes. It may be necessary to ask the difficult questions and perseverance may be required. A well-developed plan that is also well communicated is important.

PD has much to offer policy makers both in the achievement of organisational goals such as improved patient outcomes and in assisting a culture to develop that will ensure sustainable effective work practices and contribute to the recruitment and retention of staff.

Conclusion

The chapters of this book have, we hope, contributed to advancing our knowledge and understanding of PD. Since the publication of *Practice development in Nursing* in 2004 there has been much advancement in the development of theoretical and methodological frameworks to inform PD. In addition, our evidence of effectiveness has increased and become more sophisticated with increasing evidence of outcomes for individuals, teams and organisations from the adoption of PD methods in practice.

Our key challenge now is to 'shift our gaze' and convince policy makers and strategic planners of the benefits of PD to clinical redesign. To do this, we need to continue to support practitioners who are engaging in and advocating PD strategies in their everyday work. This support can come through the continuous growth in our knowledge of PD, the articulation of an evidence base and the translation of these findings/developments into practice. This final chapter has highlighted the necessity for us to include the policy arena in our gaze. As has been argued in this final chapter and reinforced by Debra Thoms, being cognisant of these global healthcare trends will enable PD methodologies and methods to become embedded in clinical redesign strategies. In addition, we would argue that PD has a role in all future strategies that claim to focus on developing patient-centred services, as well as other initiatives focused on improving the service user's experience of care services and sustaining this – all central foci of PD. This book marks a particular point in time as we advance our knowledge and understanding of PD. The engendering of critically creative methodologies in PD will help us to embrace these policy and strategically driven agendas and embody them in our ways of working, thus ensuring that the creativity of practitioners is maximised. We look forward to what the future holds.

Acknowledgements

The authors would like to thank Professor Ken Walsh for his contribution in facilitating one of the focus groups and documenting key aspects of the discussion. We would also like to thank the members of the International Practice Development Collaborative (IPDC) who contributed to the cooperative inquiry that informed this chapter.

References

Antrobus, S. (2003) What is political leadership? *Nursing Standard*. **17**(43), 40–44.
Institute for Innovation and Improvement (2007) Going LEAN in the NHS. University of Warwick, Coventry.
Manley, K., Sanders, K., Cardiff, S., Garbarino, L. & Davren, M. (2007) Effective workplace culture: draft concept analysis. In: *Royal College of Nursing, Workplace Resources for Practice Development*, pp. 6–10. RCN, London.
McCormack, B., Dewar, B., Wright, J., Garbett, R., Harvey, G. & Ballantine, K. (2006) *A Realist Synthesis of Evidence Relating to Practice Development: Executive Summary*. NHS Quality Improvement, Scotland. (www.nes.scot.nhs.uk/)

McCormack, B. & Titchen, A. (2006) Critical creativity: Melding, exploding, blending. *Educational Action Research: An International Journal.* **14**(2), 239–266. (http://www.tandf.co.uk/journals)

Piaget, J. (1955) *The Child's Construction of Reality.* Routledge, London.

Royal College of Nursing (2006) *Action Sheet 3: Developing Your Strategy for Influence.* Political Leadership Programme RCN, London.

Schneier, B. (2000) *Secrets & Lies: Digital Security in a Networked World.* Wiley Computer Publishing, Indianapolis, IN.

Senge, P. & Scharmer, O. (2000) Community action research. In: *Handbook of Action Research: Participative Inquiry and Practice* (eds P. Reason & H. Bradbury). Sage, Thousand Oaks, CA.

Useem, M. (2001) *Leading Up. How to Lead Your Boss So You Both Win.* Crown Publishing. New York.

World Health Organization (2006) *Engaging for Health Eleventh General Programme of Work 2006–2015 A Global Health Agenda.* WHO, Geneva.

Index

Page numbers followed by 'f' refer to figures and page numbers followed by 't' refer to tables

Index